A Guide to the Extrapyramidal S. ... ...ychotic Drugs

Antipsychotic drugs have revolutionised the management of major psychiatric disorders and the outcomes for those who suffer from them. They do, however, have a range of adverse effects, amongst the most frequent and distressing of which are those resulting in disturbance of voluntary motor function. Extrapyramidal side-effects (EPS) are still poorly recognised and not infrequently misattributed. Although the topic has consumed a large proportion of the research literature, clinicians have not been well served with ready sources of information bringing together both the descriptive clinical elements of these disorders and major research conclusions pertinent to routine practice. This book seeks to rectify this in the hope of increasing clinicians' awareness of the issues and acknowledgement of their impact. This is a task made more rather than less urgent by the emergence of new drugs of lower liability but which may promote subtler abnormality than standard compounds.

The author has a very readable style and provides a thorough clinical reference that is adeptly illustrated by real case histories. The book should be of particular value to trainees and established practitioners within the fields of psychiatry, neurology, primary care and geriatrics.

DAVID CUNNINGHAM OWENS is Reader in Psychiatry at the University of Edinburgh, and Honorary Consultant Psychiatrist at the Royal Edinburgh Hospital, Scotland. His major areas of research are the biological basis of schizophrenia, and the psychopharmacology of antipsychotic drugs, especially their extrapyramidal adverse effects, on which he has published extensively. Dr Cunningham Owens has for some years conducted training sessions on the recognition and standardised evaluation of drug-related movement disorders, aimed both at clinicians in routine practice and those undertaking research projects.

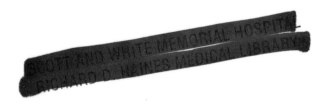

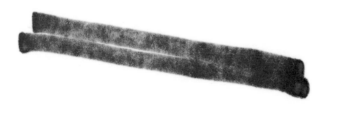

A Guide to the Extrapyramidal Side-effects of Antipsychotic Drugs

D.G. CUNNINGHAM OWENS
University of Edinburgh

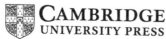

CAMBRIDGE
UNIVERSITY PRESS

PUBLISHED BY THE PRESS SYNDICATE OF THE UNIVERSITY OF CAMBRIDGE
The Pitt Building, Trumpington Street, Cambridge CB2 1RP, United Kingdom

CAMBRIDGE UNIVERSITY PRESS
The Edinburgh Building, Cambridge CB2 2RU, UK   http://www.cup.cam.ac.uk
40 West 20th Street, New York, NY 10011–4211, USA   http://www.cup.org
10 Stamford Road, Oakleigh, Melbourne 3166, Australia

First published 1999

Printed in the United Kingdom at the University Press, Cambridge

Typeset in Palatino 10/12 pt, in QuarkXPress® [SE]

A catalogue record for this book is available from the British Library

Library of Congress Cataloguing in Publication data
Owens, D. G. Cunningham (David Griffith Cunningham), 1949–
A guide to the extrapyramidal side-effects of antipsychotic drugs
D. G. Cunningham Owens.
    p.   cm.
Includes bibliographical references and index.
ISBN 0 521 63353 2 (pbk.)
1. Extrapyramidal disorders.   2. Antipsychotic drugs – Side
effects.   I. Title.
[DNLM: 1. Basal Ganglia Diseases – diagnosis.   2. Basal Ganglia
Diseases – drug therapy.   3. Antipsychotic Agents – adverse effects.
4. Extrapyramidal Tracts – drug effects.   WL 307 097g 1998]
RC376.5.O95   1998
616.8'3–dc21   98–7142   CIP
DNLM/DLC
for Library of Congress

ISBN 0 521 63353 2 paperback

Contents

Preface

History has become a legitimate field of academic study in medicine – and nowhere more so than in psychiatry. Some who stumble across the present work on a bookshelf browse might think it more rightly belongs in the historical section, as an account of how things were 'then', in the dark years BC – **B**efore **C**lozapine – but not now. For, after all, the 1990s have seen a resurgence in antipsychotic psychopharmacology, with the old generation of drugs, so strongly identified with the problems elucidated here, giving way to a new therapeutic Utopia.

If this is the reader's view, then he or she is unlikely to progress to the substance of the present volume and hence we are unlikely to share further experiences. The fact is that while these are indeed interesting times in the *evolution* of antipsychotic psychopharmacology, I – in line with many colleagues – do not feel the wind of *revolution* in the air. The new generation of drugs does seem to be pointing to a brighter future for our patients, but to interpret this as meaning that doctors can now be freed from the responsibility of acquiring the skills necessary for *comprehensive* patient care is rather like saying that with the advent of credit cards we now need know nothing about money! Extrapyramidal adverse effects are likely, in my opinion at least, to be an important aspect of medical practice for some years to come – and in those countries excluded economically from antipsychotic Utopia, for many years to come. It was in this belief that the following pages were put together.

However, a brief historical overview does start the work because it recounts events that, unknown to me, determined my career – and I am no doubt not alone in this. But it is not a story that is widely known. The substance of the volume covers in turn the major extrapyramidal syndromes associated with drug use, with a strong *clinical* emphasis, including references to examples that have crossed the author's path over the years. In saying 'drugs', what in honesty is meant is 'antipsychotic drugs', for these are the major culprits, if 'villains' there be.

However, this is only one denomination – if the largest – in an increasingly broad church, as is highlighted in Chapter 2.

In order to encourage a thoughtful use of terminology (not a strength of my profession), an account of oculogyric crises reported in association with encephalitis lethargica is included (Chapter 3), as is the question of spontaneous dyskinesias in schizophrenia (Chapter 7). This brief account of the limitations of the concept of tardive dyskinesia may be seen as of little relevance in the clinic but is, in my view, a fundamental counter to our natural tendency to view the complex as simple.

Particular attention has been paid to the examination method (Chapter 10) as such information is not readily accessible from other sources yet forms the foundation on which expertise rests. An overview of a few of the more frequently utilised tools for recording the results of our efforts is presented in Chapter 11.

The volume concludes by briefly raising some medicolegal and quality-of-care issues, especially, though not exclusively, for the psychiatrist. My depression at the increasing litigiousness of the patient body is only exceeded by that engendered by the reasons for this. In the field of the present volume, cock-ups are invariably of the 'omission' variety and the message is 'judge before ye be judged' – and record *everything*!

The potential constituency for the present work is wide. These problems are clearly part of the bread and butter of *psychiatry* – or at least should be. However, evidence presented here tends to the opposite conclusion (Chapter 2). Psychiatrists still seem unwilling or unable to give due prominence to extrapyramidal adverse drug effects. The issues are also likely to have impinged powerfully on one of the major concerns of the research community in the last decade. I have a sneaking suspicion that much of the conceptual confusion surrounding 'negativity' in schizophrenia is attributable to a simple oversight – the *subjective* manifestations of extrapyramidal side-effects (EPS), a neglected area the present volume assiduously promotes.

However, psychiatrists are not the only ones to be confronted by the sorts of neurological adverse effects described here. A great deal of neurological time is expended in this field and while *neurologists* may tend to their own sources of information, the experience of those in the trenches is not to be dismissed. With regard to EPS, psychiatrists are very much the neurological 'squaddies'. Specialists in *gastroenterology* and *care of the elderly* are also likely to confront the issues – again, perhaps more commonly than they appreciate – and with the classes of drugs implicated constantly widening, other specialists are likely to be brought into the field, the most recent affiliates being *cardiologists*. An interest on the part of *non-medical personnel* is as yet generally unexplored, but is a potentially important issue.

Increasingly, *primary care physicians* are involved in supervision and management decisions with the long-term psychiatrically ill that in the past were exclusively the domain of specialists. General practitioners are in a rather unenviable position in the present context, as decisions to treat and treatment regimes involving antipsychotic drugs are rarely theirs, yet to them increasingly falls the responsibility of longer term monitoring. In this role, the following may be of some use.

What is presented here is not intended as a reference text. Those wishing state of the art in current research will need to look elsewhere. The emphasis here is unashamedly *clinical*. There is little point in seeking the Holy Grail if you cannot recognise a cup! It is hoped that the reader drinking from the present work will emerge with a clear and durable impression that will enhance future recognition of, and sensitivity to, these frequent and frequently distressing aspects of modern medical care.

D.G. Cunningham Owens

1

The background

Introduction

It is always comforting to reflect on a 'Golden Age' – a time of optimism and hope when the barriers of ignorance and impotence tumbled before an onslaught of knowledge.

For psychiatry, the decade of the 1950s might now be seen as one such Golden Age, for the 1950s saw the explosive birth of psychopharmacology. Suddenly, those devoted to the medical management of individuals suffering the ravages of psychiatric disorder had at their disposal an ever-expanding array of therapeutic tools whose efficacy could be established by the application of scientific principle, which did not require a lifetime to show their benefits, and which were relatively cheap. No longer was the therapeutic armamentarium restricted to those who were sufficiently intelligent and articulate to utilise what was on offer, or sufficiently well-heeled to afford it. For no longer would psychiatrists need to be pseudo-physicians, misdirecting their medical skills to crude and largely ineffective physical interventions or suffocating them under a welter of unverifiable dogma. Most importantly of all, no longer were those whose misfortune it was to be afflicted by major disorders excluded from the therapeutic possibilities.

It was, of course, necessary to interpret the concept of knowledge in this 'Golden Age' in a somewhat wider than usual manner, for while it may have been clear that the increasing litany of new compounds worked, understanding of *how* they worked was rudimentary. This nonetheless had a bearing on the other exciting prospect on offer – the availability of a series of tools to explore the functionings of the human brain.

1

Table 1.1. *A chronology of 1950s' psychopharmacology*

	1949	Cade	The antimanic (and maintenance) effects of lithium salts
December	1950	Charpentier	Synthesis of chlorpromazine
December	1951	Sigwald & Bouttier	First treatment with chlorpromazine
March	1952	Hamon et al.	First publication of the efficacy of chlorpromazine
May	1952	Delay & Deniker	First systematic evaluation of chlorpromazine
	1952	Selikoff	Mood-elevating effects of isoniazid
	1954	Steck Thiebaux	First formal accounts of parkinsonism with chlorpromazine
	1954	Kline	Reserpine
	1954		Methylphenidate
	1955		Meprobamate
	1955		First trial of G22355 (Imipramine)
	1955	Delay	'Neuroleptics'
	1956	Ayd	Identification of dystonia with chlorpromazine
	1957	Kline	Introduction of MAOIs
	1957	Kuhn	First report of antidepressant effect of imipramine
	1957	Randall	Behavioural effects of 1,4 Benzodiazepines
	1958	Petersen	Thioxanthenes
	1958	Janssen	Butyrophenones (haloperidol)
	1958	Zeller	MAO inhibition
	1959		Introduction of imipramine
	1959	Sigwald et al.	First report of tardive dyskinesia
	1959		Clozapine
	1960	Cohen Tobin	Anxiolytic effects of chlordiazepoxide

The Golden Age

The onslaught of compounds introduced into clinical practice was relentless (Table 1.1). Chronologically, it actually began in 1949 when the Australian psychiatrist John Cade reported the antimanic and mood-stabilising properties of lithium salts. It has to be admitted that the theory behind the work which led to these observations was frankly awry, but the consequence was to be enormous when, in other places, the therapeutic potential was brought to clinical fruition.

The rauwolfia alkaloid reserpine, long associated with Ayurvedic medicine, was introduced into Western psychiatry by Nathan Kline in 1954, the same year that the central stimulant methylphenidate became available, though this would have to endure the controversies of several decades before it would find respectability – of sorts.

In the early years of the decade, the inappropriate elation of tuberculous patients receiving antituberculous drugs pointed to the first effective antidepressant strategy through inhibition of the enzyme monoamine oxidase, a strategy applied clinically with the introduction of iproniazid in 1957.

Meanwhile, the search for ever-cheaper, non-hepatotoxic phenothiazines led Geigy to investigate a series of iminodibenzyl derivatives for antihistamine activity similar to that of chlorpromazine. The iminodibenzyl analogue of chlorpromazine, code named G22355, was tested by the Swiss psychiatrist Roland Kuhn but with results later described as 'in some patients, quite disastrous' (Broadhurst, quoted in Healy, 1996) as the drug, although sedative, paradoxically appeared capable of promoting manic-like behaviour. In 1955, Kuhn tried it in depressed patients and in 1957 published results of remarkable effectiveness in 'vital' (endogenous) depression. Imipramine entered use in 1959.

In 1955, the first 'tranquilliser', meprobamate, became available, marketed rather quaintly under the name of the town in which it was manufactured (Miltown), and by 1957 it was the most prescribed drug in the USA. Although safer than barbiturates, it still had a rather unsatisfactory therapeutic index. In 1957, however, Lowell Randall demonstrated the behavioural properties of the 1,4-benzodiazepines, and in 1960, chlordiazepoxide became available in the vanguard of a wave of compounds that appeared to offer, at last, an instant solution to life's worries and the prospect of accommodating the public's concern that anything less than eight hours represents inadequate sleep.

It must have seemed it would go on for ever. But, of course, it did not. For the next quarter of a century or more that would essentially be it – the bubble burst and in the silence after the bang psychiatry was left to ponder, with increasing frustration and some alarm, the inadequacies of the tools with which it had been presented.

This is in no context illustrated better than by the one class of drugs omitted from the above list, and the one that is our major topic of consideration in the present volume – antipsychotics. A brief explanation of how they came to us is of some interest.

The chlorpromazine story

There is no single version of the chlorpromazine story that has percolated through the internecine squabbles about who did what and when and which perhaps inevitably followed such a success involving such disparate players. There are, however, certain indisputable facts in this tale and certain accounts that represent, to use the modern analytical jargon, truth of a more narrative than historical kind. As Mark Twain wrote, 'The older I get, the more vivid is my recollection of things that never happened', and the dramatis personae of this particular production are old men all – or dead. What personal insights can now be offered to resolve the hostilities is unclear.

The following brief account is taken from conventional sources (e.g. Swazey, 1974; Caldwell, 1978; Healy 1996) but to those who, by the revisionist nature of historical endeavour, object to the emphasis, the author presents no defence.

The development of antipsychotics could not have had less to do with the needs of psychiatry. To find their roots, we must first dig in the fertile soil of mid-nineteenth century Victorian commercialism.

The synthesis of mauve from coal tar by William Perkin in 1856 provided the fillip to a whole new industry, commercial dyeing, on the back of which flourished the new specialty of organic chemistry. In 1876, Heinrich Caro, chief chemist of the German company BASF, synthesised a new dye, methylene blue, and in 1883, August Bernthsen, a research chemist, published his analysis of its structure. Bernthsen identified the basic nucleus of methylene blue as 'thiodiphenylamin' or phenothiazine. However, it would take many years and whole new fields of research before this discovery could be brought to its potential.

One area of research was shock, specifically anaphylaxis, which led to the identification of histamine and its actions, while a pertinent strand of pharmacological investigation related to the functioning of the autonomic nervous system. By the 1930s, the existence of acetylcholine and adrenaline had been established. Since antagonists of these naturally occurring amines were known, the pharmacologist Daniel Bovet thought it 'reasonable' to postulate that there might exist substances which interfered with the chemically not dissimilar histamine. In the early 1940s, the French pharmaceutical company Rhone-Poulenc developed a series of synthetic antihistamines, some of which – such as diphenhydramine – are still with us.

Meanwhile, phenothiazine had not been neglected. The antimalarial properties of methylene blue had been established in the 1890s, and subsequently phenothiazine was shown to be an effective insecticide against mosquito larvae. However, the molecule was toxic in humans, though an antihelminthic action against swine ascaria was utilised in veterinary practice in the 1930s. In the 1940s, the American pharmacologist Alfred Gilman returned to the non-oxidised phenothiazines in search of safe antimalarials, but found these compounds to be ineffective and published his negative results in 1944.

Because of the Second World War, these results did not reach France, where a similar investigation was being undertaken by scientists at Rhone-Poulenc. This investigation succeeded in replicating the negative findings with regard to antimalarial activity, but the French group's interest in the field allowed them to observe what Gilman and Shirley had not – the potent antihistamine activity possessed by a number of these compounds. The most important product of this work was promethazine, produced in 1946.

It was clear that these new synthetic antihistamine compounds had unusual central actions. In humans they were clearly sedative, while some appeared to have beneficial effects in Parkinson's disease. In the autumn of 1950, Paul Koetschet, Rhone-Poulenc's Assistant Scientific Director, proposed a phenothiazine amine development programme, with a view to exploiting central actions irrespective of antihistamine properties. The evidence to support the proposal was flimsy, even by the standards of the time, and Koetschet admitted that it was 'difficult to know' what clinical applications there might be for whatever products emerged. The first he suggested might lie in pre-anaesthesia, while his 'hope' was for more active antiparkinson agents. 'Finally' he mused on the possibility of 'an application in psychiatry'!

Koetschet's reliance on an outcome of interest to anaesthesia was not without foundation, and brings us back to shock. For the first half of the century, the old adage that the operation was a success but the patient died was based on more than gallows humour. Haemodynamic and traumatic shock all too frequently undermined the accomplishments of even the most technically skilled surgeon. Despite a number of explanatory hypotheses, the mechanisms remained arcane. Working within this general framework was a young naval surgeon, Henri Laborit.

Laborit began his research career on a topic of concern to navies the world over – seasickness. His interest was in the possible role of cholinergic mechanisms, and in pursuit of this he and a colleague (Morand) developed a cholinesterase assay for plasma estimations. When, in 1946, it was postulated that inhibition of peripheral cholinesterase may underlie shock, Laborit was well placed to shift his emphasis. He did not accept the primacy of capillary changes in initiating shock, but was more taken with neural (i.e. autonomic) disturbances that might underlie the problem.

Laborit's views on the mechanism of shock and the cocktail of drugs he recommended to counteract it were roundly criticised in later years, but none of this is of relevance to our interest. For what cannot be denied is that Laborit was possessed of exceptional powers of clinical observation. In obviating shock, his aim was to dampen or 'stabilise' autonomic activity during and after surgery by means of a complex pharmacological regime which latterly included promethazine. This was his so-called 'lytic (i.e. sympatho-parasympatho-lytic) cocktail'.

His observations of the 'secondary' effects of promethazine were impressive, especially in relation to the affective and behavioural changes. He noted that patients became 'calm and somnolent, with a relaxed and detached expression', an effect he was clearly able to distinguish from that of morphine. Laborit's acumen is highlighted by the fact that promethazine had been tried previously in psychiatric patients but only sedation had been noticed.

Much effort has been expended in debating just how pivotal these observations were in Rhone-Poulenc's decision to proceed with the development of aminophenothiazine derivatives, and nothing can be provided here – or perhaps anywhere now – to resolve this controversy. What is fact is that proceed they did; and success came fast. Chloropromazine was synthesised by Rhone-Poulenc's chief chemist, Paul Charpentier, in December 1950, only two months after Koetschet's original proposal, and, after only three months of laboratory study, was deemed ready for clinical trial. The first samples for psychiatric evaluation, as a potentiator of barbiturate-induced sedation, were dispatched to Dr J. Schneider of the Broussais Hospital in April of 1951.

At this time, Laborit was working in the Val de Grace military hospital outside Paris on the development of artificial hibernation as an anaesthetic technique, and he apparently had no knowledge of the development of the renamed chlorpromazine. When he approached Rhone-Poulenc about the possibility of producing a more effective phenothiazine derivative than promethazine to add to his 'lytic cocktail', he was surprised to learn that one already existed. He received his first samples, as the twelfth investigator, in late June of 1951. In October of that year he was able to report 'the twilight state' that patients entered after receiving his cocktail containing chlorpromazine, and at a meeting the following December he could quote a colleague as observing that the drug 'may produce a veritable medicinal lobotomy'!

Laborit began urging his psychiatric colleagues to try it clinically, although, as the 'urging' was from a surgeon, it is perhaps not surprising that he was met with a fair degree of indifference. In early November 1951, he participated in the first administration of chlorpromazine to a normal subject – his friend Dr C. Quatri, herself a psychiatrist! Quatri described an initial period of discomfiture, supplanted later by 'an extreme feeling of detachment' in which perception was 'filtered, muted'.

In January of 1952, psychiatrists at the Val de Grace finally tried the drug, although their decision was 'without much conviction'. The patient was a young manic man with several previous admissions. The favourable results were presented orally the following month and published (by Hamon and colleagues) in March. Perhaps because of the origins of their inspiration, the authors of this first published report on the efficacy of chlorpromazine were grudging in their praise, making it clear that 'naturally' they were 'not presenting a new therapy for treating mania'!

However, it was the work of Delay and Deniker that provided the fuel for chlorpromazine's 'lift-off' through a series of reports beginning in May of 1952, although even here it seems that Laborit played a role. According to Swazey, Delay and Deniker heard of chlorpromazine from Deniker's brother-in-law, himself a surgeon, who had utilised Laborit's method.

It is hard to appreciate now how opposed the psychiatry of the time, especially in Continental Europe, was to the idea of pharmacological agents, which were seen as the antithesis of clinical science (Healy, 1996). The 'science' was in unravelling the 'tangled threads' of Bleuler's metaphor. In this context, it is not at all hard to appreciate how frostily the intrusions of a surgeon would be viewed and how, when the trophies were to be awarded, his role would become a source of controversy. But the historical record is clear that it was Henri Laborit, the surgeon, who first identified the psychotropic properties of chlorpromazine. For those offended by the suggestion that he also played a crucial role in providing an impetus for the development of the drug, it is worth recalling that when Rhone-Poulenc came to license the drug to a US manufacturer, they made it clear that they were 'very interested' in ensuring that 'the name and investigations of Dr. Laborit ... are mentioned in every scientific publication and also in the popular articles' (Swazey, 1974) – not the recognition conventionally afforded to other than a key player.

As a footnote, however, if we are looking to priority in relation to the start of the modern era of clinical psychopharmacology, this probably belongs to J. Sigwald, who, on the 28th December 1951, started solo chlorpromazine treatment in a 57-year-old chronic psychotic lady – the memorably named Madame Gob!

What, the reader might ask, is the point of all this? It is presented in the belief that those who prescribe chlorpromazine and its successors, who live with their impact and the problems they may cause, and who may even acknowledge the possibility that without them their chosen career might well have been different, may have some interest in the story. It is also presented to dispel the notion, still perpetrated in texts on the subject, that the introduction of chlorpromazine into psychiatric practice was pure 'serendipity'. The drug's development was, no matter how loosely, a result of the convergence of a number of strands of basic and clinical research with long and honourable scientific credentials, while its eventual home was built on the foundations of astute clinical observation. Its introduction may well have been empirical, but it cannot be considered serendipitous.

There is one final point to highlight from this story – perhaps one of the great ironies of medical history. August Bernthsen, the research chemist who first identified the phenothiazine ring, did so in Heidelberg, only a stone's throw from where Emil Kraepelin would soon formulate his concept of dementia praecox! It would be almost three-quarters of a century before these two powerful developments would find conjunction – years during which psychiatry was dragged through one theoretical quagmire after another and up countless therapeutic blind alleys.

In the wake of chlorpromazine

The pharmaceutical industry was not slow to capitalise on the chlorpromazine story and a series of phenothiazines was soon available. These were, at the end of the day, essentially derivative, with similar modes of action and, as would later emerge, similar sets of problems associated with their use.

The same judgement would apply to the two other drug types that emerged at this time. In 1958, P.V. Petersen, working at the Lundbeck laboratories in Copenhagen, produced the first thioxanthene. This chemical type was characterised by a carbon substitution at position 10 (the R2 position) instead of the nitrogen of the phenothiazines, the effect of which was that side-chains attached by way of a double bond. Thus, these compounds exhibited stereoisomerism, a property that profoundly affected their pharmacology.

Also in 1958, the Belgian chemist Paul Janssen synthesised haloperidol, the first of an entirely new chemical type, the phenylbutylpiperidines or butyrophenones. This was to some extent a fortuitous event as Janssen had been interested in the pharmacological properties of pethidine (meperidine) analogues modified by simple chemical reactions. Haloperidol was the first drug with relatively selective receptor actions, and hence, in terms of general side-effects, had one of the best tolerability profiles. Haloperidol was to go on to become the 'market leader' antipsychotic in terms of volume usage around the world.

Following Kuhn's demonstration of the antidepressant properties of G22355 (imipramine), other heterotricyclic compounds became of interest, and in 1958 the Swiss company Wander began a development programme of compounds which, like imipramine, comprised a seven-membered central ring structure. One of these, a dibenzodiazepine with an N-methyl-piperazine side-chain, was HF1854, registered in 1960 as clozapine.

Clozapine's success is a story of survival against the odds. Not only were its expected antidepressant actions not evident, but in laboratory animals it did not produce the responses anticipated of an anti-psychotic. However, increasing concern about its adverse effects on the granulocyte cell line culminated in 1975 with reports from Finland of a cluster of 13 cases of agranulocytosis, eight of which were fatal. This effectively terminated its development in most countries, but a lingering impression that this drug was something different led to sponsorship of a large multicentre American study of its efficacy and tolerability in a circumscribed patient group resistant to standard drugs. This study (Kane et al, 1988) has become one of the most influential trials in the history of psychopharmacology, and clozapine was the first anti-psychotic to which superior efficacy was attributed – albeit in a specific patient population. Furthermore, this and subsequent work pointed to remarkably favourable neurological tolerability.

Clozapine has radically altered perceptions of the mechanisms whereby antipsychotics bring about not only their therapeutic benefits but also their extrapyramidal effects. It has allowed us to break out of the straightjacket of single system psychopharmacology that was the inevitable lure of the classical dopamine hypothesis, and has returned us to something approaching a more realistic appreciation of neurophysiology and brain therapeutics. Clinically useful drugs that were previously denounced as pharmacologically 'dirty' are now rightly viewed as pharmacologically 'rich', and the race to find a 'safe' clozapine has promoted antipsychotic psychopharmacology once again to the first division. This may ultimately come to be seen as clozapine's lasting legacy.

Single system psychopharmacology has not left the scene entirely, however. In the mid-1960s, modification of the substituted 2-methoxy-benzamide, metoclopramide, produced sulpiride, which is chemically distinct from other antipsychotics. Although licensed in France in the late 1960s, the efficacy and especially the central pharmacology of sulpiride only came under scrutiny a decade later. It was the first highly selective dopamine D_2 antagonist and hence in effect represented the realisation of the classical dopamine hypothesis as it relates to anti-psychotic action. Furthermore, it appeared to demonstrate a dose-dependent separation of effects thought to be predictive of nigrostriatal antagonism (i.e. motor side-effects) compared to those thought to result from dopamine antagonism at mesolimbic sites (i.e. therapeutic effects). This seemed to fit with clinical observations that sulpiride might possess a lower liability to promote extrapyramidal dysfunction. Accordingly, sulpiride appeared somewhat different from other classes of antipsychotics in both its clinical and pharmacological characteristics, and hence it was the first drug to be referred to as *'atypical'*.

A range of benzamides with a range of indications is now available worldwide. What will become of the antipsychotic benzamides remains to be seen. The 6-methoxy-benzamide, remoxipride, only managed a couple of years before a reported association with aplastic anaemia curtailed its availability, but amisulpride has been available in France for some time, and raclopride has also been reported on favourably. Although enthusiasm for the highly (dopamine D_2) selective approach to antipsychotic development has waned dramatically in recent years, it may be premature to write its obituary just yet. Even 'science' has its fashions!

A new generation of antipsychotic compounds is now emerging. Thus far, all are based on a model extracted from *one* particular aspect of clozapine's 'rich' pharmacology, namely its relatively potent anti-serotonergic – specifically 5-hydroxytryptamine-$_{2A}$ (5-HT$_{2A}$) – actions. These, in combination with a lower affinity for dopamine D_2 receptors, are behind the designation of these compounds as 'serotonin–dopamine antagonists' (SDAs), although, as with standard drugs, this must not blind one to the fact that they also have many points of pharmacological difference.

This interest in the manipulation of serotonin as a therapeutic aim in psychotic disorders is *re*-newed rather than new, and revives interest of over 40 years ago. These new generation compounds are proving commercially very successful, but it may be that when their place in the armamentarium comes to be more fully established, they will be found to represent relative rather than absolute advances. It is certainly important that we do not substitute one blinkered theory for another and again condemn antipsychotic psychopharmacology to decades of derivative drugs. There are certainly other actions of clozapine awaiting investigation, such as its intriguing and complex effects on noradrenergic systems. There was once a popular theory of that in relation to schizophrenia too, which may one day again see the light of day.

Practice, theory and names

The work of Jean Delay and Pierre Deniker was instrumental in establishing chlorpromazine's therapeutic credentials in psychiatry. They began their investigations in February 1952, unaware of those of Sigwald and Bouttier or the Val de Grace group. Like most early evaluators, their approach was initially towards the drug's use in 'excited' states, regardless of diagnosis. Thus they, like others, first tried it in mania, although they soon extended it to disturbed patients of other diagnostic types. While they were enthusiastic and found some results that were 'spectacular', the wider psychiatric community was far from ready to be instantly impressed. Indeed, Deniker later recalled how, at the 50th French Congress of Psychiatry and Neurology in July 1952, his talk was scheduled for the last session of the last day, and because of an over-run, was delivered to fewer than 20 people – during the lunch break!

Initial results were, in fact, varied. This was, of course, before randomised and dose-finding clinical trials or operational diagnostic criteria. Application was of the 'try and see' variety – and cautious. The recommended dose from the manufacturer was up to 100 mg per day orally, or a maximum of 25 mg for the first intramuscular (i.m.) injection. Delay and Deniker opted for a 'very high' dose of 75-100 mg i.m. daily plus the same again orally if required, a regime they themselves were apprehensive about. In these early days, Europeans were conservative with regard to dosage. As would be repeated many times with many drugs, it was when chlorpromazine crossed the Atlantic that 'megadoses' entered practice. By the mid-1950s, doses of 1000–2000 mg per day were being used in the USA.

The first British study, reported by Anton-Stephens in the *Journal of Mental Science* in April 1954, was also of the 'try and see' variety, but the major British contribution came from the work of Joel and Charmian Elkes in Birmingham. Their study, reported in the *British Medical Journal* in September 1954, was the first controlled trial of chlorpromazine and one of the first such trials in psychopharmacology. Although providing a qualified confirmation of chlorpromazine's value, they pointed out what Sigwald and Bouttier had also emphasised: that the new drug was not 'curative', but rather produced symptomatic benefits that could be all too quickly lost on discontinuation. The seeds of maintenance were sown early!

Within two years of its announcement to an incredulous, if not hostile, profession, chlorpromazine had achieved international recognition. If this was in the vanguard of something new, however, a new name would be necessary for the class it and its successors represented. Initially, Laborit's influence was again evident in the early suggestions 'neuroplegic' and 'neurolytic'. By 1955, however, two principal effects of these drugs had been established, extrapyramidal dysfunction and so-called psychic indifference, either of which could provide a basis for classification.

The first formal report of extrapyramidal dysfunction appeared in 1954 (Steck, 1954), though the issue had been aired since shortly after the drug's introduction. This aspect of chlorpromazine's use became increasingly of interest – not concern – because it seemed to point to a possible mode of action. As early as 1953, Delay had stated that parkinsonian effects were dose related. As doses embarked on their relentless march upwards, these effects, unsurprisingly, appeared inevitable. From such an observation it was a short leap of intellect to view them as essential to the therapeutic process.

Thus, within the briefest period, the perception of extrapyramidal disorder shifted from one of adverse to necessary effect. This perception was enshrined in the term neuroleptic, coined by Delay in 1955, which literally means 'seizing' or 'grasping' nerves, and implies a more forceful and fundamental action than 'neurotropic'. The emphasis was therefore very much on the neurological component of action.

What had interested Laborit were the *affective* changes the drug was capable of producing, even after very limited exposure. The word that recurs throughout the earliest writings is 'detachment'. Chlorpromazine did not dull perception, but rather diminished the emotional response to noxious experiences. This was the so-called 'psychic indifference' that translated in behavioural terms into relative composure.

In 1955, the neurologist Howard Fabing and a classicist, Alister Cameron, coined the term 'ataraxy' to cover this phenomenon. It literally means 'without anxiety' or, as Caldwell has more figuratively suggested, 'a state of equanimity'. The drugs promoting this state would then be referred to as 'ataraxics'.

The concept of 'ataraxy' did not catch on, especially in English language psychiatry, although it has resonances in the idea of 'specific sedation' sometimes used, even now, in European psychiatry. It is interesting to speculate why this might have happened. 'Ataraxy' was, after all, a descriptive term for a characteristic mental state effect of drugs whose primary indication was by then mental state disorder. Perhaps psychiatrists had had enough of descriptive psychology, and demanded something that said more of fundamental medical modes of action. Nonetheless, it might be seen in retrospect as a source of regret that the classificatory term to receive universal recognition was one based on a pattern of adverse effects that was not unique, to the exclusion of an alternative that related to the action which set the drugs apart as special in the first place.

In the 1970s, the dopamine theory of schizophrenia was probably the most fertile source of research-testable hypotheses within what was becoming known as biological psychiatry. For some, the drugs from which this theory drew much of its empirical strength became known as 'antischizophrenics'. However, cursory awareness of previous, to say nothing of contemporary, work should have inclined those heading in this direction away from such an elementary error. What almost half a century of research has made clear is that there is nothing diagnosis specific about the effects of these drugs, at least in terms of the diagnostic categories – the syndromes – we use today.

Where these drugs do appear to exert effects that are relatively unique to them is on symptoms. They seem to act in a direct way against those features we refer to as 'psychotic'. As the means whereby they do this are not merely secondary to sedation, any reference to them being 'tranquillisers', major or any other sort, is both confused and confusing. Increasingly it seems most appropriate that all drugs which share in common these relatively unique actions against psychotic phenomenology should be classified descriptively on the basis of this lead function – i.e. as antipsychotics.

'Typicality' versus 'atypicality'

When everything seemed much the same, there was little incentive for things to be viewed differently. Even recurrent suggestions that sulpiride may have some different pharmacological actions failed to inspire, as the clinical evidence remained equivocal.

The fact of clozapine's difference is, however, indisputable. Hence, the need for a term to encapsulate the fact that this drug is indeed not typical of others in its class. The problem arises when one tries to formulate criteria by which this 'atypicality' can best be conceptualised.

The most obvious criteria are clinical ones, but there is an immediate problem in using clinical parameters. Whatever actions and effects standard antipsychotics have in common are balanced by their differences. What would need to be consistently different in clinical terms for an antipsychotic to be considered in some way separately from its peers?

There are two broad clinical areas (and within these several subcategories) by which antipsychotics might be compared (Owens, 1996). These relate to:

1. efficacy – in terms of:
    (a) acute schizophrenic symptomatology
    (b) long-term maintenance
    (c) negative schizophrenic states
    (d) treatment resistance;
2. tolerability – in terms of:
    (a) general adverse effects
    (b) neurological adverse effects.

There is *no* evidence to date that any antipsychotic compound is possessed of clearly enhanced efficacy in the generality of acute schizophrenic episodes. The concept of 'acute' schizophrenia is at best rather vague, comprising as it does the major assumption that in states in which florid, productive symptomatology predominates, the underlying pathophysiological disorders – and hence the treatment-response characteristics – are probably the same. Clinical trials of efficacy seldom distinguish first episode patients from those with florid exacerbations of long-standing illnesses, and comparative data of efficacy in these different situations are lacking. Nonetheless, even the data on clozapine do *not* point to its clear advantage in unselected 'acute' cases, although the number and quality of studies are not great (Owens, 1996). It does seem, however, that antipsychotics *cannot* have difference imparted to them on the basis of 'acute' efficacy.

With regard to maintenance, the view is also one of comparability of efficacy for standard drugs, although again formal comparative data are sparse. The evidence for advantage with clozapine in this situation is compelling, with striking improvements in quality-of-life parameters reported over 6 and 12 months (Meltzer et al., 1990; Meltzer, 1992). However, these conclusions do not emerge from randomised relapse-prevention studies but from open studies, in which neither the effects of differential attrition of the less well nor the unique circumstances under which the drug must be administered can be accounted for. It would seem rash to attribute difference on this basis.

Effective treatment of negative states is one of the most pressing requirements in psychopharmacology, and proven efficacy in this area would endow any antipsychotic agent with exceptional properties. There is evidence that such actions can be attributed to certain drugs, such as sulpiride, those SDAs for which we have sufficient data, and especially clozapine. However, the matter is not straightforward and depends, first, on conceptual issues and, second, on issues of clinical acumen.

That schizophrenia is a condition associated with impairment was the cardinal observation that Kraepelin used in delineating this disorder (or group of disorders). Like most of those of his generation, Kraepelin conceived of impairment, or decline, in interpersonal or psychosocial/occupational terms – as something to be identified longitudinally over time. In the era of psychopharmacology, however, practice is much more cross-sectional. The most 'longitudinal' the majority of psychopharmacologists extend themselves to at any one time is the four to six weeks of their current study!

When it comes to encapsulating psychiatry's position on just what are the building blocks of 'negativity', the words of Curren and Mallinson come to mind. In relation to another notoriously difficult concept for psychiatry, psychopathic personality disorder, they stated 'I can't define an elephant, but I know one when I see one'! Even a relatively perspicacious layman 'knows' a negative schizophrenic state when he or

Table 1.2. *The classification of negative features in schizophrenia. (After Carpenter et al., 1985.)*

Primary	Authentic, derived from core illness-mediated pathophysiological disturbance(s)
Secondary	Withdrawal induced by 'positive' symptomatology
	Retardation of depression or other dysphoric mood states
	Psychosocial poverty
	Bradykinesia

she sees one. However, the problems of teasing out the constituent features that comprise this complex state are legion and translate into a glaring lack of professional consensus.

Even if one could define the beast, there remains the very real issue of one's capabilities in determining confidently whether it is of the African or Indian variety – or, for that matter, a hairy mammoth. Many of the features that comprise 'negativity' lack phenomenological clarity and diagnostic specificity. Apparent improvement in negative features might, in fact, reflect improvement in outwardly similar but pathophysiologically quite unrelated phenomena.

In order to address this issue, the idea of 'primary' and 'secondary' negative features was introduced (Carpenter, Heinrichs and Alphs, 1985; Table 1.2), the former being seen as the *authentic* manifestations of the disease process, and the latter term being reserved for similar presentations whose roots are in different terrains. While this is a useful theoretical framework within which to judge clinical observations, it still makes the assumption that it is possible to identify each of these circumstances with confidence in real, living patients. This is a bold and probably spurious assumption, even in relation to any one occurring on its own. It would seem fanciful where two or more are present in the same patient. This point is worth emphasising in light of the prominence given to subjective symptomatology in some of the chapters that follow.

Thus, studies of antipsychotic efficacy in negative schizophrenic states confront Himalayan obstacles. One reviewer concluded that the conceptual and practical difficulties are such that, at present, the question of antipsychotic efficacy in negative states cannot be answered (Moller, 1993). A more pragmatic position might be that, with all of the above taken into account, there is nothing in the literature that is incompatible with the view that reported benefits from antipsychotics lie in the domains of secondary disorder, and hence reflect tolerability rather than efficacy issues. It is important to note that this general conclusion would seem to apply to clozapine as much as it does to other compounds (Owens, 1996) and, this being the case, it is very likely to apply to the new generation compounds also.

It does not, therefore, appear that antipsychotics can be separated with any confidence on the basis of efficacy in primary or authentic negative states.

The final efficacy parameter on which antipsychotics might be considered for difference is in treatment resistance. In terms of 'positive' symptomatology, the USA multicentre study showed that, by modest criteria, improvements of about 30 per cent could be attributed to clozapine compared to only about 4 per cent to chlorpromazine (Kane et al, 1988). Thus, for the first time, an antipsychotic could be credited with enhanced efficacy – albeit confined to a circumscribed patient group and not radical in degree. Clozapine is not miraculous in this regard, but its effects are sufficiently meaningful for it to be considered atypical of antipsychotics as a whole.

The general tolerability of antipsychotics is hugely diverse and as a rule is not (with one exception) a fruitful sea to trawl in search of difference. The exception is hyperprolactinaemia. Notwithstanding their diverse central pharmacologies, antipsychotics share in common the ability to block the D_2 family of dopamine receptors. This is *the* key fact in our understanding of the pharmacological basis of antipsychotic action. As a consequence of this action on the tuberoinfundibular dopamine system, the standard drugs *all* produce a sustained rise in serum prolactin levels. By contrast, clozapine and most of the newer drugs either produce no elevation of prolactin or only a transient rise.

On this biochemical parameter, clozapine and most new generation antipsychotics are not typical of standard drugs.

Without question, the single major problem associated with the use of antipsychotics is the subject of the present volume: their depressing liability to promote extrapyramidal neurological dysfunction. Any drug with a clearly diminished propensity to cause abnormalities of this sort would certainly be 'different'.

Enter clozapine! To all intents and purposes, acute dystonias do not occur with clozapine; parkinsonism appears to be at most only half as frequent; and a switch to clozapine is associated with 50 per cent or greater reductions in akathisia and tardive dyskinesia ratings. Extrapyramidal tolerability can therefore provide a clear clinical measure of 'difference' (Owens, 1996). As will be emphasised in the following chapters, the position with regard to the new drugs is unclear at the time of writing. These drugs certainly do seem to represent an improvement over standard compounds in terms of a liability to extrapyramidal dysfunction, but, whether collectively or individually, any can truthfully claim the mantle of 'the new clozapine' remains to be seen.

Thus, while the ideal would be to seek 'difference' between anti-psychotics on the basis of all of the efficacy and tolerability criteria noted above, only some are at present practical. In clinical terms, the ideal 'atypical' compound should at least have a clearly diminished liability to promote extrapyramidal adverse effects, minimal or no effects on prolactin secretion, and a detectable advantage in the treatment of productive symptomatology unresponsive to standard drug treatments.

The other set of parameters on which difference may be sought among antipsychotics is their pharmacological properties. This in some ways should represent the ideal, although only if at the end of the day it has some meaning in clinical terms. Thus far, this has not proved to be the case. Clozapine's 'rich' pharmacology offers a variety of methods for seeking difference, but these do not have ready clinical resonance. For example, it has been suggested that ratios of receptor-binding affinities to 5-HT_{2A} and D_2 sites may be a useful measure (Meltzer, Matsubara and Lee, 1989), and in this regard clozapine is certainly different, having a higher ratio than other established compounds. However, by this criterion, risperidone should be highly atypical as it has one of the highest ratios of all the available drugs, yet clearly enhanced efficacy in treatment resistance remains to be established and clinically its use is associated with a dose-dependent increase in prolactin secretion and in extrapyramidal side-effect (EPS) liability.

One established property of the standard drugs is the development of post-synaptic supersensitivity of D_2 dopamine receptors with chronic exposure. This phenomenon does not apparently occur with chronic exposure to clozapine (LaHoste et al, 1991), while chronic treatment with remoxipride is associated with upregulation (an increase in numbers) but not apparently with functional supersensitivity (Ogren et al, 1990). Remoxipride does appear to have a reduced EPS liability compared to the high-potency haloperidol, but, in comparison with other low-potency drugs, its position is less clear (Owens, 1996). Whether the ability to produce functional supersensitivity with chronic exposure is a valid basis for a dichotomous classification of antipsychotic drugs remains to be seen.

'Atypicality' is a valid concept in view of the unique clinical and pharmacological properties of clozapine but, until differences in both these areas can be meaningfully connected, it should be used with circumspection. Most importantly, 'atypical' should not be seen as a synonym for 'new'.

2

Some preliminaries

The need for vigilance

Although they are not curative agents, the beneficial effects of antipsychotics on the severest end of the psychiatric spectrum have been established unequivocally. These drugs have been the catalysts for reversing centuries-old misconceptions of madness, both lay and professional, and the tools which have made possible the implementation of humane models of care for some of the most vulnerable and misunderstood of human beings. It would be hard to over-emphasise their impact. Like all medical interventions, however, their target actions (the benefits) only come as part of a package, which includes a variety of non-target actions (the adverse effects), and while the latter issues are the primary concern of the present volume, the reader must place them in the above context.

The major impact of drug-related movement disorders is within psychiatric practice, and indeed psychiatry has more or less 'phagocytosed' the idea of EPS as its own. In terms of volume, this is justified. In no other area of medicine have therapeutic tools so crucial to practice produced such high levels of iatrogenic neurological morbidity. Any psychiatric unit and its environs provide a rich observatory of the range of ills to which the human extrapyramidal system can fall prey, and any group of people anywhere on earth may hold an example for the keen eye.

The author vividly recalls a trip to South West Java, which, although geographically close to Jakarta, remains isolated and traditional. While doing the sunset promenade in a remote mountain village, I was uncannily aware that I was not alone. Behind me stalked my 'shadow', a local lad in his early twenties mirroring everything I did. He was easily dispatched with a few rupiah and, as he left, his echopraxia left him also, to be replaced by a striking orofacial dyskinesia and a gait devoid of arm

Table 2.1. *Clinicians' recognition of drug-related*
extrapyramidal disorder. (After Weiden et al., 1987.)

	Percentage of patients given a research diagnosis
Parkinsonism	59
Dystonia	33
Akathisia	26
Tardive dyskinesia	10

swing. The local youths, for whom this all provided great – and clearly regular – amusement, knew only three words of English – 'Hello, mister' (to me) and 'Crazy' (as they gestured after the hapless lad)! Compliance can create its stigmata anywhere.

It might be accurately stated that general psychiatrists now 'see' as much movement disorder as general neurologists. With such a wealth of experience on their professional doorsteps, it might not be unreasonable to expect that psychiatrists would be adept at recognition. Would that this were so! In a revealing study a few years ago, Weiden and colleagues (1987) evaluated psychiatrists' recognition/awareness of movement disorders in relation to that of researchers trained in their identification (Table 2.1). While the clinicians in routine charge of the patients did passably well with parkinsonism, they were poor with dystonia and akathisia, and – perhaps most worrying of all – truly appalling when it came to tardive dyskinesia – and this at a time when (the mid-1980s) and in a place where (the USA) tardive dyskinesia occupied a prominent position in the research literature. It would be complacent to seek comfort in the optimistic belief that things would necessarily be better elsewhere or now.

This 'blind spot' to major physical symptomatology is perhaps explicable in terms of past traditions and current training practices. Psychiatry comes from a staunchly independent tradition, only surpassed in belief in its own expertise by that of neurology! Divergent evolutionary pathways continue to be expressed in training programmes that foster 'tramlining'- neurologists for neurology, psychiatrists for mental state. From a psychiatric perspective, this breeds practitioners with a remarkable perspicacity at inferring the damaged soul within while remaining blind to signs of the damaged body without.

'Tramlining' may also underlie a rather disconcerting failure on the part of psychiatrists even to acknowledge the impact of adverse effects on that most crucial area, compliance. This has been illustrated by Hoge

Table 2.2. *Reasons for refusal of antipsychotic medication. (After Hoge et al., 1990.)*

Patients	Percentage	Clinicians	Percentage
Side-effects	35	Psychotic or 'idiosyncratic' reasons	49
Psychotic symptomatology	30	Transference problems	11
Denial of illness	21	Side-effects	7
Stated ineffectiveness	12		

et al. (1990), who surveyed a large sample of patients refusing antipsychotic medication, the great bulk of whom (96 per cent) had received it previously (Table 2.2). Whereas some patients gave the predictable reasons based on lack of insight etc., 35 per cent stated that their refusal was based on the issue of unacceptable side-effects.

What was revealing about this study, however, was the fact that the researchers then similarly questioned the physicians in charge of the patients' care. The psychiatrists produced a fascinating array of reasons relating to 'idiosyncratic' aspects of the patients, with, of course, a liberal smattering of dynamic theory loosely presented under the heading of 'transference'. In only 7 per cent of cases did the psychiatrists consider that the reason for the patients' refusal was side-effects. Although this study did not restrict itself to side-effects of an exclusively neurological nature, the point it illustrates remains: that there exists a striking difference in perception between those who need to take these drugs and those who – like doctors – need only talk about them.

It is interesting how successful doctors can be at presenting compliance as largely, if not exclusively, a patient-based issue. When compliance breaks down, it is invariably portrayed as the patient's 'fault'. This is a cop-out. Doctors, by their recommendations, can impact on many of the factors that contribute to poor compliance, for example by simplifying regimes to something the average individual has a fighting chance of remembering, by taking time to explain the nature and purpose of treatment, and, most importantly, by recognising side-effects when they develop, acknowledging their importance and, where possible, intervening to alleviate them. Patients can forgive a lot of their doctors but not apparent ignorance or indifference. They will not be forgiving of practitioners who tenaciously seek the dynamic Holy Grail, while remaining stubbornly indifferent to the consequences of the drugs they have prescribed – nor will their lawyers. Some of the clinical

Table 2.3. *The classification of drug-related movement disorders*

Criterion			
Mode of onset/ course		Acute	Chronic
Duration of exposure	Early	Intermediate	Late
Syndromal	Acute dystonias	Parkinsonism Akathisia (acute)	Tardive dyskinesia Tardive akathisia
Relationship to pharmacological intervention	Direct/intimate neurological responsivity		Indirect/ delayed/ paradoxical neurological responsivity

and non-clinical arguments in support of a more industrious approach to the whole issue of neurological adverse effects are aired in Chapter 12.

While 'tramlining' may provide an explanation for oversight and a failure to acknowledge the impact of some of our management decisions, it can no longer provide a justification. EPS are rapidly becoming a quality-of-care issue that must be addressed within the context of management that is truly comprehensive. All those dealing with patients receiving antipsychotic and other implicated drugs – and that embraces a wide church – must be possessed of constant vigilance and, as far as doctors at least are concerned, competent assessment skills.

The classification of drug-related movement disorders

There are a number of ways in which the movement disorders associated with antipsychotic and other drug use may be classified (Table 2.3), although none is entirely satisfactory.

The first has established resonance for both neurology and psychiatry. Abnormality may be thought of in terms of the presence of movements that are not part of normal motor status, or in terms of an absence of normal motor activity – in other words, as either the 'positive' or the 'negative' manifestations of motor disorder. An alternative but similar designation might be 'hyperkinetic' or 'hypokinetic'.

The positive/negative terminology is certainly familiar and has been used in the psychiatric literature in relation to the classification of motor disorders, although not specifically those associated with drug use (McKenna et al., 1991). There is, nonetheless, a potential for confusion in its widespread adoption for there is some, albeit not consistent, evidence that 'hyperkinetic' motor disorders may relate to 'negative' mental state features, but no evidence that they correlate with 'positive' symptomatology (see Chapter 8). The merit in using such broad descriptive headings would come from them pointing to some unifying theoretical framework, which is clearly not the case. Such a simple dichotomy is further confounded by the fact that tremor, the commonest type of hyperkinetic disorder, is not considered part of the major hyperkinetic syndrome, tardive dyskinesia, but finds its natural clinical abode as a core feature of the predominantly hypokinetic syndrome of parkinsonism.

Some clinicians simply consider disorder as 'acute' or 'chronic', although the inference to be drawn is not usually stated. In medicine, these terms imply a pattern of onset as well as a time course, and whereas it is certainly the case that some types of disorder may be more likely to have a sudden onset and subsequently to run a more benign or reversible course than others, this is by no means a rule that can be generally applied. It seems, for example, perverse to call drug-related parkinsonism, which gradually evolves over months and may remain present for many years, 'acute', or to assume, as we shall see, that it is necessarily a reversible disorder.

What this system would appear to be attempting is merely the separation of tardive disorders from the rest, an endeavour that may be justified on the basis of simplicity but one that, on closer scrutiny, is negated by conceptual complexity.

A further attempt at the same separation is equally simple but frankly illogical. In recent years, some authors in the field, especially in the USA, have applied the term EPS specifically to the 'acute' end of the symptomatic spectrum, maintaining separate usage of tardive dyskinesia. The term EPS carries nothing more than a general pathophysiological inference with a hint of localisation. There is no suggestion – not even from those who adopt this terminology – that tardive motor disorders are mediated by anything other than disruption of so-called 'extrapyramidal' mechanisms, and as such they are just as legitimately considered EPS as anything else. A classification based on 'EPS' versus 'tardive dyskinesia' is confusing and unsound, and should be avoided.

Perhaps the most satisfactory means of classifying drug-related movement disorders is on the basis of the relationship their onset bears to the duration of exposure to the implicated drug. Disorders may, therefore, be considered as genuinely 'acute' and 'chronic' in relation to both their onset and their course, with an 'intermediate' category for abnormality most likely to emerge subacutely and to have a variable course.

The major merit of this system is that it relates to readily identifiable syndromes and thus has clinical, and possibly pathophysiological, validity. It must be appreciated, however, that the duration of exposure criteria can only be specified in the most general terms, because of the interposing effects of a range of variables that will be encountered as we progress.

At a practical level, the symptomatology of disorders at the acute or intermediate end of the classificatory spectrum should retain an intimate relationship to pharmacological interventions. Features should be swiftly appeased by specific drug treatments or decrements in dose or potency of the implicated drug or exacerbated by dose or potency increments. In tardive or chronic disorders, the inference is that these intimate pharmacological relationships are *lost*, strikingly compromised or paradoxical.

One final point is to note an exclusion from the present work. Recently, some authors have included neuroleptic malignant syndrome in the category of drug-related movement disorders along with the syndromes to be discussed below. This is not a convention adopted here. While extrapyramidal motor disturbance is certainly a cardinal feature of this rare and mysterious disorder, it is but one aspect of a complex and ill-understood state which sits uncomfortably in the relatively 'pure' taxonomic environs of the present volume. An exposition on neuroleptic malignant syndrome is best left for a specialist monograph, one which the author will not be in a position to produce. After more than 20 years of practice specialising in the management of schizophrenia, I have yet to see a definite case – but of this, more later!

The villains of the piece

Much of the aforegoing – and most of the following – is slanted heavily towards antipsychotic drugs as the pharmacological 'villains' (although, as we shall see, this may be to put too thin a veneer of understanding on things). This emphasis is deliberate: not only does the author's background as a clinical psychiatrist make it inevitable, but the overwhelming association in the literature is with this class of drugs. Indeed, in suggesting above that the term EPS had been more or less purloined by psychiatry, the author was in fact referring to this association. It would be a mistake, however, to assume that these were the only type of drugs with which extrapyramidal neurological adverse effects have been reported. The words are chosen well, for observing an association is not the same as establishing a cause-and-effect relationship, and some of these associations may represent chance occurrences. The major associations, along with some of the less frequently reported, are shown in Table 2.4 and are presented here in order to highlight the need for a breadth of awareness of the issues throughout modern medical practice and to emphasise that, while antipsychotics may be one of the most persistent offenders, they are not the only extrapyramidal delinquents in the pharmacopoeia.

Non-antipsychotic phenothiazines continue to be widely used for their antihistamine properties and are sometimes recommended as anti-allergics, antimigraine treatments and as medications to combat travel sickness. A number of years ago, the student counsellor at a local college referred to the author a young man recently arrived from West Africa, who she believed to be experiencing 'cultural disassimilation'. In response to any attempt at conversation, the student stuck out his tongue, grimaced and, to any reasonable ear, appeared to parody the speech or others, a response which inevitably bred a certain indignation. It transpired, however, that the young man was a poor traveller and in order to try to ensure an incident-free journey, had taken proprietary antitravel sickness pills, which he had continued on arrival to help him sleep. His instant 'assimilation' was effected via a 'stat' dose of anticholinergic!

The widespread inclusion of phenothiazines in proprietary preparations must not be overlooked. Many proprietary cold cures and cough remedies available 'over the counter' contain antihistamines and such preparations have been reported as causing acute dystonic reactions, especially in children (Rainier-Pope, 1979; Etzel, 1994). Indeed, one might wonder if in the very young this is not a more common occurrence than the literature would suggest, as such episodes may easily be confused with seizures.

These types of provoking agent are seldom taken long enough for anything apart from acute dystonias to emerge in terms of EPS although tardive orofacial disorder has been described with prolonged ingestion of antihistamine decongestants (Thach Chase and Bosma, 1975). Anti-emetics used in gastrointestinal practice may, on the other hand, be taken long term and may be associated with the same spectrum of extrapyramidal disorder as antipsychotics. The major 'culprit' here is metoclopramide, which is probably the single most frequently implicated agent after antipsychotics, especially in relation to tardive dyskinesia (Ganzini et al., 1993). Onset of tardive dyskinesia following commencement of metoclopramide is often rapid, with a mean duration of exposure in one review of only 14 months (Harrington et al., 1983). This perhaps relates to the fact that patients tend to be older and may also be suffering from major physical illness, factors that, as we shall see,

Table 2.4. *Drugs associated with the development of movement disorders*

	Frequent	Established but infrequent	Rare or poorly documented
Acute dystonias	Standard antipsychotics Metoclopramide	Prochlorperazine SSRI antidepressants Amoxapine Antimalarials Antihistamines	Tetrabenazine Mefanamic acid Oxatomide Flunarizine Cinnarizine
Parkinsonism	Standard antipsychotics Metoclopramide Prochlorperazine Reserpine Tetrabenazine	Clozapine SSRI antidepressants Amoxapine Ca channel antagonists Methyldopa Pethidine (meperidine) Toxins: MPTP manganese cyanide carbon disulphide alcohol withdrawal	Phenytoin Lithium salts Cytosine arabinoside
Akathisia	Standard antipsychotics Metoclopramide Reserpine Tetrabenazine	Prochlorperazine SSRI antidepressants Amoxapine Dopamine agonists Flunarizine Cinnarizine	Ethosuximide Methysergide Trycyclic antidepressants
Dyskinesias choreiform	Standard antipsychotics Metoclopramide Dopamine agonists: L-dopa Apomorphine Bromocriptine Lisuride	Antihistamines Prochlorperazine Anticholinergics Amoxapine Oral contraceptives Alcohol withdrawal Phenytoin (toxicity)	Ethosuximide MAOI antidepressants Tricyclic antidepressants Methyldopa Methadone Digoxin Flunarizine

Table 2.4. (*cont.*)

	Frequent	Established but infrequent	Rare or poorly documented
	Pergolide Amphetamines Methylphenidate Amantadine Pemoline Fenfluramine	Cocaine	Cinnarizine Volatile solvents Carbamazepine (toxicity) Lithium salts (toxicity) Phenobarbital (toxicity)
Dyskinesias dystonic	Standard antipsychotics Metoclopramide L-dopa	Direct dopamine agonists: Apomorphine Bromocriptine Lisuride Pergolide Phenytoin (toxicity)	Flunarizine Cinnarizine Carbamazepine (toxicity)
Dyskinesias tics	Indirect dopamine agonists	Direct dopamine agonists Standard antipsychotics	Carbamazepine Dopamine agonist withdrawal in Parkinson's disease
Dyskinesias myoclonus	L-dopa Anticonvulsant (toxicity)	Tricyclic antidepressants Clozapine	
Tremor	Standard antipsychotics Lithium salts Tricyclic antidepressants Alcohol withdrawal L-dopa Na valproate Amphetamines Caffeine Thyroid hormone Sympathomimetics Steroids Hypoglycaemics Bronchodilators	Amiodarone Cyclosporin A	

seem to be of importance in a psychiatric context too. Metoclopramide's predilection to promote EPS comes as no surprise in view of the fact that it is a substituted benzamide with the D_2 antagonist properties shared by that group; but this is easy to overlook, particularly in non-specialist settings. Nonetheless, patients prescribed this compound should be monitored just as closely as those receiving antipsychotics.

Antidepressants have hitherto remained remarkably untarnished, but this favourable appraisal now needs some revision, with possibly interesting ramifications. Tricyclics as a group may, in a small percentage of patients, produce a degree of excitement associated with restlessness and agitation – especially in the first few days of exposure – sometimes referred to as the 'early tricyclic' or 'jitteriness' syndrome (Pohl, Yeragani and Ortiz, 1986). Only rarely has this been linked conceptually to akathisia, and it remains unclear whether these are the same or different phenomena. It is certainly the case that tricyclics can cause tremor, probably noradrenergically mediated. A handful of reports have described dyskinetic abnormalities developing in the course of tricyclic treatment (Fann et al., 1976; Dekret et al., 1977), but such reports are so rare in the context of the widespread international use of these drugs for 40 years that they must be seen as aberrations, probably reflecting incidental spontaneous dyskinesias. This is supported by the one formal investigation of the question. In an elderly population, Yassa et al. (1987) found a dyskinesia prevalence of 6 per cent, which is comparable to the rates reported for spontaneous disorder.

However, one exception to the general rule is worth noting. Amoxapine is a dibenzoxazepine with a very close structural similarity to the standard antipsychotic loxapine. Its active metabolite, 8-hydroxyamoxapine, has potent dopamine antagonist properties which, from radioreceptor bioassays, are probably comparable to those of standard antipsychotics. It is therefore not surprising that this drug can be associated with the development of EPS and in particular tardive dyskinesia (Lapierre and Anderson, 1983).

Of interest, however, is the evidence that has started to accrue in recent years that the selective serotonin re-uptake inhibitors (SSRIs) may cause extrapyramidal dysfunction. The first report appeared during the evaluation phase of fluoxetine (Meltzer et al., 1979), although the bulk of reports have only emerged since 1989 following the widespread clinical introduction of these drugs (Messiha et al., 1993; Arya, 1994). The most frequently implicated agent has been fluoxetine, but this probably reflects nothing more than this drug's widespread use, particularly in the USA, from where most case reports have emanated. Fluvoxamine, paroxetine and even the early member of the group, trazodone, have also been implicated and it seems likely this is a *group* phenomenon. The gamut of extrapyramidal disorder is represented in these reports, i.e. acute dystonias, parkinsonism, akathisia and dys-kinesias. Some cases had received coincidental or prior antipsychotics, and it does appear that this may increase the likelihood of precipitating disorder. Nonetheless, it seems clear that SSRIs can promote these changes *on their own*.

One young, non-psychotic patient of the author's developed a chronic torticollis coinciding with several months' treatment with paroxetine, which showed no resolution after 12 drug-free months. The only other medication he had been prescribed previously was amitriptyline and diazepam, the latter of which he undoubtedly aug-mented from illicit sources. Treatment of this disabling disorder required local injections of botulinum toxin, although with only partial success. This may, of course, have been a chance association, but it does illustrate the need for open-mindedness in appraising the neurological risks of long-term exposure to these compounds.

The real interest of the observations concerning SSRIs lies in what they may tell us about the relationship between dopaminergic and sero-tonergic mechanisms and the role of the latter in the control of motor function, although a detailed understanding of these issues is some way off. Other compounds with exclusive or significant 5-HT actions have also been rarely implicated in the causation of extrapyramidal dysfunc-tion, such as ondansetron, a highly selective 5-HT_3 antagonist, fenflu-ramine, a putative 5-HT agonist, and buspirone, amongst other things a partial 5-HT_1 agonist, although the last two of these also exert effects on dopamine systems.

Intrusive, course tremor is a well-described side-effect of lithium treatment affecting around 10 per cent of patients (Lyskowski et al., 1982). It is predominantly adrenergically mediated and may respond to beta-blockers. Lithium has in addition been linked with the emergence of other forms of extrapyramidal dysfunction, including dyskinesias, although this has usually been in patients in whom some predisposition can be discerned, such as those with pre-existing Parkinson's disease or Alzheimer's disease. Lithium's complex and ill-understood pharma-cology precludes an understanding of these observations at present.

Drug-related parkinsonism was first described with the rauwalfia alkaloids and can be readily induced by the presynaptic monoamine depleting agents, reserpine and the synthetic, reversible and short-acting analogue, tetrabenazine, although both these compounds are now infrequently used. The antihypertensive methyldopa has similarly been around for many years but is now seldom prescribed. It can induce parkinsonism, possibly by acting as a false transmitter, and several cases of choreiform disorder have been described which have been linked to its interference with the conversion of 5-hydroxytryptophan to serotonin.

A more direct effect on dopamine mechanisms may underlie the extrapyramidal reactions reported with calcium channel blockers, the predominant manifestation of which is, thus far, parkinsonism (Padrell et al., 1995; Daniel and Mauro, 1995). In view of the increasing use of these drugs in older, physically unwell, and hence perhaps more vulnerable, patients, the association must be borne in mind. Cinnarizine and flunarizine – calcium channel antagonists with antihistamine properties – have been similarly implicated (Micheli et al., 1987). Heightened susceptibility may also underlie the few reported associations with the H_2 antagonist cimetidine.

Hyperkinetic disorders can be a well-recognised manifestation of phenytoin toxicity (Chadwick, Reynolds and Marsden, 1976), and although these have been reported infrequently in patients whose blood levels were within the therapeutic range, it again seems that such a scenario can best be explained by the presence of an underlying predisposition (Nausieda et al., 1979). Extrapyramidal symptomatology emerging during carbamazepine treatment (Joyce and Gunderson, 1980; Schwartz et al., 1986) and, rarely, with valproate (Sasso et al., 1994) probably has a similar basis.

The first report of choreiform movements developing in conjunction with the contraceptive pill appeared in 1966 (Fernando and Chir, 1966). Since then, this association has been well documented. The presentation is similar to chorea gravidarum, with onset usually in the first few months of starting the pill and resolution complete one to two months after stopping. The hormonal climate of pregnancy created by contraceptives provides an obvious pathophysiological parallel, with the dopaminergic sensitising effects of oestrogens as a common mechanism. However, there is evidence that, once again, involuntary movements only develop in the presence of subtle organic change. Contraceptives may therefore operate in the dual role of producing the microvascular and ischaemic changes in the basal ganglia that provide a predisposing substrate, while also being the source of the increased oestrogen load that acts as provoking agent.

A major therapeutic challenge in Parkinson's disease is the hyperkinetic disorders that occur in the course of treatment with L-dopa. These comprise choreiform, dystonic and myoclonic dyskinesias that emerge in association with either peak or trough plasma levels (Comella and Tanner, 1992). Peak dyskinesias during the 'on' phase of maximal L-dopa effectiveness are the most common and are to be found in up to half of those on treatment. They can vary in severity from mild, unobtrusive abnormality to the potentially life threatening. Patients may be profoundly distressed, or strikingly unconcerned.

A few years ago, the author asked a neurologist colleague for patients with Parkinson's disease in order to make a teaching video. On arrival in the department, one middle-aged woman who had been thought suitable by my colleague was not at all what was expected, as she had a severe, generalised dystonia. She admitted to 'a bit of a shake', but this did not bother her as it was only present 'sometimes'. Her neurologist was surprised to see the results of the video as she had never demonstrated anything like that in the clinic nor made any complaint. It transpired that she had taken her L-dopa immediately before coming for the video, as she wished to be mobile and 'do well' for the students. Her routine outpatient appointments, however, were in the afternoon, some time after her last dose and certainly nothing worth making a special effort for!

L-dopa-induced dyskinesias can also be associated with 'off' phases when plasma levels are lowest. In this situation, dystonias predominate. One manifestation of this type of disorder occurs with trough levels on waking in the morning.

L-dopa dyskinesias can be indistinguishable cross-sectionally from tardive dyskinesia. However, their cyclically fluctuating course is strikingly different and, on detailed analysis, they also have more of a peripheral distribution (Gerlach, 1977; Karson et al., 1984). Also, whereas tardive dyskinesia is, as we shall see, strongly associated with advancing age, L-dopa-related disorders are more of a problem in patients with a younger onset of their Parkinson's disease.

It is easy to forget that extrapyramidal symptomatology is not only associated with prescribed medications. A number of drugs used for recreational purposes can have similar consequences. Choreoathetoid and tic-like movements can be produced by excessive use of amphetamines and their analogues, which act as indirect dopamine and noradrenaline agonists (Mattson and Calverley, 1968). A similar phenomenon can occur when these drugs, and the related compound methylphenidate, are administered to patients with hyperactivity/ attention deficit and narcolepsy (Lowe et al., 1982; Erenberg Cruse and Rothner, 1985). Similarly, excessive recreational use of cocaine can produce a restless-appearing choreoathetosis, referred to in the colourful parlance of the streets as 'crack dancing' (Daras, Koppel and Atos Radzion, 1994). There is, in addition, evidence that recreational use of cocaine may exacerbate the abnormal movements of Gilles de la Tourette's syndrome (Factor, Sanchez-Ramos and Weiner, 1988). Choreiform movements have been described rarely with methadone use (Wasserman and Yahr, 1980), and parkinsonism with solvent abuse (Utti et a., 1994).

In the early 1980s, four cases of sudden-onset, severe parkinsonism occurred in young people in a geographically discrete area of California (Langston et al., 1983). It transpired that each of the victims had taken a 'designer' drug contaminated by 1-methyl-4-phenyl-1,2,5,6-tetra-hydropyridine or (MPTP.) This compound has opened the door to the most satisfactory model for Parkinson's disease to date. Although it was originally thought that this was itself the toxic agent, it subsequently became clear that the sequence is more complicated. MPTP is readily absorbed from nasal mucosa but is metabolised by monoamine oxidase-B (MAO-B) to 1-methyl-4-phenylpyridine (MPP+). This in its turn is taken up into dopaminergic neurons in the substantia nigra, where it exerts a selective toxicity in the zona compacta, resulting in the development of parkinsonism with a risk proportionate to the degree of cell loss.

Many individuals other than those who presented initially were exposed and it is to be expected that they will in effect have advanced their risk of developing the syndrome, both in terms of their overall likelihood and their age of onset, as the effects of age-related cell loss become added to those inflicted by the drug. Thus, an amateur chemist with an illicit still and a mission to alter minds unwittingly altered medical research instead by opening a whole new door on one of medicine's great mysteries. He may further have shed light on the mechanism of the parkinsonism very occasionally encountered with the narcotic analgesic pethidine (meperidine) which may result from formation of MPTP.

Finally, there is, as always, alcohol. The association here is not, for once, a positive one but more, as it were, a 'negative' one. Individuals suddenly withdrawing from prolonged, excessive intake may develop generalised choreoathetoid movements (Mullin, Kershaw and Bolt, 1970). These are not associated with deficiency states or other overt physical disorders and are invariably transient. The author has seen only a single case, in a 27-year-old man in whom rudimentary, flitting perioral and upper limb movements emerged 48 hours after he was persuaded to abandon a protracted 'bender' he had pursued with particular diligence. The movements resolved spontaneously over the subsequent two days. Recently, reports have also described parkinsonism developing transiently during alcohol withdrawal (Luijckx et al., 1995). One's assumption is that both hyperkinesis and parkinsonism emerging in the course of withdrawal from alcohol must be comparatively rare in view of the infrequency of reports in the literature, although again it may be that greater awareness will dispel this view.

Thus, when evaluating disturbance of voluntary motor function, drugs *must* nowadays be a major consideration and the list to be borne in mind is substantial and expanding. All clinicians, regardless of specialty interest, must be alert to these disorders. However, working from a psychiatric perspective, and by the old adage that the bird on the rooftop is more likely to be a sparrow than a cockatoo (except possibly if one lives in Australia), the rest of our deliberations will be restricted almost exclusively to antipsychotics.

A small caveat

Much of the thrust of what follows is towards a heightened recognition of disorders that are often frankly bizarre in patients who usually are, or have been, seriously psychiatrically unwell. The expectation is that such recognition will retain the reader well and truly within a biological (i.e. neurological) frame of reference and dissuade him or her away from the wilder frontiers of dynamic speculation. If this aim is achieved, there will be no surprise that the diagnostic differentials periodically noted do not as a rule refer to psychological/psychiatric causes of movement disorders.

The omission is deliberate. No-one practising in the field of clinical neuroscience will need to be reminded of the problems speculative dynamics have caused in the past, and nowhere more so than in the field of movement disorders. Nonetheless, in recent years a number of reports from expert sources have highlighted the rare but valid diagnosis of psychogenic movement disorders (Factor, Podskalny and Molho, 1995; Marjama, Troster and Koller, 1995). One does not need to get bogged down in terminology here, but the inference is that the root of the problem in these cases resides in disturbed psychological rather than neurological mechanisms.

The author has experience of only a solitary case in which a severe, generalised and outwardly very convincing dystonia emerged in an unhappy woman. The patient developed a 'stiff neck', for which she sought relief from an osteopath – who indicated she had dystonia! She then spent the two years prior to specialist referral as a stalwart of the local branch of the Dystonia Society, where she 'learned' much. Notwithstanding her impressive symptomatology, there were concerns that the origins of her disorder may not have been neurological, not least because of its rapidly generalised distribution. Psychogenic dystonia was subsequently confirmed from video by a world authority in the field of movement disorders. A comprehensive psychiatric management plan was then implemented, with good results.

There were two lessons for the author in this case. The first was the necessity of being confident about such a diagnosis in order to make the treatment plan effective, a confidence that would have been attenuated without the back-up opinion of a world authority. The second was the truth of the old adage about the dangers of a little knowledge!

In the group of patients at risk of developing drug-related movement disorders, it is unlikely that a psychogenic diagnosis would be a frequent or reasonable consideration. The present caveat is offered mainly to complete the differentials that follow. In raising it, the earnest hope is that far from fostering dynamic tendencies, it will further help dispel them, for such disorders are extremely rare and the stuff for super-specialists.

3

Acute dystonias

Introduction

Movement disorders developing in the early phase of exposure to antidopaminergic medication or following dose increments are overwhelmingly dystonic in type. However, it must be borne in mind that acute dystonias are not the only motor disorders that can occur at these times. There may be myoclonic jerks of face, neck and limbs as well as jerky tongue protrusions, lip smacking, blinking, tic-like shoulder shrugging and even writhing, choreoathetoid-type arm and leg movements. Such disorders have been referred to as *initial dyskinesias* (Gerlach, 1979). They are certainly a relatively uncommon reaction to antidopaminergic introduction or increment, although how uncommon is unclear. Similarly, although transient, their relationship to other extrapyramidal syndromes is unknown. Over a few days, some of these disorders may blend into the features of akathisia.

From our point of view, however, the vast majority of the early and incremental disorders that we shall have to deal with will be of dystonic type, and it is to this area that we shall devote our attention.

The concept of dystonia

Before embarking on a discussion of acute dystonia, it might be of value to review the basic concept of dystonia itself.

The term 'dystonia' is one that has caused a certain grief to both psychiatry and neurology (Owens, 1990). Its generic meaning obviously refers to a primary abnormality of voluntary muscle tone. This was the sense in which Kinnier Wilson used it, i.e. 'any variability of muscle tone'. On the other hand, such abnormality has outward expression, and some authors used the term to emphasise the postural abnormalities that resulted from the tonal disturbance. Thus, the American neurologist Denny-Brown understood dystonia as 'an abnormal degree of fixity of any attitude owing to sustained muscular contraction', which could be applied to the consequences of spasticity following corticospinal lesions, decerebrate rigidity, or even the flexion of Parkinson's disease. Dystonia, however, had longer and more specific antecedents than such general usage would imply.

In 1871, the American physician W.A. Hammond described two stroke patients who developed distorted postures and muscle 'spasms' affecting the limbs. Because of the inability to maintain the limbs stable, Hammond referred to this as 'athetosis' (literally 'without fixed position'). In 1908, W. Schwalbe published his 28-page doctoral thesis 'A Peculiar Case of Tonic Cramp with Hysterical Symptoms', in which he described three siblings of a Lithuanian Jewish family who developed progressive 'cramp-like' movements from the age of seven. Hysteria was one of some nine differential diagnoses he proposed. The children's father had at one point left for Africa, at which time their distressed mother shook and trembled, an 'insight' based on imitation that even Schwalbe found unconvincing. The cases had too many features of an organic nature and, in a prescient statement, he noted that 'hysterical' features were frequently to be seen in neurological conditions.

Hermann Oppenheim, a powerful force in German neurology, had no doubts. In 1911, he added some more cases to the literature and proposed two suitably imperious names to root the condition well and truly in the neurological field. His first, dysbasia lordotica progressiva, emphasised the pelvic and bizarre gait disturbances, but his second, focusing descriptively on the fluctuating muscle tone, christened the condition with the name by which it is still known, dystonia musculorum deformans (DMD).

Also in 1911, Ziehen published a case report in which he emphasised the rotational quality of the abnormalities the movements produced – that is, the element of torsion. In proposing the term 'Torsionsneurose', however, he combined this clinical observation with an aetiological inference. Although the concept of neurosis then was somewhat different from what is generally understood by the term now, a dominant role for speculative psychological mechanisms went beyond what neurology could accept, and Flatau and Sterling's 'torsion spasms', proposed in the same year, provided a preferable, if clearly neurological, alternative.

Thus, the concept of dystonia was debated widely in the context of a serious, chronic and often hereditary disease, but from the early 1920s, neurology achieved a certain unanimity. Nonetheless, the 'hysterical' cat was out of the 'dynamic' bag, and with the widening of 'dystonia' from a term for a specific disease to a more general syndromal usage, a parting of the ways was inevitable. For neurologists, any sustained abnormal posture would forever be a dystonia; for psychiatrists, it became a mannerism or something else in need of interpretation.

It might be instructive for generations not immersed in psycho-analytic ideology to be apprised of where this orientation could lead in relation to dystonia. An example comes from the writings of Wilfred Abse, who in his 1966 text *Hysteria and Related Mental Disorders*, described the case of a 44-year-old man who developed a 'severe' spas-modic torticollis, progressive over a year or so. The essential elements of the analysis focused on the fact that this had developed during a period of worry about his only son's health and very heavily on the fact of his wife's withdrawal from sexual relations after the birth of this child. Further analysis revealed that all these years he had in fact resented this 'unwelcome intruder' (i.e. his son) who had so selfishly destroyed his relationship with his wife. Indeed, it was discovered that he had unconsciously wished the lad out of the way. The fact that nature almost did just that heightened his guilt and anxiety and broke down his ability to repress his sexual impulses. It transpired that, on 'closer investigation', the torticollis was a disguised expression of his uncon-scious sexual wishes (Abse, 1966; p. 23):

> The movements of his neck were of an auto-erotic nature; that is to say, he had pleasurable sensations on account of them. The neck had come to represent the erected genital organ, was a symbol for it; vasomotor dis-turbances resulted in swelling, and the rhythmic movements aped those in coitus.'

Perhaps it is necessary to have at one's disposal a more extensive experience of the varied anatomy of the male sexual organ than the author has managed to acquire in order fully to appreciate this inter-pretation. On the other hand, maybe such 'insights' are only worthy of recall as a historical footnote to a general silliness that characterised former times, in which psychiatry was an eager participant if not a prime mover.

Recent years have seen a degree of convergence, with the neurolog-ical perspective on dystonia (the syndrome) engendering less indignant opposition, if not total acceptance, in psychiatric circles (Owens, 1990). This in part undoubtedly reflects the general decline of analytical influ-ence within psychiatry itself, although it may also reflect a more com-prehensive and convincing reappraisal of dystonia on the part of neurology.

The above clearly refers primarily to chronic or persistent dystonia, something that is returned to in Chapter 7. However, the acute, drug-related variety does not differ phenomenologically, and an understanding of the evolution of the concept as a whole is valuable in placing the present focus of our attention in context.

Dystonia – the abnormality

Dystonia refers to involuntary motor activity in which the muscle action is sustained at the point of maximal contraction, for however short a period. This latter point is important because there is a widespread belief that dystonias are slow or ultra-slow movements, a perception enshrined in a previous definition that stated that contractions should be maintained for at least 1 second to qualify (Fahn, 1984). This is not now thought to be the case. The spectrum of rapidity from maintained through to fleeting can be encountered, with very rapid movements, such as those sometimes referred to as myoclonic dystonia (Obeso et al., 1983), presenting an almost choreiform appearance.

A further characteristic is that as a consequence of the disconnection between agonist action and reflex antagonist inhibition, movements frequently result in a twisting or 'torquating' distortion of the affected part.

Perhaps the most useful way of considering dystonia from a psychiatric point of view is that proposed by Wechsler and Brock (1922). In effect, they considered dystonias in terms of the 'movement' versus the 'disorder'. They referred to those abnormalities in which repetitive or recurrent dyskinesias predominated as 'kinetic' dystonias, while those sustained disorders in which a disturbance of attitude or postural relationships was the dominant abnormality, they called 'myostatic' in type.

The value of this for the non-neurologist is that it forces one to bear in mind the common pathology behind two clinically different presentations. Acute dystonias are overwhelmingly *myostatic* in type, although, like most things in medicine, this is not an absolute and kinetic disorders can sometimes be found.

Acute dystonias comprise a syndrome and it is in the syndromal context that neurology tends to consider dystonia in general. As shall be seen later (see Chapter 6), for our purposes we can also view dystonia at a sign level.

Clinical features

Standard accounts of the clinical presentations of acute dystonias often omit two obvious and crucial points. The first is that acute dystonias present with a spectrum of severity, and the second is that they have a strong subjective component. These two factors are not unrelated.

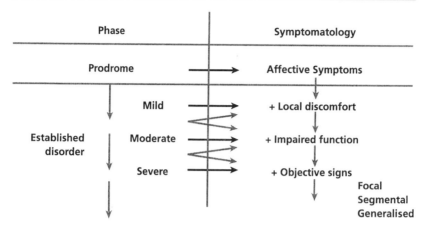

Phase		Symptomatology
Prodrome		Affective Symptoms
	Mild	+ Local discomfort
Established disorder	Moderate	+ Impaired function
	Severe	+ Objective signs
		Focal Segmental Generalised

Fig. 3.1. The spectrum of acute dystonic symptomatology.

Symptoms

Prodromal symptomatology is exclusively subjective (Fig. 3.1) and so apparently unexceptional that it can usually only be detected in experienced patients who, in the light of previous events, latch on to what is happening. Complaints are of no more than a progressive restlessness, unnerving anxiousness or inability to settle, or the sense of an impending 'something'. Even the site at which the 'something' might occur may not be appreciated, but the perception of change is clear. It is easy to dismiss these vaguest of complaints as a crude and half-hearted attempt to squeeze some anticholinergic medication out of gullible staff – as, indeed, on occasion it may well be. However, they may also represent a genuine prodrome and hence provide for the astute the ideal situation in which to achieve some serious prevention.

It is important to bear in mind that the manifestations of truly mild disorder are not twisted muscles or distorted postures but also comprise purely subjective symptomatology (see Fig. 3.1).

Patients who progress beyond the prodromal phase may start to experience tension in affected body parts, or feelings of stiffness or frank pain. Involvement of the tongue may result in feelings that the tongue is swollen or cannot be controlled properly, or progressive recruitment of disorder in the neck may cause an aching discomfort, usually clearly distinguishable from a simple headache, or the bizarre feeling that the head is 'too heavy' to be held upright. As things progress, the complaints become more of impairment of function. Movements in affected muscles are no longer executed without thinking, but seem to require conscious effort, yet to the patient they feel increasingly crude and clumsy.

At this stage patients usually develop characteristic behavioural signs, when they can be seen to 'exercise' the affected part with slow, deliberate, rotational shoulder and head movements, or jaw opening and rotation and repeated grimacing etc. These are not involuntary movements but willed and understandable efforts to relieve their discomfort. While initially restrained, such efforts can become increasingly frantic as the condition evolves.

Associated with the motor symptoms is a usually escalating level of affective symptoms. Patients become anxious, agitated and frankly fearful. Their behaviour can develop a demanding, importuning or dependent quality, which, in the absence of an appreciation of what is going on, can be trying. It is clear that to some extent these features might be an understandable response to the relatively sudden onset of impairment of function, often occurring in vital muscle groups such as those subserving swallowing, posture and so on. Patients may feel they are falling victim to stroke or other serious illness. However, even experienced patients who are well aware of the nature of the problem invariably describe acute dystonic symptomatology as profoundly unpleasant, and it is fair to conclude that affective disturbance is an integral part of the phenomenology of the full-blown syndrome.

This sets a trap for the unwary because this pattern is usually evolving early in the course of treatment (see below), at a time when the professional focus is on the mental state disturbance, which is likely to be maximal anyway. It is all too easy to misattribute such acute extrapyramidal symptomatology to an escalation in the psychiatric condition rather than to the effects of treatment given for it. A further snare in the trap is that these early features, in common with the overt manifestations of the syndrome, often fluctuate in intensity, not merely hour by hour but minute by minute. The unwary and the blinkered can all too readily divine 'hysteria' at work, a snare that attaches itself to all dystonias, as shall be seen.

The temptation is therefore to seek only psychiatric explanations when comprehensive assessment would demand inclusion of a neurological one as well. Failure in this regard can have far-reaching consequences. A policy of non-intervention or attempting to set boundaries may allow a full-blown dystonia to develop later, while in the meantime the patient continues to suffer, awaiting the inevitable or, worse still, a decision may be made to increase medication, thereby precipitating the full syndrome. The author is aware of the case of an adolescent male admitted for assessment and treated initially with haloperidol. He subsequently became loud, restless and apparently threatening in his behaviour and was given further haloperidol and placed in seclusion. During a routine check, he was found to have amputated the anterior half of his tongue. It is as easy to see the unfortunate repercussions of such an event for staff as well as for the patient.

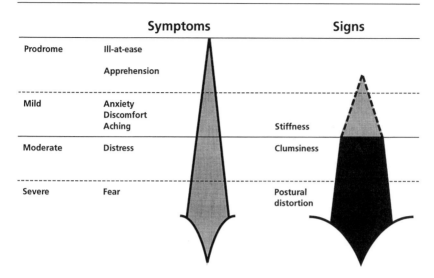

Fig. 3.2. The balance of symptoms and signs in acute dystonias.

Doctors cannot always be held responsible for not detecting this mild or early symptomatology as patients may not themselves provide clear clues. The extrapyramidal features may be genuinely buried in the generality of behavioural and affective disturbance. Alternatively, this phase may be traversed so rapidly that no-one – not even the patient – has the opportunity to register what is happening prior to the development of clear objective signs. However, considerable distress to patients may be ameliorated and a few catastrophes averted if the mandatory high index of suspicion necessary in relation to all EPS is extended to these manifestations of dystonia as well.

Signs

Once objective signs become evident, the problem is of at least mild–moderate severity. This symptom/sign balance is illustrated in more detail in Figure 3.2. Signs usually develop rapidly over a few minutes and have a distribution that, like idiopathic dystonia, is dependent on age. Thus, acute dystonias tend to be more extensive in younger patients and, especially in children, may be generalised, while in adults they are more likely to be restricted to the postural muscles of head and neck, perioral and intrinsic tongue muscles and extrinsic ocular and periocular muscles.

The best data on the frequency of different presentations in adults comes from the Boston Collaborative Drug Surveillance Program, which extracted data on 1152 cases (Swett, 1975). The best is not, however, strong. Data were based on retrospective interviews of physicians by nurse monitors, which would be likely to focus on the dominant abnormality as opposed to a detailed regional evaluation. Furthermore, only a first episode of acute dystonia was considered when more than one occurred. The figures must therefore be treated with circumspection. Nonetheless, they indicate that the commonest adult presentation is a torticollis, accounting for approximately 30 per cent of cases. Torticollis tends to be used clinically as a somewhat imprecise term for any dystonic distortion of the neck, so presumably this figure includes the variants of laterocollis- and anterocollis and, what from clinical experience is probably the most common neck displacement in this context, retrocollis.

The next commonest abnormality was 'swollen tongue', which one assumes refers to the exclusively subjective manifestation noted above, since there is no suggestion that the tongue actually does swell in the course of an acute dystonic episode. However, all the other features cited in this study are signs. Of interest is the fact that trismus, or forced jaw closure from masseter spasm, comprised 14.6 per cent of cases, probably making this a more common abnormality than most people would imagine.

Only 6 per cent of cases comprised what the study referred to as 'oculogyric crises'. This low prevalence of eye signs to some extent flies in the face of popular wisdom, as this is *the* one manifestation of acute dystonia that every nurse and every trainee, to say nothing of every experienced patient, knows about. The striking presentation of this variant and the indelible impression it leaves on those who experience it have no doubt contributed to its prominence in the professional consciousness, but its relative infrequency in a formal study is probably compatible with the clinical reality. The question of whether we have adopted the correct terminology for this phenomenon is one that shall be addressed further at a later stage.

In the Boston data, 3.5 per cent of cases were of opisthotonos (arching of the back), and just under 30 per cent were made up of disorder affecting a range of sites not specified, some of which presumably included limbs.

As was noted, young adults, adolescents and particularly children are more likely to present a picture of generalised dystonia (Owens, 1990). Thus, there may be truncal involvement which, if bilateral, will give rise to opisthotonos. If truncal dystonia has a predominantly or exclusively unilateral distribution, the patient develops a one-sided lean with a backward rotation which brings forward the shoulder on the opposite side. This is probably a more frequent manifestation of chronic dystonia, although it can present as an acute sign as well, especially in the elderly. It is often referred to as the Pisa syndrome – for obvious reasons – or as one of Dr Ekbom's three eponymous syndromes. This is, however, merely one manifestation of a segmental dystonia and does not appear to have any unique characteristics or correlates that would justify its separate consideration. Notwithstanding psychiatry's hunger for syndromes and eponyms, the terms Pisa syndrome and Ekbom's syndrome are best dropped (Owens, 1990; van Harten, 1992).

Signs in the upper limbs include typical dystonic hyperpronation of the forearms with flexion at the wrists and metacarpo-phalangeal joints combined with finger extension, frequently resulting in bizarre posturing and 'accusatory' pointing. In the legs, the hips and knees are held in extension with the ankles tending to plantarflexion, while the dominant action of the powerful adductors forces the legs together or even to cross. The impact of these changes on gait is obvious, with the patient either attempting to walk on 'tip-toe' or developing a so-called 'scissor' gait where each foot is forced across the path of the other with each step.

In recent years, a number of reports have highlighted two uncommon but potentially dangerous manifestations of acute dystonia, namely laryngeal adductor spasm giving rise to respiratory distress, frank stridor and asphyxiation, and supraglottic and pharyngeal dystonia resulting in profound dysphagia, choking and inability to swallow even saliva (Flaherty and Lahmeyer, 1978; Newton-John, 1988; Stones, Kennedy and Fulton, 1990).

In fact, sudden, unexpected asphyxial death in patients receiving anti-psychotics was reported shortly after the introduction of these drugs (Hollister, 1957), as was death resulting from what was subsequently described as a 'bulbar palsy-like syndrome' (Solomon, 1977). It is very likely that acute dystonias involving pharyngeal/laryngeal musculature might have been implicated in at least some of these tragedies.

These latter facts should go some way to dispelling the widely held belief that although distressing, acute dystonias are not serious. They can be – albeit it rarely. Forget that in any one patient and he or she will, of course, be the very patient who develops major complications. Furthermore, it is not just internal involvement that can cause problems. The muscle contractions produced by acute dystonic spasms can be *very* powerful, sufficiently so to produce damage to teeth and more serious complications such as dislocation of the jaw and even rhabdomyolysis (Cavanaugh and Finlayson, 1984). Forced jaw closure contemporaneous with forced tongue protrusion clearly produces the fateful combination behind amputation, as in the case mentioned above.

It is certainly clinical experience that varying degrees of trauma to the tongue are not uncommon as a result of acute dystonic episodes, and may follow from any lingual involvement regardless of whether or not trismus is present. The literature does not, however, make anything of frank amputation. Nonetheless, in addition to the case noted, the author has been apprised of another example involving amputation of the anterior quarter, which also resulted in considerable disfigurement. Combining this with the relative frequency of trismus, one does wonder if such major trauma is more common than the literature would suggest. Both of the cases cited here were the subject of litigation, which may go some way to explaining a failure of material of this sort to reach publication. After the tortuous and demoralising shenanigans of the legal process, most clinicians will be understandably reluctant to parade their misfortunes before their colleagues. If this is the case, clinicians have our sympathy, but must be reminded (tactfully) of their duty to inform.

There is one further point concerning the clinical aspects of acute dystonias that is worth mentioning. Recently, a pattern of diurnal variation has been reported with a predominance in the afternoon and evening (Tan et al., 1994; Mazurek and Rosebush, 1996). In Mazurek and Rosebush's sample, 80 per cent of disorders occurred between the hours of 12 noon and 11 p.m. Patients were on a twice-daily medication regime and acute dystonias were four times more likely to emerge in the four hours before the night dose than in the four hours before the morning one (at 11am). This finding was not simply attributable to fatigue, and despite the relatively late administration of the morning doses, it was also concluded that the time elapsed from the last dose of medication could not provide the explanation.

This finding is of interest in light of the fact that it has been known for many years that a similar diurnal pattern of expression can be seen with idiopathic chronic dystonia – that is, disorder more frequently manifest in the second half of the day. Indeed, in the earlier stages of this condition, patients are often completely symptom free on waking, with disorder only emerging as the day progresses. Furthermore, this corresponds to the pattern that was seen with oculogyric crises in patients with encephalitis lethargica (see below).

This diurnal pattern may have important training implications as afternoons and especially evenings are times when medical cover on the wards tends to be at its lowest and by the most inexperienced. More effort in training nursing colleagues in the recognition of these disorders might therefore be a sound investment of time.

It will by now be clear that acute dystonias invariably cause patients distress and occasionally can have consequences that may cause doctors very great distress as well. These varied and not infrequent disorders deserve to be viewed in a manner commensurate with these facts.

Diagnosis

It is easy to appreciate how such bizarre presentations might be diagnosed as anything other than what they are. They provide fertile ground for the practitioners of conviction medicine whose first consideration is their only one. In the past, patients have been diagnosed as suffering from tetanus, meningitis or other intracerebral infections, epilepsy and of course hysteria – and these are only the ones that have reached the literature. Benighted sufferers have on occasion had to be rescued from intensive care units and even from tracheotomies.

An appreciation of the source of such an error does not, however, make the error itself forgivable. Patients, their relatives and most especially their lawyers, are becoming most unforgiving of such diagnostic errors. In addition to the case noted above, the author has, over the years, come across a number of others. One teenage girl developed signs at the home of relatives, to which she had absconded for a premature and illicit pass. She was taken to the emergency department of an august psychiatric unit but was told that her 'hysterical' behaviour would have to be dealt with at her own hospital. As a result, she was transported across London in the rush hour with an opisthotonos that converted her body into an almost perfect semicircle. This four-hour nightmare journey was only possible at all because her relatives had a van into the back of which she 'curled' nicely!

Another example was that of an Iranian student whose appearance sitting was quite unexceptional, but who, on attempting to walk, became acutely and embarrassingly camp. He walked ballerina-like on point, his arms pronated with flexed wrists held tightly over his genital area. His gait and postural abnormalities, recurrent over 24 hours, were believed by his doctor and his family to be a ploy to prevent him returning home to do his bit for the Revolution, at that time in full swing. In fact, after some intravenous anticholinergic and a limited continuation of his antipsychotic, it subsequently proved impossible to prevent him returning home to do his bit, even though he remained quite clearly psychotic.

The following is presented in order to dispel any impression that the author may have created that he has, throughout his career, been immune to such errors. The patient was a student in his early twenties in his second episode of illness and four days into treatment. The nurses said he had started turning in circles, which indeed he had. Every few seconds, he would rapidly define a tight circle in a clockwise direction, following his outstretched left arm. After consultation with a junior colleague (now an eminent academic), the consensus was the young man was 'at it', and after a procyclidine 'buzz'. Being budding scientists, we determined to prove the point by giving him a blind injection of normal saline, a practice that would now be considered unethical but that was not uncommon at the time. Needless to say, this made not a whit of a difference, a point established to everyone's satisfaction when the nurse in charge of the ward, who had successfully avoided previous turns, failed to duck in time and landed a stout blow to the lower jaw. Procyclidine did the trick!

The author's experience of working in a multi-ethnic setting has often raised the very real concern that such misattributions may be more readily made in those from ethnic minorities, especially if their indigenous culture is seen as perhaps more inherently 'extrovert' or alien. While there are no data available to support such a hypothesis, it is a legitimate possibility and as such urges particular care when operating in these contexts.

There can be no excuse nowadays for considering acute dystonias as 'hysterical', and those who cannot suspend their dynamic prejudices in the face of even such gross motor disturbances must be prepared for the consequences.

The watchword is 'bizarre'. The sudden onset of any unusual subjective complaints along the lines described, or of movements, postures and attitudes that are weird and require the exercise of fancy to 'understand', should raise the question. Indeed, the very bizarreness of the signs is something that should take you towards, not away from, the diagnosis.

Within broad boundaries – and bearing in mind the point raised above regarding the potential for involvement of *all* striated muscle – the distribution is fairly predictable and, especially in adults, a useful guide. Young children presenting with the combination of generalised disorder and an inability to articulate subjective distress require particular consideration, especially since the picture can resemble a fit. Seizure activity can be excluded by the retention of consciousness, although if a diagnosis is being sought on the basis of history alone, as in the very young or those with learning disability, this can be a difficult differential. Hence, the greater reason for a high index of suspicion in paediatric practice.

A further point of value is what neurologists sometimes refer to as the sign–time curve – that is, the development of features over time (Fig. 3.3). There are few – if any – other situations in which such gross motor disturbance evolves so rapidly, particularly in an age group in whom the risk of vascular disease is slight.

A confirmatory history of ingestion of an 'offending' drug is important but not essential information. Patients may not have any clear idea of precisely what they have taken or may only mention what they believe to be of importance, not what actually is. Distraught parents, for example, may only think to mention prescribed medication such as antibiotics but omit the 'cold cure' they bought themselves. Most obviously, victims may simply not wish to be too forthcoming in this regard. Also, of course, with extensive lingual, oropharyngeal or laryngeal involvement, they may not be able to talk at all. Thus, the diagnosis – and hence

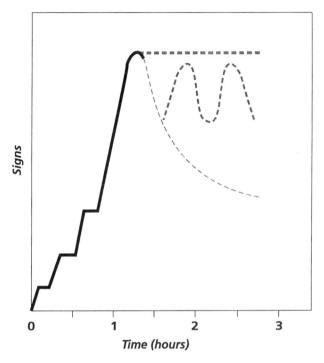

Fig. 3.3. Acute dystonias: the 'sign–time' curve.

the decision to treat – must *not* be dependent on establishing the details of the drug history.

A wide range of disorders, mostly neurological and mostly rare, can be associated with the development of dystonia. These are essentially chronic conditions presenting dystonia in chronic form and are mentioned in Chapter 7. A thorough evaluation of acute dystonia should nonetheless encompass at least an awareness of these.

This section began with an exhortation to avoid a diagnosis of hysteria with all its inferences of arcane subconscious conflicts, but it is appropriate to end it with a reminder of the fact that acute dystonias can be simulated – quite a different kettle of psychological fish. All the many motivations behind this are as relevant in this situation as they are in any situations in which specific behaviours are simulated – but one is important above all others, and that is a desire to achieve the 'buzz' anticholinergic medication provides. Anticholinergics are euphorogenic and subject to abuse. Anyone who doubts their currency has not discussed with their patients the goings on behind the social club of an evening! The author has not infrequently come across patients, usually young males, wilfully and sometimes skilfully simulating acute dystonic episodes in order to get anticholinergics, especially intravenously. The message is: beware the experienced patient!

Epidemiology

Figures on the epidemiology of acute dystonias have in the past been scant, and provided contradictory information that has been frankly misleading. The topic, for whatever reason, attracted little in the way of systematic investigation, and such original research as was undertaken was retrospective. Because of the nature of the clinical problem, acute dystonias are particularly unsuited to retrospective data collection. They are transient, and may not be reported to staff and, if they are, may be given varied interpretations, all of which militates against a case-note entry. So retrospective methodology is likely to result in significant underestimation.

One possible reason for an unjustified absence of acute dystonias from the research literature might have been a deep-seated belief that these are infrequent occurrences, a perception fostered in no small part by a mis-understanding of the findings from a particularly influential report. In one of the first formal studies of the subject, Ayd (1961) reviewed the prevalence of each of the extrapyramidal syndromes in a large group of 3775 patients treated with antipsychotics. He reported that acute dyston-ias affected 2.3 per cent of the sample – a figure that for a generation of psychiatrists became the fact. This figure was, however, based on a hier-archical and mutually exclusive method of calculation in which parkin-sonism 'trumped' akathisia, both of which 'trumped' acute dystonias. Thus, the figure of 2.3 per cent referred to those who developed *only* acute dystonias and no other signs of extrapyramidal disorder. Nonetheless it does seem clear that prevalence rates in general were lower then.

The past, it has been said, is like a foreign land – things are done differently there. One of the psychiatric 'things' that was done differ-ently was antipsychotic prescribing. Average doses were clearly lower and patterns of usage more eclectic, with less emphasis on high potency compounds, especially in the USA, where most of this work was – and continues to be – done. Also, while the antidystonic effects of anti-cholinergics may have been known, a similar action of other coin-cidentally administered drugs, such as barbiturates, may have been underestimated. It is further worth keeping in mind that at a time when part of the object of these studies was to define the boundaries of toler-ability, the threshold of awareness for these bizarre disorders among patients as well as staff may have been less precise than now.

More recent studies have suggested higher prevalences more conso-nant with current clinical experience (Table 3.1). Nonetheless, it is quite

Table 3.1. *The prevalence and incidence of acute dystonias*

Study	Frequency (%)	Comment
Ayd (1961)	2.3 [P]	Retrospective Acute dystonias as sole manifestation of EPS
Addonizio & Alexopoulos (1988)	31.0 [P]	Retrospective
Singh et al. (1990)	34.0 [I]	Fluphenazine: fixed dose Objective criteria: 'clear-cut and impressive increase in muscle tone'
Chakos et al. (1992)	36.0 [I]	Fluphenazine: variable but fixed at 20 mg for 6 weeks Objective criteria: 'verified by a physician'
Aguilar et al. (1994)	60.0 [I]	Haloperidol: fixed dose (15 mg)+variable Objective criteria: 'nursing observation or patient's relatives' complaint'

P=prevalence study; I=incidence study.

clear that figures still vary. As discussed below, the prevalence of acute dystonias is directly dependent on a series of largely idiosyncratic and treatment practice variables. Any or all of these can exert such a strong independent influence as severely to limit the idea that there is such an entity as *the* prevalence. (We shall encounter this crucial point in relation to each of the syndromes discussed in these pages, especially those at the 'acute' end of the spectrum.) This proviso notwithstanding, it would seem reasonable to conclude from the more recent retrospective literature that acute dystonias can affect up to one-quarter to one-third of adult patients treated with standard antipsychotic drugs.

The emphasis on 'standard' drugs is important, for only a single clinically recognisable case has been reported with clozapine use (Kastrup, Gastpar and Schwartz, 1994), and even this was not typical in that it developed during established treatment, as opposed to at the start of treatment. This figure is (at the time of writing) in total exposures to clozapine approaching one million worldwide. The unique circumstances in which clozapine is licensed means, of course, that treatment is currently confined to patients who are antipsychotic veterans by the time they receive it, and this in itself may bias things in favour of

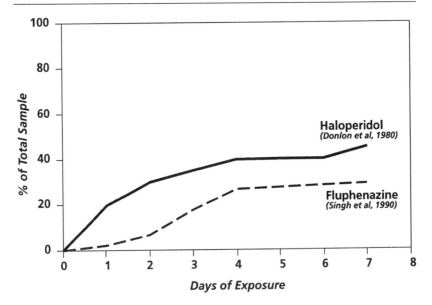

Fig. 3.4. The incidence of acute dystonias.

clozapine. Nonetheless, even if the day of publication of the present work coincides with an avalanche of reports of an association, this will not undermine the remarkable fact of clozapine's dramatically reduced – and in reality probably non-existent – liability to promote acute dystonic episodes. This clinical conclusion is supported by work in primate models, in which clozapine has been unable to produce acute dystonias (Goldstein, 1995).

Only recently – after over 30 years of awareness – has the literature addressed the issue of incidence in prospective studies with acute dystonias as a primary focus, although even now these remain few and far between and continue to concentrate on populations treated with high-potency compounds (Table 3.1). In attempting to estimate the incidence of acute dystonias it is essential to try to control for those variables over which one can exert some influence, and the studies listed are those which utilised a fixed dose design. As is clear, with close observation, the risk of acute dystonic episodes in current practice using high-potency standard antipsychotics is not insubstantial, running in the range of 30–40 per cent (Fig. 3.4). This estimate comes from studies that have used solely *sign*-based criteria for establishing the diagnosis, and it may be that including patients who do not progress beyond the symptom stage would inflate these figures even further.

Two issues and a question are raised by all of this. The issues are firstly, that acute dystonias are *not* uncommon and the risk during early

Table 3.2. *Factors predisposing to acute dystonias*

Drug related	Non-drug related
Potency	Age (inverse)
Dose (especially initial)	
Rate of increment	?First episode
?Naivity	?Stress

phase and incremental treatment can be considerable; and secondly, that clinicians and nursing staff must be alert to the problem that has to be appraised in the context of treatment choices, i.e. the agents and regimes being used.

The question is why on earth has psychiatry become so favourably disposed to the use of high-potency antipsychotics?

Predisposing factors

The first group of risk factors (Table 3.2) to be considered comprises pharmacological and treatment practice variables which constitute a trio that will be encountered with each of the acute/intermediate syndromes. The development of acute dystonias relates to antipsychotic potency, to dosage and, as importantly, to rates of dose increment.

The relationship to potency has been long known and is one of the most reproducible of findings in the literature. Thus the National Institute of Mental Health (NIMH) Collaborative Study (1964) found an incidence rate of 1.1 per cent with thioridazine, 4.5 per cent with chlorpromazine, and 6.6 per cent with fluphenazine. In a review of the earlier antipsychotic studies, Cole and Davis (1969) calculated a combined figure of 0.88 per cent associated with thioridazine and up to 8 per cent with fluphenazine. The modern literature seems to take this relationship as established, although its lack of further exploration may also reflect a decline in the frequency of comparative studies, only recently revived with the introduction of the new generation of antipsychotics.

The author accepts this association as fundamentally valid – with one qualification that the reader must also insinuate into the corresponding comments for parkinsonism and akathisia. This relates to the persuasive evidence that, considering antipsychotic equivalence, high-potency drugs are used in substantially *higher* dose regimes than low-potency compounds (Baldessarini et al., 1984). Thus, while the principle may be sound, the magnitude of the potency effect may be less than is generally believed.

A positive association with dose is also well established, and has been confirmed prospectively (Khanna, Das and Damodaran, 1992). This, however, seems to reflect a more complex set of circumstances than at first sight. One might reasonably suppose that a relationship with dose would reflect a similar relationship with blood levels, but this does not appear to be the case (Tune and Coyle, 1981). Those who develop acute dystonias cannot be differentiated from those who do not on the basis of antipsychotic blood levels. No studies to date have evaluated plasma levels at the actual time of the dystonic episode but even so, it must be taken that blood levels are not in themselves the important factor.

Where dose may be more relevant is in determining the membrane-bound concentration of drug (Rupniak et al., 1986). Rapid dose escalations may result in more rapid membrane saturation and hence accumulation of antipsychotic at critical brain sites. There is some supportive evidence for this using a red blood cell model, but whereas the clinical observation of an association with antipsychotic dose is valid, the explanation of the relationship remains obscure.

Some years ago, the use of ultra-high antipsychotic doses had a vogue, associated with which was the observation that prevalences of acute EPS, including dystonias, appeared to decline above certain critical levels (Keepers and Casey, 1986), probably because of other receptor-binding properties coming into play. Such practices have, however, rightly been abandoned because of the other inherent short-term and long-term problems associated with their use.

The other practice variable of importance is the rate of dose increments. The more rapidly doses are escalated, especially early in treatment, the more likely acute dystonias are to develop. Surprisingly, this is not an issue the literature has addressed systematically and it is somewhat dogmatically presented here in the absence of hard evidence. Recently, experts in the field have started to emphasise this point based on their experience, and the present author is doing likewise as it is certainly his. It is, furthermore, in keeping with the idea of rapid membrane saturation noted above. To state the obvious, the starting dose of any medication represents the most rapid escalation of all, hence the need to keep this low.

The other clear factor predisposing to acute dystonic reactions is age. These reactions are more frequent in young adults than in older patients. The point is illustrated in the study of Addonizio and Alexopoulos (1988) who found a rate of 36 per cent in those under 60 years of age but of only 2 per cent in those over 60. Whether or not this relationship is linear is unknown, but it is likely that it is not. It seems more likely that a cut-off exists between the high-risk and low-risk periods, although where such a putative cut-off might lie is speculative.

It is certainly likely to be considerably below 60, and it would seem reasonable on the basis of clinical experience to propose that these types of abnormality are strikingly less frequent after the fourth decade. However, it does not seem that one can extend this inverse age relationship backwards and conclude that children are at particular risk, although, as we shall see, the data on which this conclusion rests are scant (see Chapter 9). Again, it must be remembered that these statements refer to *objective* disorder.

It does remain possible that the relationship with age is not primarily with prevalence but rather with severity. Thus, it could be that within the population there exists a group of individuals predisposed to antidopaminergic-related acute dystonias by virtue of genetic, pharmacokinetic or other factors. What age might then do is to determine the severity with which this predisposition is expressed. In children and young adults, expression is severe and generalised, while in older people it may only be expressed in mild, subjective symptomatology, easy to miss or misattribute. In line with such a formulation is the suggestion that acute dystonias may occur more frequently in those with a family history of acute drug-related dystonia or, of greater significance, dystonia musculorum deformans (Eldridge, 1970). It is clinical experience that some predisposed individuals develop recurrent episodes of dystonia with the cycles of treatment that accompany repeated episodes of florid relapse, and indeed a similar phenomenon has been described in some patients after each depot injection. What is unknown, however, is whether such recurrent disorders diminish in intensity over recurrent treatment cycles.

For whatever reason, the immature brain seems to possess an impaired ability to exercise a protective or counter action against the dystonia-producing potential of antidopaminergic drugs, a function apparently acquired with maturity or with the superimposition of ageing. The mechanisms underlying this are in need of exploration.

Another consideration, however, is the impression that acute dystonias are predominantly phenomena of the drug-naive, the greatest risk (or possibly the greatest severity) being at first exposure. This remains a largely clinical observation, although an association has been reported with first episodes of illness (Singh et al., 1990), which is probably the same thing expressed in a slightly different way. Those who comprise the bulk of the 'at-risk' population are individuals suffering from psychotic illnesses, which of course tend to show themselves first at relatively young ages and to be recurrent thereafter. Hence, a further factor that age correlates with in such patients is a likelihood of past and chronic exposure to antipsychotic agents. It may be that receptor changes consequent upon cumulative drug exposure may also operate 'protectively' and contribute to the declining risk.

It is widely held that young males are at particular risk of developing acute dystonias, with gender operating as an independent risk factor (Ayd, 1961; Swett, 1975). This is certainly the almost unanimous consensus of the retrospective literature, and the observation has assumed the level of fact not in need of challenge. This always troubled the author for the most valid of reasons: it did not seem entirely to reflect his own clinical experience in a practice not noticeably dominated by masculine women. Prospective studies have *not* confirmed this association (Singh et al., 1990; Chakos et al., 1992; Aguilar et al., 1994). Indeed, in the study of Chakos and colleagues, females were significantly more likely to develop disorder of this type than males.

This striking discrepancy between the findings of the retrospective and the prospective literature could clearly do with an explanation. The obvious one is probably also the most pertinent: young males are treated differently from young females. We have just seen how the risk of acute dystonias increases with increasing antipsychotic doses and with the rate of dose increments. It is a very tenable proposition to suggest that in routine clinical situations males – especially young males – are not only treated with higher absolute doses but, equally importantly, may have them increased more rapidly, especially in the face of challenging behaviour, or the threat of it.

But does this help us interpret the finding of Chakos et al.? An important aspect of this study was that its design incorporated a period of fixed antipsychotic doses. While this would ensure that absolute milligram dosages were comparable in both genders, it would equally ensure that relative dosages in terms of milligrams per kilogram of body weight were higher in females. In addition to establishing a relationship with dose, Singh et al. (1990) found the mg/kg dose to be relevant. The difficulty with generalising this explanation is that Singh and colleagues did not themselves find a significant gender difference in a study that also adopted a fixed dose design!

A further joker in the pack complicating the interpretation of these data is the role of body fat. It might be that there is less opportunity for rapid membrane saturation at central sites in females, with their relatively higher body fat, or the adipose, because of greater immediate distribution to fat stores. Chakos and colleagues do not tell us whether or not their females were particularly anorectic!

The ubiquitous 'stress' has also been implicated, which in reality means an association with anxiety. While this would be in keeping with what is known about idiopathic dystonias and what the historical record reported for oculogyric crises (see below), one would have to be sure in evaluating anxiety that one was indeed dealing with a genuine independent precipitant and not mild but established dystonia at the symptom-only stage.

Recently, particular vulnerability has been claimed for patients undergoing a rapid switch from clozapine to risperidone (Radford, Brown and Borison, 1995). Clozapine has potent inherent anticholinergic actions, whereas risperidone is virtually devoid of these, and one possible explanation of this phenomenon might therefore be a sensitising effect imparted via the withdrawal state sometimes encountered with sudden cessation of powerfully anticholinergic agents, a proposal for which there is some evidence in the early literature (Simpson and Meyer, 1996). Risperidone is also, of course, a potent central dopamine D_2 antagonist, whereas clozapine is relatively weak in that department, which may provide a simpler explanation. Simplest of all, however, is that in the relevant case the patient had in addition to antipsychotics been receiving the SSRI sertraline. This is nonetheless a possible association worth bearing in mind.

As will be clear, acute dystonias harbour many mysteries still to be unravelled. Any trainee psychiatrist in search of a career-enhancing research project could do worse than attempt some unravelling in this area.

Onset, course and outcome

The great majority of those who are going to develop acute dystonic reactions will do so in the four to five days after initiation of antidopaminergic medication or dose increments. Ayd, in his 1961 review, estimated that approximately 90 per cent of cases manifest themselves within five days, a finding re-affirmed in other retrospective studies and, more recently, prospectively too (Fig. 3.5).

Onset has been reported to be both brought forward and delayed with the use of depot formulations, findings that need not be contradictory. The suggestion of an earlier onset (Ayd, 1974) came from the USA at a time when the only depots available were of fluphenazine. Fluphenazine decanoate appears to be pharmacokinetically unique amongst depots in that administration is followed by a rapid post-injection rise in plasma levels, maximal in 12–24 hours, after which levels fall to around one-third peak at four days or so, with a gradual decline thereafter (Marder et al., 1989). Other depot preparations by contrast, attain peak plasma levels more sedately over four to seven days. Even allowing for the strictures of the discussion presented above, these pharmacokinetic differences may hold the explanation to an apparent contradiction.

While this pattern of early onset is important to bear in mind in order to maintain a mandatory high level of awareness, it must be emphasised that 90 per cent is not 100 per cent! Some cases of acute dystonia may

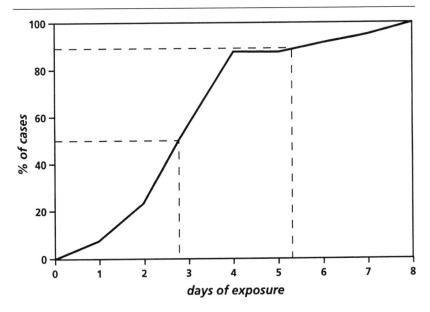

Fig. 3.5. Onset of acute dystonias. (After Singh et al., 1990.)

occasionally emerge in the context of long-term and established anti-psychotic exposure, often as a recurrent phenomenon. Tan et al. (1994) found that during a two-month observation period, 1.7 per cent of a large inpatient population experienced episodes of oculogyric spasm which were recurrent in more than half the sample. Notwithstanding the fact that patients had been on maintenance medication for anything from five months to three years, these events appear, by the ultimate criterion laid out above (see Chapter 2), to have been 'acute', in that they swiftly and completely responded to anticholinergic. In line with the study of Tan et al., it is the author's experience that this delayed and recurrent pattern of 'acute' disorder is confined largely, if not exclusively, to oculogyrus.

The onset of acute dystonias is, as we have seen, sudden (see Fig. 3.3). The time from first awareness of subjective symptomatology to the development of full-blown postural distortions can be alarmingly swift – only a few minutes. More usually, features emerge over 30–60 minutes in a stuttering pattern of dramatic escalations interrupted by brief, ill-sustained periods of appeasement.

The natural history of the unmodified state can take one of three main forms: sustained, fluctuating and episodic (see Fig. 3.6). Motor abnormalities may relentlessly progress and reach a plateau of severity that is sustained without amelioration for the duration of the natural history. Alternatively, a fluctuating level of intensity may be evident during which symptomatology waxes and wanes, although without

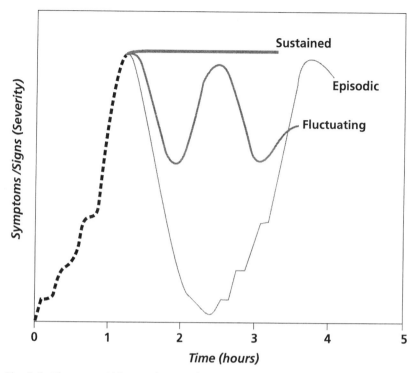

Fig. 3.6. The natural history of acute dystonias.

ever really disappearing. Finally, features can completely resolve only to return dramatically and unpredictably in recurrent episodes of diminishing intensity.

The natural history varies enormously in its duration from individual to individual, though typically an unmodified period of disturbance is likely to last a few hours. Rarely, especially with an episodic course, disorder may be recurrent over several days before spontaneous resolution occurs.

The unmodified course of drug-related acute dystonias is something that should not now be seen, as treatment is immediately and predictably effective.

Treatment

Many treatments have in the past been proposed for acute dystonias, although only three have held the course.

Antihistamines have been advocated but, for the reasons mentioned above, must be chosen with care. Diphenhydramine is the one usually recommended, given in a dose of 10 mg i.v. or orally. Especially in the USA, this is a widely used strategy, although it is less popular in the UK. However, this drug has itself been implicated in the production of dystonic disorder (Etzel, 1994).

Benzodiazepines have also had their advocates (Korczyn and Goldberg, 1972; Rainier-Pope, 1979). Diazepam 5–10 mg orally or i.v. can be effective.

In the UK, anticholinergics are overwhelmingly the preferred treatments. There appears to be little to choose between them, although in general it is better to stick to more M_1-selective compounds (see Chapter 4) in the management of drug-related side-effects, in order to minimise some of the side-effects of the side-effect treatment! By this criterion, biperiden should be the first choice (2.5–5 mg i.v. or 4–6mg orally) as it is the most M_1 selective, although by custom procyclidine is probably the most frequently used. Its relative selectivity also makes it a reasonable choice. Given in a dose of 10 mg by slow intravenous infusion over a minute or two procyclidine is rapidly effective and safe. An oral dose of 5–10 mg can also abolish disorder quickly, especially when of milder degree.

Following intravenous administration, symptoms should start to ease within a few minutes, and with oral use after 15–30 minutes. It is only if resolution fails to take place after *intravenous* injection that one should reconsider the diagnosis.

Mild subjective symptomatology without signs that is associated with minimal distress can be treated with oral medication, especially if everyone is alert to the problem or it has been experienced before, but as a general rule, once objective signs have emerged, one should proceed straight to intravenous administration. In pharmacokinetic terms, intramuscular injections offer little advantage over the oral route for any of these drugs and with, for example, diazepam may actually be less advantageous by being associated in certain circumstances with slower and more unpredictable absorption. The major indication for intramuscular administration is the patient's wish to have it. The author has found many patients over the years who simply believed a medication for an acute medical problem was no use unless it was in the form of an intramuscular injection. When dealing with the psychiatrically unwell, it is never advisable to challenge such confidence, no matter how misplaced. You may need it later!

A first acute dystonic episode is *not* in itself an indication for regular prophylaxis. Following intervention, antipsychotic doses should be stabilised for a few days before attempting increases, which should subsequently be cautious.

Should a second episode occur, this would then be the indication for more definitive action. In this situation, one should perhaps be more phlegmatic about the use of antihistamines and benzodiazepines and, on both a practical and evidential basis, anticholinergics are the most satisfactory tools. They can be started orally on a regular basis and maintained for five to seven days – e.g. procyclidine in a dose of 2.5 mg twice or three times daily, increasing if required – after which they can be slowly discontinued over a few days.

The great majority of patients will not require indefinite treatment, which is to be avoided for reasons that are expounded in Chapter 4. Longer term treatment is only necessary on the rare occasions when problems recur on stopping brief prophylaxis, and even in this situation should be time-limited to the period of escalating doses or at the most four to six weeks, whichever passes first. However, before longer term treatment of this sort is undertaken, antipsychotic potency, dose schedules and incremental regimes should be reassessed and modified whenever possible. There are few patients in whom such treatment variables cannot stand a degree of modification or deceleration, and many in whom this may be beneficial.

There is now clear evidence that introduction of anticholinergics at the start of antipsychotic treatment does reduce the likelihood of acute dystonic episodes, and this has been used as a basis to argue that concurrent use of both drugs should be the standard in clinical practice (Keepers, Clappison and Casey, 1983; Sramek et al., 1986; Arana et al., 1988). This evidence, however, pertains particularly to the use of antipsychotics of high potency for which the risk is inherently greater. With careful use, only a minority of patients will develop acute dystonias, even with these compounds, and to expose the majority to unnecessary drugs which have major side-effects of their own (see Table 4.9) in order to avoid a problem that can be better avoided by more thoughtful management, would seem to advocate perversity as the standard. It is not a general principle the author, in line with most commentators in the field, would recommend. A possible exception is in cases where, for reasons of clinical imperative, it is essential to avoid dystonias or other acute/intermediate EPS at all costs, such as in those with physical disability or in young patients in whom acceptance of recommendations and subsequent compliance are deemed tenuous. In such patients, however, it might now be considered more appropriate to proceed straight to a new-generation compound.

An outline of these recommendations for management is shown in Figure 3.7.

Pathophysiology

The pathophysiology of acute dystonias is not understood, and the expanding list of implicated compounds, some of which, such as

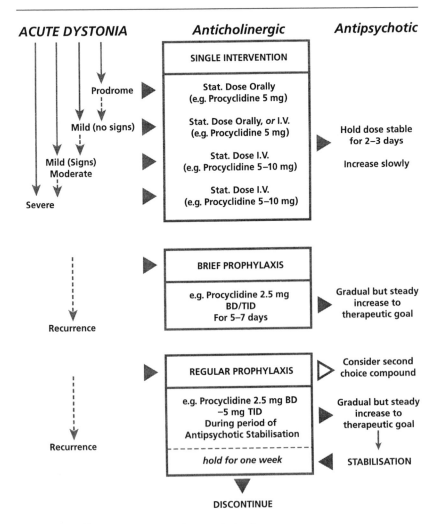

Fig. 3.7. Outline management of acute dystonias.

SSRIs, have little or no primary actions at dopaminergic systems, has added to the complexities.

One of the obstacles in exploring pathophysiological hypotheses has been the difficulty in identifying standard animal models. Although disorders recognisable as dystonias have been described in non-human primates, species differences are evident. Thus, while some New World species such as Cebus and squirrel monkeys seem particularly vulnerable, dystonias do not appear to be the earliest manifestation of extrapyramidal disturbance in them. It is necessary to 'prime' these species for some time before acute dystonias with characteristics similar to those encountered in humans develop. However, such 'priming' may not be necessary in baboons. Primates are complicated and expensive to work with, but it has not been possible in rodents to reproduce early dystonic disorders recognisably comparable to those of humans.

Clinical observations may offer some potentially useful clues which point to an imbalance between dopaminergic and cholinergic mechanisms in the basal ganglia. Dystonias are the commonest manifestation of lesions in the striatum, which is in line with laboratory data that focus the site of the drug-related disruption in neurotransmission to this area. The evidence is that, notwithstanding their basic pharmacological diversities, all drugs associated with the problem act either directly or indirectly on dopamine systems and this is, of course, particularly the case for those compounds most implicated, antipsychotics. Furthermore, antipsychotics of high propensity also tend to possess low anticholinergic activity. The time relationships are highly characteristic. Acute dystonias occur significantly earlier in humans than the other drug-related extrapyramidal disorders and tend to undergo a clear degree of tolerance with continuous exposure.

The final clinical clue lies in the swift, predictable and complete response to anticholinergics. In certain primate experiments, cholinergic agonists may induce dystonias, as may focal intrastriatal application of acetylcholine or carbachol, and acute administration of antipsychotics has been shown to produce an increase in striatal acetylcholine release.

This evidence strongly suggests that the proximate pathophysiological event underlying the production of acute dystonias is an increase in striatal cholinergic activity. Where the evidence diverges is in relation to the dopaminergic context in which this cholinergic excess is operating. There are data to support both the view that it is increased *and* that it is reduced (Rupniak, Jenner and Marsden, 1986).

The strongest support at present is for dopaminergic excess, although this does raise an obvious paradox – namely, how do compounds whose primary action is dopamine antagonism bring about an increase in dopamine transmission?

Central dopaminergic systems undertake two main manoeuvres in an attempt to overcome the effect of the blockade inflicted by standard antipsychotics (Fig. 3.8). The immediate response is the triggering of a compensatory increase in dopamine turnover – that is, via a feedback mechanism more dopamine is manufactured, released and metabolised. This process can readily be detected by an accumulation of metabolites such as homovanillic acid (HVA) and 3,4-dihydroxyphenylacetic acid (DOPAC). However, this 'attempt' to restore the status quo is short lived and rapidly undergoes tolerance to be replaced by the second and more durable mechanism, post-synaptic receptor supersensitivity.

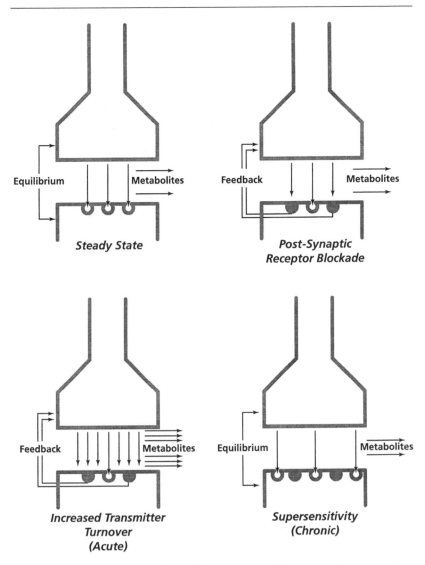

Fig. 3.8. The acute and chronic adaptive processes of dopaminergic systems to post-synaptic receptor blockade.

Increased turnover is certainly taking place within the clinical time sequence of acute dystonias. This initial phase of exposure is pre-steady state so is further characterised by escalating and, more importantly, rapidly declining antipsychotic blood levels (Marsden and Jenner, 1980). These two facts have given rise to what has been referred to as the 'mismatch' hypothesis, which proposes that acute dystonias are a result of increased release of striatal dopamine (from increased turnover) onto post-synaptic receptors that are inconsistently occupied and become 'unblocked' as antipsychotic levels fall (Kolbe et al., 1981; Rupniak et al., 1986).

This theory accommodates a number of clinical and laboratory observations concerning acute dystonias but may be incomplete in ignoring the fact that, in rodents at least, emerging supersensitivity can be detected within 48 hours of a single antipsychotic dose (Christensen, Fjalland and Nielson, 1976). It may be, therefore, that increased dopamine is not only bombarding receptors 'freed up' from blockade by falling blood levels but may also be hitting some already developing the properties of functional supersensitivity (Kolbe et al., 1981).

One objection to this formulation might be that if acute dystonias are a consequence of combined cholinergic and dopamineric excess, then it might be anticipated that the effect of administering anticholinergics might be merely to convert dystonic-type abnormality into dyskinesias in general, for which an underlying dopaminergic excess has been proposed. This is something that clearly does not occur. However, there is evidence that anticholinergics impede the increased turnover in striatal dopamine induced by antipsychotics (Rupniak et al., 1986). Thus, the efficacy of anticholinergics in acute dystonias can be accommodated within this theory, as can possibly their role in short-term prevention and prophylaxis.

This elegant theory does not have it all its own way for it has also been argued that acute dystonias emerge in a context of dopamine *deficiency* (Neale, Gerhardt and Liebman, 1984). The amine synthesis inhibitor alpha-methyl-para-tyrosine (AMPT) and the presynaptic depleting agent reserpine have been found to block the development of acute antipsychotic-related dystonias in certain primates, although AMPT and the other amine depleter tetrabenazine have also been reported to *produce* these disorders in other studies and – most importantly – in humans. Similarly, L-dopa has been shown in primates to reverse antipsychotic-related dystonias, as has apomorphine. However, the actions of dopamine agonists are contradictory. L-dopa, for example, may promote severe dystonias in patients with Parkinson's disease but dramatically improve those associated with the autosomal dominantly inherited condition dopa-responsive dystonia, and apomorphine has dose-dependent presynaptic as well as post-synaptic actions.

Despite their limitations, these observations do prevent an uncritical acceptance of the 'miss-match' theory as being applicable to all situations. An additional hurdle is that, as formulated, this would not account for acute dystonias caused by exposure to SSRIs. There is now evidence that serotonergic systems do modulate dopamine function in the striatum and other brain areas, and the clinical observation of an enhanced liability to acute dystonias with serotonin agonism has been confirmed in non-human primates (Arya, 1994). However, the evidence to date is that serotonin systems *inhibit* dopamine function.

It is likely that acute drug-related dystonias are a clinical destination at which patients arrive by a number of routes. A more detailed map of the complex chemical terrain of the striatum will be necessary before these paths can be identified with certainty.

Addendum: acute dystonias and oculogyric crises

It is always useful to challenge accepted wisdom, especially when the wisdom has superficial roots. We have already seen that, contrary to popular belief, so-called 'oculogyric crises' are a relatively uncommon manifestation of acute dystonic abnormality, comprising less than 10 per cent of examples. The question is whether they are even as common as this.

Oculogyric crises were first described in 1695 by J.P. Albrecht, who wrote a pamphlet on what he called 'Lethargia Epidemica' which had, as a striking part of the clinical presentation, eye signs. He described the daughter of an 'honest citizen' who developed the symptoms of a febrile malady 'the most notable (of which) was an extraordinary propensity to sleep'. He went on to record:

> In the period of temporary improvement of health, there was plainly noted a distortion of the eyes, which propelled the pupil toward the upper eyelid, showing the white of the whole half of the lower eyeball.

Other large-scale epidemics of encephalitic influenza-like illnesses have been described throughout recent history, though whether these represented similar or totally different disorders remains unclear.

The flu pandemic of this century began amongst American troops in 1918 and the encephalitic condition was sometimes referred to as von Economo's disease after the Viennese physician, Constantin von Economo, who first described in Austrian soldiers the novel characteristics of the illness. It is now generally recalled as encephalitis lethargica. It has been estimated that over 30 million people died of flu worldwide, with countless millions more invalided before the pandemic faded. Sporadic cases diagnosed as encephalitis lethargica on the basis of a similar clinical picture are still occasionally described, but as the nature of the encephalitis of three-quarters of a century ago remains uncertain, despite many theories, the view that these represent the same condition must to some extent remain conjecture.

The first modern accounts of oculogyric crises were published in 1921 when Oeckinghaus and Frigerio reported separately on the development of eye signs in patients who had suffered from encephalitis

Table 3.3. *The characteristics of oculogyric crises*

Prodrome	'Warnings' (affective)
Precipitants	Extreme emotion
	Sensory stimulation
	light
	heat
	touch
	noise
	Exercise
	Fatigue
Pattern	Diurnal variation (late afternoon)
Neurological	Conjugate (upward) eye deviation
	Neck displacement (retro-/torticollis)
	Other dystonias
	Autonomic overactivity
	hyperhidrosis
	seborrhoea
	tachycardia
	pupillary dilatation
Psychiatric	Affective symptoms (anxiety/depression)
	Altered consciousness
	Stupor
	Speech disorders
	mutism
	logorrhoea
	palilalia
	echolalia
	stereotyped phrasing
	'Made'/obsessional phenomena
	thoughts
	perceptions
	utterances
	forced shouting (Benedek's klazomania)

lethargica (Wilson, 1940). So, what were the features of oculogyric crises in the context in which they were originally described (Table 3.3)?

These episodes were not a part of the acute illness, but rather emerged as the features of post-encephalitic parkinsonism developed usually some years afterwards, though for onset to be delayed for more than six or seven years was exceptional. Reviewing the topic in 1929, the American psychiatrist, Smith Ely Jelliffe, provided a pertinent caution:

> The kind of oculocephalogyric crises that follow in the wake of epidemic encephalitis, while standing out as striking and apparently isolated phenomena, are really but parts of a much enlarged general picture ... out of which the oculogyric crises are artificially dismembered and intensively studied.

Indeed, he went on to add that 'The oculogyric crises, as such, rarely, if ever, occur alone.' (Jelliffe, 1929).

A series of 'warnings' was described such as malaise, vertigo, headache and anxiety. Indeed, high levels of emotional arousal seem to have frequently augured a full-blown attack – the 'usual beginning' as Jelliffe called it – but this was most often interpreted as an emotional state precipitating the episode. As mentioned above, however, in connection with drug-related acute dystonias, these states may have represented prodromal or early disorder itself, an interpretation in line with the view that 'psychogenic factors are of very minor importance in originating the phenomena' (McCowan and Cook, 1928).

Other precipitating factors included heat and bright light or other sensory stimulation to, especially, the face, noise, pungent smells, vigorous exercise and fatigue, although the disorder could also emerge without any identifiable precipitating experiences.

Onset was sudden, but often preceded by a brief period of fixed forward staring described as 'trance-like' or ictal-like dissociation. In severe cases, patients would fall to the ground. The oculogyric component comprised paroxysmal conjugate upward deviation of the eyes, most often with an emphasis to the right, though this could be in any direction. A degree of neck displacement commonly accompanied the eye movements, which most frequently comprised a retrocollis, usually with a degree of rotation in the direction of the gaze deviation. This combination of eye and neck involvement was the oculocephalogyric symptomatology referred to by Jelliffe (above). He described these displacements as often being painful – 'Jesusly painful' to quote one of his patients – but Wilson (1940) says only that 'pain is seldom remarked', though these two impressions are not necessarily contradictory.

However, a wide range of additional symptomatology was also described. Kinnier Wilson, the neurologist, commented that 'numerous crises are virtually monosymptomatic', but was referring strictly to the extent of the neurological signs (Wilson, 1940). Other signs evident in complex examples included forced mouth opening, blepharoclonus and spasm, spasm of frontalis, contractions of tongue, pharyngeal muscles and larynx as well as respiratory muscles and sometimes limbs. These were usually of 'tonic' (i.e. dystonic) type but the complete range of movement types was also to be expected.

Autonomic overactivity could be evidenced in tachycardia, hypertension, hyperhidrosis and pupillary dilatation (what Bumke called 'terror pupils'). Furthermore, a wide range of mental state disorders was considered an integral part of the syndrome. Significantly, altered conscious levels were frequently noted during, not just at the start of, episodes, with levels of awareness ranging from 'full vigilance to complete psychic blocking or even to unconsciousness' (Jelliffe, 1929). The affective state was dominated by what this author described as 'great anxiety', and depression was frequently of sufficient degree to be associated before or afterwards with suicidal ideation and acts. Misperceptions of all kinds were noted, but especially auditory hallucinations, which could be imperative, a further cause of the heightened suicide risk.

Complex disturbances of thought were almost invariable. These could take the form of an inhibition of spontaneous thinking ranging from true 'blocking' to bradyphrenia or, as Jelliffe called it, 'stickiness' of thought. Alternatively, thinking could be disrupted by a wide range of what we might nowadays refer to as 'positive' features. Suspiciousness, extending sometimes to frank persecutory delusions, was common, as were automatic or forced thinking, described in the terminology of the day as 'compulsive', palilalias and other verbal and motor stereotypies (van Bogaert, 1934) and bizarre forced utterances that went by the name of Benedek's klazomania (Wohlfart, Ingvar and Hellberg, 1961), a concept recently revived under the Baconesque term, 'the screaming tic' (Bates et al., 1996).

It was said that the only thing that was certain about post-encephalitic oculogyric crises was the uncertainty of each presentation (Wilson, 1940). Episodes comprised a constantly varying constellation of features across patients and in the same patient at different times. Some 'tricks' were described that could either abort, at least temporarily, or modify the symptomatology. Thus, full episodes may have been prevented by the patient adopting a prone position, or forcibly closing the eyes for a period (McCowan and Cook, 1928) or by what Wilson described as 'powerful extrinsic stimulation'. Episodes could last for a few minutes to several days and usually came in runs interspersed with longer periods free from abnormality. After an attack, patients would often sleep for long periods.

The overall prevalence was estimated at 17–20 per cent of post-encephalitic cases (Wilson, 1940). Although young adults were supposedly preferentially affected, age does not appear to have been identified as a striking factor in determining development. Furthermore, descriptive accounts do not suggest that the extent of the symptomatology depended on the age of the subject. A pattern of diurnal variation with an emphasis in the later part of the day was repeatedly commented on, and invariably taken to reflect the cumulative effects of exertion and fatigue (McCowan and Cook, 1928; Jelliffe, 1929; Wilson, 1940).

Thus, it is clear that oculogyrus was only but one part of a complex neuropsychiatric syndrome, the rest of which laid most of the claim to comprising the 'crisis'. The question to be considered is the extent to which the picture seen in present-day psychiatric practice resembles this.

Clearly, some of the similarities extend beyond superficially shared symptomatology. The prevalence figures, the possibility of a greater risk in young adults, and the pattern of diurnal variation have echoes in acute drug-related dystonias. Alteration of the clinical presentation by engaging in certain 'tricks' bears a passing resemblance to the situation encountered in idiopathic dystonia (see Chapter 7). There are, however, no data on environmental or sensory factors that may precipitate or promote acute drug-related dystonias, apart (possibly) from the ubiquitous 'stress'. Certainly, there is nothing at all to suggest that acute dystonias are in any way associated with alterations in conscious level. Indeed, as was pointed out, patients are usually 'hyper-alert'. The only cognitive disturbances thus far attributed to the drug context are impaired attention and, rarely, fixed and distressing ruminations of obsessional type (Leigh et al., 1987), which might be seen as something at least akin to the 'forced' or 'made' phenomena described in post-encephalitic states.

In recent years, several case reports have described isolated auditory and occasionally visual misperceptions occurring in the context of episodes of ocular deviation or, in one instance, preceding it (Chiu, 1989; Sachdev and Tang, 1992; Thornton and McKenna, 1994). However, these examples are few and have referred to cases on established anti-psychotic treatment and hence with neurological disorder appropriately classified as tardive. (Tardive oculogyric spasms are mentioned in Chapter 7.)

Acute dystonias are difficult to study for both practical and ethical reasons but the frequent role they play in clinical experience would suggest that those who encounter them – doctors *and* patients – should by now have been able to construct a more comprehensive profile of symptomatology were such symptomatology there to be constructed into a profile.

The author's experience of something he would be comfortable with calling a genuine 'crisis' extends to a single case – possibly. At grand rounds, a colleague presented the case of a 64-year-old chronic psychotic man in long-term care and receiving high-dose Modecate monthly. For some months, in the week following his injection he showed episodes of disturbed and aggressive behaviour interspersed with unresponsive periods, during which he had a clear retrocollis, opisthotonos and oculogyrus, and was sweaty, tachycardic and hypertensive. These spells would last for anything up to several days, with intermittent remissions, although he would eventually emerge from them as rapidly as he had sunk into them in the first place. Anticholinergics were ineffective. He could give no account of his mental state content during these episodes, which was in line with the fact that he could give no account of it at any other time either. The colleague's video was extremely convincing that the signs were those of an extrapyramidal state. The spanner in the works in attributing this entirely to drugs was that the patient had a vague but nonetheless suggestive history of 'encephalitis' a few years previously.

It may well be that differences between the oculogyric crises of yesteryear and those events we now call by that name are merely ones of degree – what was seen before was simply more severe. However, it is questionable whether physicians of the 1920s and 1930s would acknowledge the problem of our patients as anything but a pale shadow of what afflicted theirs. Calling things that have superficial resemblance by the same name is potentially dangerous, implying that they are the same. Until we can be sure that acute drug-related dystonias are usually or frequently possessed of hidden symptomatic depths hitherto untapped, the deception of understanding is best avoided and, in the absence of supplementary symptomatology, those involving the extraocular musculature are best referred to descriptively as what they are – namely, extraocular (or oculogyric) spasms or dystonias.

4

Parkinsonism

Introduction

Parkinsonism associated with drug use was first described by De in 1944 in Indian patients treated with rauwalfia alkaloids. In this situation it was observed to be a common occurrence that could be readily reversed by atropine. This was clearly seen as an adverse effect but, presumably because of its easy treatability, was not commented on as a source of clinical concern.

Those psychiatrists who had early access to chlorpromazine noted similar symptomatology associated with its use too. Patients were, as mentioned above, initially treated symptomatically for 'excitement' as opposed to by diagnosis, and were noted to become 'retarded' and to develop 'wooden' expressions and difficulties with gait and balance. Delay and Deniker noted features of this sort as early as 1952, but again the unmistakable impression one is left with is that this was not considered an issue of concern. At the first Largactil Symposium held in Basel in November of 1953, in response to questions from the floor, Staehelin (quoted in Caldwell, 1978) stated that:

> 'This parkinsonoid syndrome occurs more or less developed depending on dosage but also on predisposition or previous brainstem disease. Usually the syndrome quickly recedes if dosage is reduced; so far we have never seen persistent parkinsonism after discontinuation of Largactil.'

The fact that this appeared to be readily manageable allowed it to be dealt with in a passing manner.

The first formal report of extrapyramidal dysfunction with chlorpromazine appeared in 1954, when Steck pointed to the similarity between the parkinsonian symptomatology that could develop on this drug and that which could be found in patients receiving reserpine (Steck, 1954). Further descriptive reports followed but, for those of a theoretical

68

persuasion, the shift of emphasis from adverse to necessary effect had already begun. As early as 1953, Fluegel had suggested that therapeutic response was contingent upon not just the development but in fact the 'production' of extrapyramidal symptomatology. The influence this debate had on the name by which this new class of drugs became known has already been mentioned.

By the 1960s, the necessary role of extrapyramidal symptomatology in therapeutic effectiveness had been fairly comprehensively debunked, although not, it must be said, on the basis of specific clinical trials. However, the evidence from mainly efficacy studies conducted until that time did not support the hypothesis.

An alternative view, that extrapyramidal signs represented not merely adverse but frankly toxic effects, was explored within a context still mooted in some circles, that of the 'neuroleptic threshold'. The advocates of this view, most notably H.J. Haase in Germany, proposed that the departure of antipsychotic blood levels from the therapeutic to the toxic range was marked by the development of subtle features of parkinsonism, such as characteristic distortions of handwriting. Haase postulated that a reduction of 30 per cent in the area of the page occupied in writing a poem or passage allowed one to infer that the hypothesised threshold between therapeutic and toxic had been crossed and that the desired dose would be found by cautious reduction. Recent attempts to validate this hypothesis using tremor as the criterion have suggested some theoretical but hardly practical utility, but handwriting appears too varied within and across individuals to be of value (Shackman, van Putten and May, 1979; Gilmour and Bradford, 1987).

The history of parkinsonism in relation to antipsychotic drug use is one of fading interest. The first 20 years were characterised by an awareness that, apart from a brief period of theoretical excitement, was tainted by a certain lack of professional concern. In the second 20 years, even the awareness seemed to fade. To some extent, parkinsonism was near terminally suffocated as a research topic by the sheer weight of the hysteria that surrounded tardive dyskinesia. Yet it is now becoming clear that such neglect is not only clinically reprehensible, it is foolish. The major selling point of new compounds could well be enhanced efficacy should some lucky pharmaceutical company find the needle in the psychopharmacological haystack. Failing such a long-awaited miracle, it is most likely to be an improved profile of extrapyramidal tolerability – and in the first instance that means a reduced liability to produce parkinsonian symptomatology. Even if doctors think little of these features, patients do not. They may be the single most memorable aspect of their first contact with antipsychotics, and their abiding and life-long dread of continued exposure. If we are aiming to offer genuinely comprehensive patient assessment, we must know parkinsonism in *all* its guises.

Terminology

From the start, there was a reluctance on the part of psychiatry to name names. The early writers referred only to a *similarity* between the features of drug-related parkinsonism and those of idiopathic disease. This probably reflected the fact that the clinical emphasis in the former seemed somewhat different, with the bradykinesia that was initially described as 'retardation' predominating in the relative absence of other features. For this reason, much of the early descriptive literature refers to the problem as 'pseudoparkinsonism' or 'Parkinson-like syndrome'. It is now generally accepted, however, that the major features that comprise Parkinson's disease can also be found in the drug-related state, even if the emphasis may indeed be somewhat different, as we shall see.

Neither of these terms has anything to commend it. The syndrome is certainly 'like' Parkinson's disease but we already have an adequate term for this in 'parkinsonism' – which, as a simple descriptive term, is without aetiological or other implication. In the interest of avoiding nominal clutter, we do not need another descriptive term to say the same thing in a different way.

Pseudoparkinsonism is still favoured by neurologists, mainly to cover two conditions sometimes mistaken for Parkinson's disease – essential tremor and anteriosclerotic pseudoparkinsonism, also referred to as lower body parkinsonism (Quinn, 1995). In the former, it is the diagnosis that is 'pseudo' and, in the latter, the pathological implications that flow from the diagnosis. The idea of 'pseudo-Parkinson's *disease*' would seem to avoid the smack of illogicality that surrounds 'pseudoparkinsonism', but neither has any particular merit in the present context.

From our point of view, the drug-related states encountered in psychiatric practice are but one form of secondary or symptomatic *parkinsonism* and this simple descriptive term should suffice.

Finally, there is an idiosyncrasy of the author's that has perhaps become apparent and is worth explaining. The conventional terminology for parkinsonism associated with drug use is 'drug-induced '. The implications of this are certainly not wrong but hint at associations that are straightforward and in need of no further comment. As will become clear, this is not necessarily the case, and the author's preference is for a term which merely encapsulates the relationship without any further inferences – hence the term 'drug-related ' which the reader will find throughout the present work. This, furthermore, provides consistency with other syndromes, especially the tardive ones, for which the nature of the relationship with medication is altogether more complex.

Clinical features

General concepts/core features

The core features of parkinsonism of whatever cause are the same: namely, the triad of bradykinesia, rigidity and tremor.

Bradykinesia

Bradykinesia also goes by the names of hypokinesia and akinesia. Purists might object to use of the prefix 'a', because total as opposed to relative abnormality is clinically the exception. Akinesia is nonetheless sometimes used by neurologists as a sort of generic term. Essentially, however, these terms all mean the same and since in the context of drug use, disorder is always relative, bradykinesia will be used throughout the present work.

Bradykinesia refers to a loss or absence of voluntary motor activity. This has four principal manifestations:

1. diminution or poverty of background motor activity;
2. slowed execution of movements associated with difficulty in initiation;
3. progressive fatiguing and diminishing amplitude of repetitive alternating movements;
4. an interruption to the flow of consecutive movements.

Combinations of these phenomena make a major contribution to the clinical presentation of parkinsonism, though the mechanism underlying the disorder remains unclear. Bradykinesia is in fact a symptom complex, something which in classificatory terms sits ill in medicine. It has been pointed out that while features of this sort can represent a primary 'core' disturbance, similar symptomatology can result from the consequences of rigidity (i.e. 'secondary' bradykinesia) and that these two manifestations of outwardly similar disorder may have different anatomical localisations (Narabayashi, 1995). In the present context, however, such distinctions will be ignored, partly to avoid confusion but also because, as rigidity is a relatively junior symptomatic partner in drug-related disorder, the distinction has little practical merit.

Some commentators have taken a grand taxonomic sweep by classifying bradykinesia together with other states of motor poverty, of which the two most obvious in a psychiatric context are the retardation of

depression and the apathy/anergy of negative (especially schizophrenic) states (Bermanzohn and Siris, 1992). However, this is a risky
mind-set. Oedema may indeed result from leaks in the legs but one's
expectation of medicine is for a somewhat more profound understanding of its many causes than that! There is as yet no evidence that
merit flows from considering these phenomena as similar in any but the
most superficial, descriptive way.

Rigidity

Rigidity is an increase in resting muscle tone evident on passive
movement. That of parkinsonism exhibits a predominantly central to
peripheral spread, usually being evident first in the large axial and
proximal limb girdle muscles.

Two types of rigidity are described in association with extrapyramidal disease. The first affects agonist and antagonist muscles equally and
results in an even resistance to passive movements throughout the
range. This is the so-called lead-pipe variety. In the second type, resistance gives at regular intervals, to be rapidly re-established as the
motion is pursued. This conveys a jerky, ragged feel throughout the
range of movement and is aptly referred to as cog-wheel rigidity. The
pathophysiological basis of cog-wheeling is complex and poorly understood and the proposal that it results from nothing more than the
combination of rigidity with coincidental tremor may be an oversimplification. This challenge to a professional truism is particularly
justifiable in drug-related cases, where cog-wheeling is a relatively
common, if mild, abnormality whereas high-amplitude/low-frequency
tremor is uncommon.

Tremor

Tremor is the regular, rhythmic or oscillatory involuntary
movement of a body part, usually about a joint. Neurology's relationship with the classification of tremors, especially at a clinical level, has
tended to be somewhat vague and not always consistent. Essentially,
however, tremors can be defined in terms of their frequency, technically
expressed as Herz, or the number of excursions or cycles per second.
Alternatively, they can be described more simply in terms of the circumstances in which they occur.

Two types of tremor are found in parkinsonism. The first is the
characteristic 'paralysis agitans' type everyone knows about. This is a
tremor of high amplitude and low frequency, in the range of 4–6 Hz
(cps). It is, furthermore, a tremor that shows itself predominantly at rest
and disappears during active movement of the affected part.

What is often forgotten is that parkinsonism is also associated with
tremors that are predominantly postural. These are tremors of low

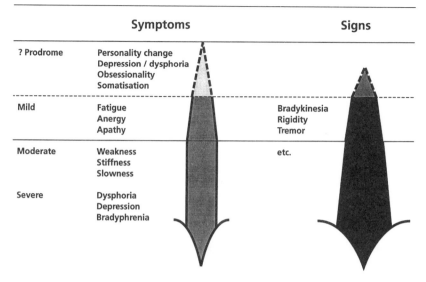

	Symptoms	**Signs**
? Prodrome	Personality change Depression / dysphoria Obsessionality Somatisation	
Mild	Fatigue Anergy Apathy	Bradykinesia Rigidity Tremor
Moderate	Weakness Stiffness Slowness	etc.
Severe	Dysphoria Depression Bradyphrenia	

Fig. 4.1. The balance of symptoms and signs in parkinsonism.

amplitude and high frequency (8–10 Hz) which emerge in the context of sustained motor activity and abate in the passive state. They are best observed in the upper limbs with arms outstretched. The third type of tremor, referred to as 'action' or 'kinetic' because of its intimate relationship to the dynamic of movement itself, is *not* a feature of extrapyramidal disorder. Clinically, however, the distinction between postural and action tremors can sometimes be blurred.

In addition to the core symptomatology, a series of other features indicative of disruption of autonomic and reflex functions complete a complex picture that will now be pursued in more detail.

Symptoms

One of life's little paradoxes relates to psychiatry's approach to drug-related parkinsonism. The specialty whose expertise resides in aspects of the mental state has seemed content to view the problem of parkinsonism related to drug use almost exclusively in terms of neurological *signs* – another consequence of 'tramlining' (Fig. 4.1).

No-one could really claim that the neurological literature showed us how things ought to be done, but as early as the 1950s those involved in the first tentative steps at standardised assessment of parkinsonism were aware that objective or purely sign-led methods could be relied upon to provide only a partial picture of disability. There was an increasing acknowledgement that the illness had an impact on the patient and that comprehensive evaluation needed to embrace this. As a result, the literature began to focus on what were called the activities of daily living (ADL) – those basic practical motor skills that, by erosion, could severely compromise the patient's quality of life.

In addition to these consequences of motor disturbance, it has also been known for some time that mental state changes may be part of Parkinson's disease. The obvious ones are depression and, in the later stages, dementia (Dooneief et al., 1992; Lees and Smith, 1983). Furthermore, certain 'pre-diagnosis' psychological features have been described as typical, if not characteristic, including premorbid obsessionality (or anankastic personality type), depressive disorders and a typical type of cognitive slowing referred to as bradyphrenia (Rogers et al., 1987). There is also a suggestion that neurotic and psychosomatic illnesses may be significantly more frequent in the years prior to diagnosis in those with Parkinson's disease than in control patients without it (Rajput, Offord and Beard, 1987).

None of the studies exploring these issues is free from criticism, especially since most have been of necessity retrospective. However, this does represent an extensive and sustained effort to pursue the wider boundaries of the condition. Seen in this light, psychiatry's efforts in drug-related disorder look paltry and unimaginative.

Psychiatry might have been forgiven for failing to take these clinically very justifiable moves on board on the basis that the severity of abnormality encountered within its jurisdiction was not of the same order as in patients with idiopathic disease, or the coincidental mental state abnormalities made uncontaminated appraisal difficult. This will hardly do though, and it remains distressing that the psychiatric literature has so resolutely ignored or at least de-emphasised the subjective symptomatology of drug-related parkinsonism.

Patients with Parkinson's disease do not, as a rule, present to the neurological outpatients department sounding off about their 'cogwheeling' or the like. Those signs diagnostically important for the doctor are features the patients themselves are at this stage unlikely to be aware of. The commonest presenting complaints are usually of weakness and fatiguability. What patients are likely to have noticed is that routine tasks require increasingly greater effort because of a subjective awareness of fatigue developing prematurely in the affected muscles, most often in the limbs initially. This becomes associated with a general tiredness and inability to sustain effort.

The author recalls being asked by a general practitioner (GP) to see a 47-year-old man with just such complaints, particularly that he found it 'tiring' to hold his infant daughter for too long, something both his wife and G.P. interpreted as loss of interest. I was acceptably convinced of the presence of some psychiatric disorder (although would be prepared to admit now that I might have been hard pressed to specify precisely which one!). As the man walked me to the door, it was evident that he had strikingly reduced arm swing on the left. A hastily extended examination in the hallway confirmed the presence of rigidity.

A further feature patients may become aware of is stiffness. Thus, they may experience an aching discomfort, especially in axial and proximal limb muscles and characteristically most evident on waking. This tends to ease as they 'get on the go' but may become evident again following spells of exertion. This obviously must be distinguished from orthopaedic causes of similar symptomatology.

As was mentioned, there is now an extensive literature linking Parkinson's disease to formal affective disorder, especially depression, and although this mainly refers to patients with established disease, those in earlier, including prediagnostic, phases may similarly experience affective symptoms. While in some cases this may conform to operational criteria for a formal depression, in others it can perhaps be more accurately thought of as dysphoria. Patients may feel listless, anergic and apathetic, with a decline in their initiative and interest in the external world. They may not say they are sad as such, but rather that they are just not happy.

Some exceptions to the psychiatric neglect of the subjective side of drug-related extrapyramidal symptomatology have been lodged in mainly the American literature (van Putten, 1974; Rifkin, Quitkin and Klein, 1975). The merits of these efforts have, however, frequently been off-set by the inclusion of idiosyncratically broad or needlessly dynamic concepts. Rifkin and colleagues pointed out that 'akinesia' was indeed a 'poorly recognised drug-induced' extrapyramidal disorder, but defined the abnormality in vague behavioural terms and stated that its presence represented drug toxicity. Van Putten and May (1978) provided accounts of the subjective complaints of patients with mild 'akinesia' in terms of them feeling 'listless', 'tired' and without 'interest, life or ambition'. They also found 'akinesia in pure culture' (i.e. without other EPS) in 30 per cent of their sample which, as it developed, was associated with increased ratings of depression. Both the 'akinesia' and the 'depression', which was mild, invariably resolved with anticholinergic medication. For this latter situation, the authors coined the term 'akinetic depression', largely on the basis of a dynamic evaluation of the patients' own statements. This terminology still appears in the American literature but, in the light of the present account, this would seem a confusing complication.

If we accept the general principle that *all* the features of Parkinson's disease can be expressed in the drug-related condition, we must extend this to the subjective symptomatology as well. We must be aware of the emergence of weakness, fatiguability, muscle stiffness, anergy, apathy and diminished interest and initiative in patients exposed to antipsychotics as potentially subjective manifestations of extrapyramidal dysfunction.

There is, of course, a major problem here in that all or any of these may be indistinguishable from features of the mental state disorder for which the drugs are being given in the first place. Nonetheless, it is crucial to bear in mind the *possibility* of a drug-related component to any such symptomatology in patients receiving antipsychotics.

As the condition becomes more established, patients may become aware of particular aspects of their symptomatology in a highly individualistic way. Indeed, such awareness may lead to the initial medical presentation of idiopathic disease. Movement in affected parts loses its automatic quality and becomes increasingly laboured. Motor actions are no longer fluid and consecutive but seem ponderous, course and disjointed, and routine tasks can no longer be taken for granted. One man's problem came to light when his wife kept nagging him that he was not shaving the right side of his chin properly, while the friend of a former nursing sister commented that she made a funny noise with her left foot when she walked. 'I'd just got new shoes,' she said. 'I thought it was the shoes.'

The impact of drug-related symptomatology on patients' functional capacity has not concerned psychiatry hitherto. There is quite simply no substantive literature on the topic of ADL in this population. This is undoubtedly an omission, though how much of an omission is impossible to say. The effect on personal hygiene of cups of tea dribbled from a shaky hand is self-evident and a common enough sight in chronic psychotic patients, as are the burn marks from dropped cigarettes that are all too easy to attribute to a generally deteriorated self-concern. One must, in addition, wonder about the extent of problems such as difficulty in doing up buttons, combing hair, shaving, tying shoe laces, or using domestic implements like cutlery or tin-openers, which are never explored and seldom volunteered. These are questions that could do with posing to patients receiving anti-psychotic drugs, as the answers cannot be taken for granted.

For all the above, it is undoubtedly easy to see parkinsonism in exclusively sign terms – but important that this tendency is constantly countered. Even when the balance of symptomatology tips the scales very much in the sign direction, this is *not* to say that subjective symptoms evaporate (see Fig. 4.1). It merely means one has to counteract all the more consciously one's inclination for assessment to be carried along by the lead features.

Signs

The clinical presentation of parkinsonism is a complex picture (Table 4.1) that varies in severity and distribution across individuals and over time. Its detail cannot be appreciated in a passing glance.

Bradykinesia affecting the facial muscles gives rise to so-called hypomimia (sometimes referred to as amimia) or the characteristic 'masking'

Table 4.1. *Summary of the major features of parkinsonism*

Symptoms	Signs
Weakness	Facial mask
Fatigue	Glabellar tap
Anergy	Sialorrhoea
Apathy	Speech disturbance
	loss of pitch
Tiredness	loss of power
Stiffness	loss of tone
Aching discomfort	loss of articulation
Slowness	Slowing of movement
Clumsiness	Loss of background movement
	gesture
Shakiness	interactive posture
	Impaired dexterity
	Impaired initiation
	Interruption
	freezing
	Loss of pendular arm swing
	Posture disturbance
	trunk flexion/hyperextension
	arms flexion–abduction
	legs flexion
	Impaired postural reflexes
	instability
	Gait disturbance
	slowing
	reduced step length
	reduced step height
	festination
	Rigidity
	cogwheel
	leadpipe
	Tremor
	postural
	resting
	Autonomic disturbance
	seborrhoea
	(sialorrhoea)

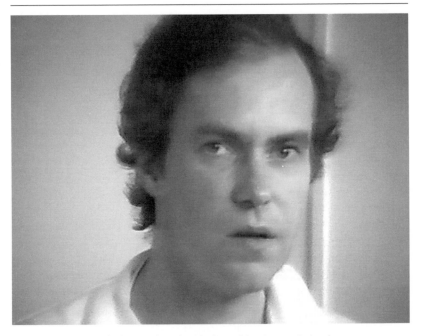

Fig. 4.2. Facial mask. (Reproduced with the subject's permission.)

of facial expression. The term 'masking' is a good one for it emphasises that it is the apparatus of expression that is damaged, not affect itself. The subtle ebb and flow of facial expression that is the normal accompaniment of thought, speech and social interaction is lost, with only a fixed and relatively immobile facies to take its place. Gradations of affective display diminish, the signs of laughter, when they do appear, flashing on suddenly to disappear as quickly. The patient often has a somewhat 'gormless', vacant appearance (Fig. 4.2). This comes not only from the flattening of the facial contours but from the rather wild, staring quality imparted to the eyes owing to a reduction in blink rate (sometimes referred to as the 'reptilian stare') and from the fact that the mouth is held slightly open.

The facial masking of parkinsonism can be difficult to distinguish from the two differentials that recurrently confuse diagnosis of the manifestations of bradykinesia, namely the retardation of depression and the affective flattening of, especially, schizophrenia. The latter two features – reduced blink rate and the aimlessly parted lips and open mouth – can be helpful in attempting the distinction.

A positive glabellar tap, or Myerson's sign, is the sort of striking feature of established idiopathic disease that neurologists like to demonstrate to students and that students like to remember. While this can be present in drug-related cases, it is rarely so in marked degree and, at the level at which it tends to show, is a fairly non-specific and unhelpful finding in psychiatric patients. A failure of blink rate to habituate on tapping the glabellar ridge can be found in patients who are anxious and tense or otherwise hyperaroused or, perhaps most importantly of all, when the examination technique is clumsy and incompetent, something that is addressed in more detail in Chapter 10.

A further reason for de-emphasising the glabellar tap in patients with major psychiatric disorder is that, even if clearly present, its origins may *not* lie in the drug-related parkinsonism but in the underlying psychosis. A positive glabellar tap is one of a series of so-called 'primitive reflexes' reported to be present and to carry possible diagnostic weight in Parkinson's disease (Vreeling et al., 1993). Others include the snout, palmomental, nasopalpebral, suck and grasp reflexes. The presence of such signs can persist into adulthood in some otherwise unexceptional individuals, but their presence in disease states appears to correlate with the degree of cognitive impairment. Hence, these features may be a clinical manifestation of diffuse brain disorder. Similar findings, and a similar explanatory hypothesis, have also been reported in schizophrenia (Quitkin, Rifkin and Klein, 1976; Johnstone et al., 1990).

There is, therefore, reason to doubt, firstly, how prominent a feature of drug-related parkinsonism a positive glabellar tap actually is, and, secondly, even if present, whether this sign can be validly attributed to a drug effect.

Sialorrhoea literally means excessive salivation and can be a prominent and distressing part of parkinsonism. The patient may, in mild or early cases, simply have a sensation of moistness in the mouth, but as the problem progresses, an imbalance between production and clearance of saliva results in pooling in the floor of the mouth and eventual drooling. Sialorrhoea is not, however, an entirely objective sign. Patients vary considerably in the distress they experience from apparently comparable degrees of abnormality and this affective overlay can make the feature hard to evaluate. Perhaps the nearest to an objective parameter is moistness on the pillow on waking as a result of nocturnal drooling. A further pointer is the patient who, Pavarotti-like, carries a handkerchief in his or her hand constantly.

Although the term sialorrhoea implies excessive production of saliva, it is by no means clear that this offers a universal explanation. It is probably the mechanism underlying the phenomenon in patients on clozapine, a drug with a strikingly reduced liability to promote extrapyramidal dysfunction overall (Owens, 1996), but with standard compounds it seems more likely that the problem is less an autonomic one but rather one of impaired swallowing consequent upon bradykinesia of the oropharyngeal musculature.

Involvement of the pharyngeal, lingual and laryngeal muscles affects speech and articulation. Pitch, power and intonation are all progressively affected so the voice becomes deeper, more monotonous and softer, with ultimately only a barely audible, hoarse whisper possible. Added to this is the fact that phonemes are incompletely articulated, with adjacent sounds running into one another, resulting in thickness and slurring. The combined effect of these is to render communication difficult and, in severe cases, incomprehensible.

Bradykinesia of the systemic musculature results in observable slowing of voluntary movement. Activity takes on a graceless, awkward and rather stilted quality which, with progression, becomes associated with visible signs of impairment. In conversation there is a lack of interactive posture and gesture, with the individual seeming distant and uninvolved. Initiation becomes difficult with, for example, two or three attempts necessary to get out of a chair. Tasks that demand rapidity and complexity of movement are increasingly impaired, which shows most clearly in loss of manual dexterity. As a result, the sort of domestic skills noted above may be compromised. Disruption to the flow of consecutive movements may become evident, with actions appearing hesitant, disjointed and incapable of initiation or completion – so-called 'freezing'.

Bradykinesia also produces a characteristic loss of arm swing on walking. Pendular arm swing is not something instilled in childhood by parents demanding their offspring 'march like soldiers', but an automatic function whose action is to stabilise the body's shifting centre of gravity as weight shifts with forward motion. There is, however, an idiosyncratic element to this in that people achieve the goal by way of a range of excursions and personal peculiarities. With the onset of parkinsonism, the arms, instead of moving freely on walking, describe an increasingly restricted arc and eventually come to be held immobile by the sides.

Progression sees the combination of loss of swing with changes in attitude. Increasing flexion and abduction become evident, which as they develop are associated with advancing pronation. The arms, instead of hanging loosely by the side, come to be flexed and abducted with the knuckles rotated through 90 degrees and ending up 'facing the front'.

Reduction of pendular arm swing is a frequent and sensitive indicator of antipsychotic exposure. Indeed, in the author's experience, it is one of *the* most sensitive of all the clinical signs of drug-related parkinsonism and, despite the element of variability in the basic function, can be detected in the majority of patients, especially in the early phases of drug exposure when doses are increasing.

Postural changes are seen in more general and progressive adoption of a flexed attitude. This is usually evident first in head/neck, then involves trunk and, as already noted, upper and finally lower limbs. This pattern of flexion of the trunk, arms and legs is often referred to as 'triple flexion' and is characteristic of advanced idiopathic disease. The attitude adopted may, however, be towards hyperextension, with the patient standing or walking 'bolt' upright with a 'poker' spine or even a slight backwards lean. This is relatively uncommon in idiopathic disease but more typical of drug-related disorder.

By pushing the centre of gravity forward, the flexed attitude of parkinsonism contributes to the instability that can be so incapacitating for such patients. However, the major factor in this is impairment of righting reflexes, which are essential for maintenance of the upright position. Patients cannot bring into play rapidly enough the changes in tone in the antigravity postural muscles that are the necessary pre-requisite to sustaining a secure position in a dynamic motor situation. Patients may be aware of this before much in the way of objective features is detectable and may present it in what at first glance seems to be psychological terms, such as a lack of confidence when outside, without specifically articulating a basis for this. One lady attributed the restrictions in her life to the fact that she could no longer go out as she could not cross the main road beside her house. A more detailed enquiry revealed that she could in fact manage out *and* cross the road but having got to the other side could not turn with confidence in the direction she wanted to go, so ended up following the crowd, even if this was in the direction opposite to her planned route. 'I'm thoroughly fed up with this,' she said, 'so I just stay in'.

Subsequently, patients experience difficulty with any change in position, such as turning corners, without feeling they might fall. Having managed to overcome the initiation problem in rising from a sitting position, they may then feel uncomfortably unsteady standing.

Some patients with Parkinson's disease may eventually become totally dependent and wheelchair bound, unable to stand unaided or to support an erect posture when sitting. This degree of disability is, however, usually only found during the 'off' phases of motor fluctuations. The so-called 'wheelchair sign' of permanent dependency is more commonly associated with causes of parkinsonism other than Parkinson's disease (Quinn, 1995). It should not be seen in drug-related disorder.

Disturbance of gait is evident not only in a slowing of pace but also in a reduction in both the length and the height of step. The breadth of base, on the other hand, is not affected. The normal sequence of walking – namely, heel to the ground first followed by the ball of the foot – is inverted so that the patient walks initially flat-footedly and subsequently ball-to-heel, which has the effect of reducing the forward propulsive force of each step. This combination of inverted sequence, with short, shallow steps gives rise to a shuffling gait which, as in the lady mentioned above, has an audible component. It is sometimes referred to descriptively as *marche a petit pas*. Forward momentum can acquire an almost impelled quality which makes patients look as if they are running – so-called 'festination'. Finally, an inability to bring antagonist muscles into play appropriately prevents the patient from exerting instant control on forward and backward movement, so having started they may not be able to stop, giving rise to anteropulsion when the motion is in a forward direction and retropulsion when it is backwards.

A further abnormality of walking can make for a rare if well-described presentation of Parkinson's disease (Poewe, Lees and Stern, 1988) which, although of little relevance to drug-related presentations, has been encountered in general clinical work by this psychiatrist. The author was approached by an orthopaedic colleague in the canteen one day asking for an opinion on a middle-aged woman who had developed an 'hysterical' gait. When the woman walked, her foot inverted. A built-up shoe had been ineffective and the woman was becoming 'understandably depressed'. I was, of course, delighted to see a case of 'hysteria' as at that point I had been waiting some 15 years of my professional career to meet one! I was on this, as on so many other occasions, to be disappointed since, on the day of her appointment, in walked the woman with her built-up shoe still revealing a foot dystonia – plus a masked facies, an absent arm swing etc. The orthopaedic surgeon was surprised by my formulation, as he had accepted the initial referral complete with 'hysterical' diagnosis – from a neurologist!

The writing of patients with parkinsonism becomes smaller, a phenomenon known as micrographia. This affects not only the vertical size of the script, but also the horizontal dimension. Thus, the area of page utilised for any writing task can be strikingly diminished (Fig. 4.3). This can be disproportionately disruptive, even when other manifestations of disorder are slight. The author recalls a 25-year-old legal secretary with a delusional disorder who improved somewhat symptomatically, and not insubstantially in terms of overall well-being, on pimozide. During a routine follow-up appointment she told me, almost in passing, that she had had to give up her job 'because I can't write properly'. A detailed examination, done at the behest of my alarm, revealed only a mild bilateral postural tremor, and slight reduction in arm swing and dexterity on the right. Her truly microscopic hand-writing did not enlarge much on anticholinergics, and only resolved in the six to eight weeks after pimozide was stopped. Somewhat surprisingly, she had not herself made the connection between her changed script and drug treatment and blamed her inability to write on 'tiredness'.

The two types of rigidity found in extrapyramidal disease have been

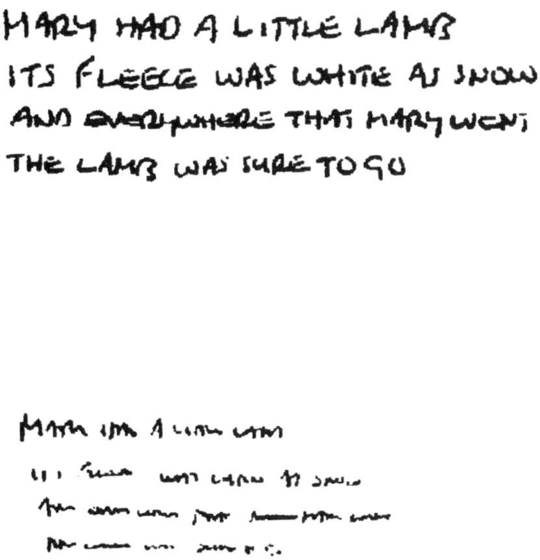

MARY HAD A LITTLE LAMB
ITS FLEECE WAS WHITE AS SNOW
AND EVERYWHERE THAT MARY WENT
THE LAMB WAS SURE TO GO

Mary had a little lamb
its fleece was white as snow
and everywhere that mary went
the lamb was sure to go.

Fig. 4.3. Micrographia: handwriting samples six weeks apart. (The patient had been on pimozide 6 mg.)

mentioned above. There is a widespread view, particularly in psychiatric circles, that only cog-wheeling has any significance in drug-related cases. This is incorrect. Both types are of equal significance and diagnostic import. The earliest signs of increased tone are to be found in the proximal limb muscles, although disorder is invariably easier to elicit distally. Rigidity is also to be found in axial musculature as a resistance to passive whole-body movements.

Conventional wisdom has it that there are no changes in tendon reflexes associated with extrapyramidal disorder. However, this is not so. An increase in jerks has been reported in up to one-third of patients with Parkinson's disease, especially evident on the more prominently affected side, although not apparently correlated with the overall severity of disease (Hammerstad et al., 1994). Whether or not similar changes are to be found in drug-related parkinsonism has not been explored, although this is not an oversight about which psychiatry need feel too embarrassed: it took neurology 175 years to explore the question systematically!

Tremor, too, can have a wide distribution. Resting tremor is seen in the limbs and although a similar course tremor can also be present in the head, typical 'affirmation' ('yes–yes') and 'negation' ('no–no') tremors are more characteristic of essential tremor.

Postural tremor, as already noted, is best seen in the outstretched hands but its influence can also be detected in writing or in a spiral

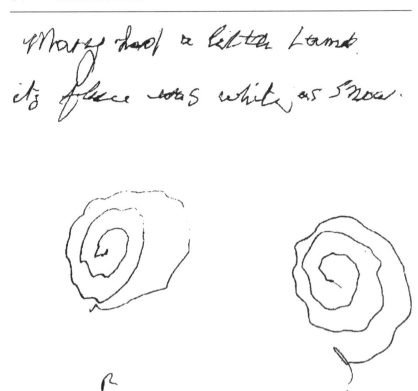

Fig. 4.4. Tremor in parkinsonism.

drawn by the patient (Fig. 4.4). It can be observed elsewhere too, such as in the eyelids with the eyes closed or in the protruded tongue. Although the clear distinction elaborated here between high-ampli-tude/low-frequency resting and low-amplitude/high-frequency pos-tural tremors has general validity, it is not absolute. Tremors evident at rest may carry over into other situations as well. One woman with a marked resting tremor of the right leg had almost a dancing quality to her walk from the intrusion of the tremor into her gait also.

A considerable deal has been made in some quarters, especially in North America, about the occurrence in some patients on antipsychotics of an isolated, vertical, perioral tremor, particularly in the upper lip, referred to as the 'rabbit' syndrome (Villeneuve, 1972; Casey, 1992). This, according to its advocates, may present either as a solitary phenomenon or in combination with other features, usually tongue tremors, and appears to have the electrophysiological characteristics of high-ampli-tude/low-frequency tremor (Jus, Jus and Villeneuve, 1973). Although only a handful of case reports of this 'syndrome' has been published, an epidemiological survey suggested an overall prevalence of around 3 per cent (Yassa and Samarthji, 1986). It has also been reported that the disorder is not to be found in patients on anticholinergics. The present author cannot impart to the reader any expertise on this topic as he has never encountered a case for which he considered such isolated symptomatology sufficiently noteworthy to be worthy of note! It would hardly seem to justify separate consideration as a 'syndrome'.

Autonomic disturbances can also become evident in the course of parkinsonism. Excessive sebaceous secretions give rise to seborrhoea, which imparts a waxy quality to (especially) the skin of the face. This, combined with the pallor which is a consequence of autonomic change, can bestow on the patient an almost spectral appearance. Impaired autonomic function can result in a compromised capacity to maintain blood pressure, particularly in the face of postural change, and also to disturbed bowel, bladder and sexual function. Its possible role in sialorrhoea has already be mentioned.

With the exception of seborrhoea (and sialorrhoea if, indeed, autonomically mediated), signs of autonomic dysfunction are usually to be found in cases of advanced idiopathic disease or other extrapyramidal syndromes, and whether they occur as an integral part of severe drug-related disorder is not known. This would be a hard question to address in view of the intrinsic anti-autonomic actions of many antipsychotics. No studies have been undertaken of autonomic function in patients with marked parkinsonism from high-potency antipsychotics which possess minimal anti-autonomic actions.

The clinical presentation of parkinsonism is therefore complex and comprises features that, by the unwary, can be confused with those of mental state origin. Furthermore, it must be remembered that many of these features may initially present *unilaterally*. Indeed, a unilateral emphasis at first presentation and throughout the course is the norm in idiopathic disease (Quinn, 1995), which probably reflects a combination of anatomical and pathological factors. A similar clinical asymmetry in drug-related disorder presumably reflects more purely anatomical asymmetry in the dopamine systems on which the pathophysiological process is focused. This issue was a source of some interest in the psychiatric literature a few years ago in relation to drug-related disorder, with the suggestion that abnormality was more likely to show on the dominant side, though, even if true, this has not taken our understanding any further forward.

The author has come across a memorable example of unilaterality in a 47-year-old man with a relatively late onset (or late diagnosed) schizophrenic illness, who developed a striking tremor of his left arm on antipsychotics. Although he consistently denied it, this seemed to the outside observer rather incapacitating. It was associated with mild

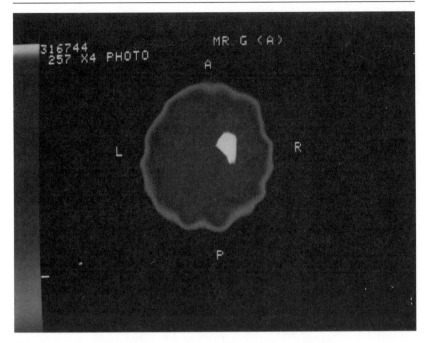

Fig. 4.5. Unilaterality of basal ganglia function (SPET).

rigidity and moderate bradykinesia on the same side but no other abnormality. In the course of his long-term follow-up, the patient, a pleasant and helpful man, volunteered for an imaging project utilising single photon emission tomography (SPET), which revealed him to have *no* detectable function in the striatum on the right. The assumption was that his strikingly low dopamine endowment on the right side was probably congenital.

A further interesting dimension to this man's case was that he was dyschondroplasiac (though with incomplete penetrance as evidenced in muted stigmata of the phenotype) and in addition had cranio-cleido-dysostosis. If this triad of developmental disorders has not hitherto been recorded – orthopaedics being by now a somewhat distant memory – the author would like to abuse the pages of the present volume to claim priority!

However, to raise the theme of 'It ain't necessarily so', a further case was that of a 26-year-old man whose SPET scan (Fig. 4.5) showed a similar gross asymmetry of striatal function. Clinically, however, he demonstrated no unilaterality of neurological signs. His features comprised a constant, high-amplitude jaw tremor and marked flexion of neck and upper back – i.e. central signs. What the future holds in this case is for the future to tell.

The potential for a unilateral distribution of drug-related parkinsonian symptomatology is of considerable clinical importance and again shouts loudly for examinations that are comprehensive. Not only might the obvious features of tremor, rigidity and a number of the manifestations of bradykinesia, such as reduced arm swing, be evident unilaterally, so too might a variety of the symptoms and less obvious signs such as postural instability.

Parkinsonism is, of course, a disorder that affects actions of a predominantly willed nature. In the early stages of idiopathic disease, however, patients may 'learn' that by recruiting the involuntary or overlearned component of motor activity, they can help, at least temporarily, to overcome some of their disability. They may, for example, hum a military-type tune or beat a rhythm in their head. In an interview given early in his illness, the comedian Terry-Thomas recalled how glad he was that he had started his career as a soft shoe shuffler. As his Parkinson's disease progressed, he found it difficult to get over a step at the entrance to his house, but discovered that by implementing his old dance routine a few yards from the door, he was able to mount the step without difficulty. As a result, he was still able to get out and about even in the face of advancing disability.

In the author's experience, this phenomenon is rarely, if ever, found in patients with drug-related parkinsonism, perhaps because the condition is seldom severe enough or perhaps because the superimposition of a major psychiatric illness, combined with some of the other adverse effects of treatment, precludes the expression of such ingenuity. There is a single case that comes to mind. The author and a colleague were videotaping patients on a long-stay ward with a view to recording their movement disorders. As is usually the case, the radio was on in the background, tuned to the mandatory 'easy listening' station. One rather disengaged middle-aged man, with admittedly only mild signs of EPS, was asked to walk the length of the ward and back as the final part of his assessment just as the disc jockey was announcing the result of the station's weekly competition. To herald this great event, on came 'Pomp and Circumstance No.1' (Land of Hope and Glory), at which point the patient threw back his shoulders and got into stride with a gait and an arm swing that would have done credit to any guardsman! When the music faded, so did he.

This is given only as a 'possible' example, for not only did our man perk up physically, he grinned from ear to ear during every one of his few seconds of triumph. Perhaps this deeply entrenched piece had stirred some long-forgotten memories of happier times or perhaps a severely damaged and not over-sophisticated man was just getting into the spirit of the 'game'. Either way, the effects of the music might have been on his mental state as much as on his motor function.

Idiopathic versus drug related – a case for difference?

The above clinical outline is mainly predicated on the (general) assumption that what is sauce for the idiopathic goose is sauce for the drug-related gander – the widely accepted view that there is nothing unique about the symptomatology of the drug-related state. While the author would not wish to challenge this as a general principle, it still leaves open the possibility that the *balance* of symptomatology may differ. This is certainly his – and others' – belief. The following, summarised in Table 4.2, is not, however, based on experimental data – for there are none of quality – but on clinical experience.

The UK Parkinson's Disease Society Brain Bank has operationalised diagnostic criteria for Parkinson's disease (Gibb and Lees, 1988). In this system, bradykinesia is the core 'core' feature, and neurologists agree that bradykinesia in the upper part of the body *must* be present in order to make the diagnosis (Quinn, 1995). In drug-related parkinsonism, bradykinesia is not only present, it forms the dominant symptomatology. As noted, loss of pendular arm swing is an early and sensitive sign well worth looking for. It must not be assumed that this is always a purely objective sign. One young man in his early twenties became remarkably unadventurous about leaving the house. 'I get embarrassed,' he said. 'I've developed the mental hospital walk.' – and indeed he had!

Corresponding postural changes in the arms are not infrequent, but marked truncal flexion is uncommon. Indeed, a mildly hyperextended 'poker' spine is more often encountered. The classical 'triple flexion' is not – or, perhaps more accurately, *should not be* – a feature. If this does develop, one ought to be seriously considering treatment schedules or the presence of underlying pathology. The same might be said for gait disturbance, which is usually a manifestation of heavy, rapid dosing of dubious therapeutic merit.

On the other hand, postural instability, usually a late development in Parkinson's disease, is undoubtedly common. Like most psychiatrists, the author never used to examine for this but has now changed his ways. What is distressing is to find often quite marked degrees of this – degrees associated with subjective morbidity – in young people who rarely, if ever, complain.

It is not only the young who do not complain, however. One of the most effective and appreciated interventions the author implemented was in an elderly psychotic woman, symptomatic but controlled on the same medication for 30 years. As a result of a catalogue of physical illness, she was able to do little, and could no longer make her weekly visit to the local shopping centre with her husband, which had been her sole pleasure in life. A series of falls had severely compromised her confidence. She felt that, as a result of her medical problems, she had just become too frail.

Table 4.2. *Clinical comparison with Parkinson's disease and drug-related parkinsonism*

	Parkinson's disease	Drug-related parkinsonism
Bradykinesia	Essential feature in upper body	Dominating symptomatology
Rigidity	Marked, progressive usually evident without reinforcement	Mild/moderate severity Often requires reinforcement Usually does not correlate with level of bradykinesia
Tremor	Majority at presentation Virtually universal with progression	Resting: infrequent late feature Postural: common early manifestation
Posture	Predominantly flexion	Disturbance uncommon and may show as mild hyperextension
Gait	Reduced speed Decreased length and height of step Shuffling	Uncommon late or severe manifestation
Glabellar tap	Frequently positive	Infrequently positive (?not a part of the disorder)
Distribution	Unilateral emphasis	Unilaterality may be evident but tends to general distribution, especially in younger patients

On examination, the woman's postural instability was such that it seemed a breath would have knocked her to the ground. It was, however, possible to implement a management strategy for this tricky problem which resulted in the restoration of her weekly sojourns, an improvement in her quality of life beyond measure, and almost embarrassing praise for its architect. This 'magical' treatment comprised a reduction in the thioridazine she had been taking for years from 200 to 100 mg per day! Even pseudo-magic requires some genuine 'knowledge'.

Although a 'core' feature of parkinsonism in general, rigidity is by no means an invariable component of drug-related parkinsonism and, if present, is usually mild and may require reinforcement to elicit. It is certainly unusual to come across the severity of abnormality that is frequently to be seen in idiopathic disease. At a clinical level, the severity of rigidity does not seem to correlate with the severity of bradykinesia, although systematic data on the issue are lacking.

Tremor is present in approximately 70 per cent of Parkinson's disease patients at presentation and only rarely does it never emerge at all (Quinn, 1995). In the majority, this takes the form of the characteristic high-amplitude/low-frequency resting tremor. In drug-related disorder this pattern is uncommon, affecting probably no more than 10–12 per cent of patients (Hausner, 1983). When it does occur, it is almost exclusively a late development after many years' exposure. On the other hand, postural tremor is, as has been emphasised, a relatively early and common finding, though comparative studies of this feature in idiopathic disease are lacking.

These comments on tremor prevalences are based on clinical observations, and more sensitive instrumentation methods may reveal a slightly different picture. Tremorographic studies in older patients without apparent signs of extrapyramidal disease but receiving antipsychotics found that 28 per cent demonstrated low-frequency tremors of less than 7 Hz (Arblaster et al., 1993). Again, this raises the question of the relationship between drug-related and idiopathic disorder in the middle aged and elderly but nonetheless, as a clinical observation, the original point on tremor stands.

One final difference lies in the pattern of symptomatology at onset. Although the possibility of a unilateral distribution for drug-related disorder has been noted, this is in fact the exception in younger patients at least, of whom about 70 per cent exhibit bilateral signs (Hausner, 1983; Montastruc et al., 1994). This is the opposite from Parkinson's disease where the majority of patients present with a clear unilateral emphasis which is usually maintained to some extent throughout the course (Quinn, 1995). However, here too, the general principle may be modified by age, in that it has been found that about one-third of older patients with drug-related disorder have notable asymmetry (Sethi and Zamrini, 1990).

Whether or not such observed differences of emphasis tell us anything about pathophysiological differences or merely reflect differing severities or the generally non-progressive nature of drug-related disorder is unclear. It could, furthermore, be that what they actually reflect is differences in either age or age of onset. In one of the few comparative studies, no difference in presentation of idiopathic versus drug-related parkinsonism was evident, though no standardised recording instrument was used. This study comprised a geriatric population (Stephen and Williamson, 1984).

Nonetheless, accepting the widespread view, shared by the author, that such differences do exist, the importance of highlighting them lies in the necessity of ridding psychiatrists of the stereotype of parkinsonism recollected from undergraduate days. The advanced case of Parkinson's disease with a full house of signs and progressive disability that was seen as a student is unlikely to cross one's path in psychiatric practice – except possibly on the road to the law courts! The issue one must be far more alert to is that of mild, early and perhaps largely subjective change that superficially may bear more than a passing resemblance to some disorders of the mental state.

In approaching drug-related parkinsonism from a psychiatric perspective, it is necessary to abandon the stereotypes of the past and derail oneself from the 'tramlining' of personal and educational bias.

Diagnosis

Parkinsonism is a guise for many pathologically distinct disorders (Table 4.3) the commonest of which is Parkinson's disease. This can be a difficult condition to diagnose confidently, with about 25 per cent of cases diagnosed in life failing to show characteristic changes at post-mortem (Hughes et al., 1992).

Parkinsonism is always a diagnostic option in 'at-risk' psychiatric patients. For our purposes, that means essentially those on antipsychotics, but drug-related disorder is nowadays such a frequent consequence of many prescribing decisions (see Table 2.4) that *all* practitioners must operate a high index of suspicion.

The rule of thumb in psychiatric practice is *always* to assume the presence of such features, never their absence. One should not wait for them to emerge or allow them to lurk in dark corners undetected, but from the start hunt them out.

The major differentials for the psychiatrist to consider have already been mentioned: the retardation of depression and affective flattening. While neither of these is diagnostically specific, it is the context of schizophrenia that is our particular focus here (Table 4.4).

Psychomotor retardation shares many superficial characteristics of bradykinesia. Subjective symptomatology such as apathy, anergy, fatiguability etc. can be indistinguishable, as can signs such as motor slowing, diminished activity, and altered posture. There may even be a diurnal pattern of symptom expression common to both.

The first thing to focus on in attempting a distinction is mood itself. Despondency or dysphoria associated with bradykinesia is usually a

Table 4.3. *Differential diagnosis of parkinsonism*

Idiopathic Parkinson's disease
Drug-related disorder
Multi-system atrophy
   striatonigral degeneration
   olivopontocerebellar atrophy
   Shy–Drager syndrome
Progressive supranuclear palsy (Steele–Richardson–Olszewski
   syndrome)
Diffuse Lewy body disease
Alzheimer's disease
Corticobasal degeneration
Parkinson–dementia–amyotrophic lateral sclerosis complex of Guam
Hydrocephalus
Wilson's disease
Pick's disease
Dementia pugilistica
HIV-related encephalopathy
Huntington's disease
Neoplasms
Carbon monoxide intoxication
Post-encephalitis (lethargica)
Heavy metal (manganese) intoxication
Alcohol withdrawal
MPTP toxicity

supplementary symptom that may make life more difficult and less enjoyable but seems to lack the all-pervasive and overwhelming quality of the mood change of major depressive symptomatology. The patient with bradykinesia will characteristically experience a mild dulling which modulates both the range *and* depth of affect with an expression that is correspondingly gentler and more muted than normal. Hopelessness and suicidal ideation are uncommon, as are the so-called biological features of depression such as disturbed sleep and impaired appetite. On the other hand, the depressed patient with retardation invariably has a striking limitation in the range of emotion while depth is retained and indeed intensified into a profound, if single, feeling state that can be strikingly contagious.

The posture of depression is one of passive rather than active absence. A fluid, erect and appropriately interactive posture cannot be maintained because the patient lacks the initiative or will to do so. With bradykinesia, the patient is much more 'locked in' by a state that is

Table 4.4. *Some clinical points of comparison between major manifestations of parkinsonism, depression and chronic schizophrenia*

	Bradykinesia	Psychomotor retardation	'Affective flattening'
Facial expression	'Masked' Loss of facial contours Loss of gradations of expression Eye contact preserved Staring gaze from reduced blink rate Parted lips	Downcast Facial contours accentuated – 'haggard' Gradations of expression retained, variety restricted Avoidance of eye contact Outer eyebrows elevated, inner eyebrows depressed Vertical glabellar furrowing Horizontal forehead furrowing Angles of mouth inverted	Fixed through emotional range 'Empty' Avoidance of eye contact Gradation maintained, variety lost
Mood	±Dysphoria Range and depth retained	Depth (usually) retained and heightened Range restricted	Range and depth restricted
Speech	Loss of pitch, power and intonation Impaired articulation Spontaneous generation of words unimpaired	Loss of power and intonation Articulation preserved Reduced word usage	Loss of intonation Articulation preserved Reduced word usage
Posture	Flexion 'Actively' imposed abnormality	'Crumpled' Head bowed, round shouldered 'Passive' abnormality	No characteristic change May be avoidant ('aversive') and awkward
Engagement/rapport	Preserved	Preserved–heightened	Impaired–the 'brick wall'

actively imposed. Gradations of postural change are more seamless but less extensive for the depressive, while bradykinesia is characterised by peaks and troughs, relatively suddenly alternating.

The most striking difference is perhaps in facial expression. The typical depressed patient is literally 'downcast', with a bowed, avertive gaze, and a pained expression. The outer parts of the eyebrows are elevated, while the middle third is lowered. Vertical furrowing is evident between the brows, with horizontal furrowing of the upper forehead. The angles of the mouth sag. The characteristic appearance of hypomimia has already been described. The eyes of the bradykinetic, on the other hand, may be a key to their alertness, for behind the stare they may reveal the more outgoing and active mentition that lies beneath the softened facial contours and bland, unemotive exterior.

So-called 'negative' states are not, of course, unique to schizophrenia but are considered characteristic of this condition in a way that perhaps they are not of the other disorders in which they can be found. The problems of cross-sectional evaluation of 'negative' schizophrenia have already been referred to. A major weakness of the whole evaluative process is that, for purely practical reasons, the recognition of 'negativity' is rarely something that occurs in ignorance of the basic schizophrenic diagnosis. It is not usually the case that one is in the position of evaluating the presence of a set of features and therefore concluding that the issue is one of 'negative' schizophrenia, but rather that one sees a patient known to be schizophrenic, as a consequence of which certain features are acknowledged as 'negative'. This is the inverse of the diagnostic process and the opposite of what is usually undertaken in evaluating the significance of both bradykinesia and depression. To have legitimate diagnostic power, 'negative' states also require to be appraised non-prejudicially.

Patients afflicted with authentic 'negative' mental state disorder may feel what they do not betray. Thus they may be aware of their listless non-involvement and of a dulling in the appreciation of pleasurable experiences. They may even acknowledge the 'laziness' others accuse them of. Similarly, they may feel the absence of creativity and spontaneous, original thought. One woman confessed: 'I'm an empty barrel. There's nothing in my head.' Exploring this subjective element is always important.

Whereas depressed individuals may retain the ability to respond to conducive external stimuli, as may patients with bradykinesia, the 'negative' schizophrenic patient can at best react in only a partial way and indeed may actively withdraw in the face of such stimuli. These patients become creatures of habit, the tapestry of life's experiences reduced to the lowest common and least emotionally demanding denominator. Posture is unlikely to be primarily affected, though in interpersonal contexts it may tend to be socially incompetent and aversive. Facial expression is bland, befitting the 'empty barrel' so poignantly described above. Although concentration and other cognitive parameters are usually clearly damaged in schizophrenics with negative symptomatology, other biological functions such as sleep and appetite are usually healthily preserved.

A final tip in the evaluative process is that while bradykinesia can frequently, and depressive retardation sometimes, be a 'spot' diagnosis, affective flattening *never* is. If you can make the diagnosis confidently on purely observational information, what you are seeing is unlikely to be a negative state. Psychiatry can rue the day that the teachings of a previous generation were forgotten and 'negativity', especially in relation to schizophrenia, began to be seen as something rateable on purely cross-sectional evidence.

If the reader is left with the impression that the above is an inadequate attempt to articulate what are, at the end of the day, little more than 'gut reactions', he or she would probably be correct, for in a clinical context of mild pathology or, especially, multiple co-existing disorders, that may be about the level of one's 'diagnostic' formulations. The important issue is that comprehensive evaluation of such scenarios requires consideration of the neurological as well as the psychological. In clinical situations where no confident distinctions can be made, a trial of specific treatments may need to be undertaken and can be heartily recommended. However, one must remain aware of the range of the diagnostic differential before such a trial can be adequately comprehensive.

Having hammered home this point once again, it must be remembered that variations on the neurological theme also need to be considered. A detailed knowledge of the weird world into which the differential diagnosis of bradykinetic-rigid extrapyramidal symptomatology might lead one (see Table 4.3) is hardly necessary for the jobbing psychiatrist. It will suffice to remember once again that a differential diagnosis *does* exist and to bring to mind the most obvious – and hence the most easily overlooked – possibility, namely coincidental Parkinson's disease.

The conjunction of Parkinson's disease with the condition most likely to be associated with antipsychotic drug use (i.e. schizophrenia) is theoretically awkward, but has nonetheless been established as a definite, if infrequent, occurrence (Crow, Johnstone and McClelland, 1976). We have already touched on the issue of medication acting to promote a tendency already established in the patient, especially older individuals. However, the question of idiopathic disease developing in patients exposed to antipsychotics is one sometimes posed in younger people who develop either unexpectedly severe extrapyramidal disorder or disorder that strikingly deviates from the clinical emphasis outlined above. This can present a potential source of contention between psychiatrists and neurologists which can erupt with Vesuvian force.

The author is speaking personally of the case of a man in his forties who first became psychotic in his early twenties. Although at one point he had been heavily treated with antipsychotics, for many years he had, largely at his insistence, been managed with modest but adequate doses. I was asked to see him by a psychiatric colleague because of his parkinsonism, on virtually every feature of which he scored a full house. He 'trotted' everywhere with a festinant gait and crashed into obstacles regularly, including passersby, and was so tremulous he could hardly eat or drink. His medication had been 20 mg Depixol four weekly for some years, but his parkinsonism had only emerged over the previous two years. His depot was stopped and clozapine commenced, but life being as it is, his white cell count went into an almost instant nose-dive. A small dose of sulpiride (200 mg per day), along with an anticholinergic, was commenced but, after a few letters of bizarre content, the sulpiride was increased to 300 mg per day. During this time, his gait did improve to the extent that he could at least walk about without risking a charge of assault, though he remained precarious, but the rest of the features held more or less static.

Incidentally and unknown to the author, the patient's GP referred him for a neurological opinion which related the problem to drugs, all drugs and nothing but drugs. The antipsychotics were duly stopped. His parkinsonism remained unchanged, though his psychosis alas did not and, after some months without drugs, showed itself in a barrage of correspondence which, through the thought disorder, seemed more than vaguely pornographic. The neurologist could not be persuaded to a 'two syndromes' view and stated that as the patient was being re-commenced on antipsychotics, by then an ethical if not legal necessity, his expert opinion was being ignored and he had no further role to play – a communication paraphrased here to spare the reader!

However, by chance, during an admission to stabilise the patient, another eminent neurologist happened to be visiting the ward to see someone in the adjacent bed. Afterwards he asked the author, somewhat awkwardly, if our friend had drug-related disorder. 'I don't think so,' I replied. 'Neither do I,' said the neurologist, with an audible sigh of concurrence!

A final point worthy of remembering is one that has been alluded to and will be returned to later (see Chapter 8). This is to what extent detectable extrapyramidal disorder can in fact be directly attributed to illness-related causes. In evaluating the role of medication in the production of extrapyramidal symptomatology, it must be borne in mind that such signs can also be found in patients with certain psychiatric disorders *prior* to their exposure to antidopaminergic drugs. The most obvious example of this comes from certain types of dementia (see Table 4.3) in which the co-occurrence of cognitive and extrapyramidal impairments can form a basis for clinical classification. In addition, however, extrapyramidal features, especially rigidity, have recently been reported in around 16–20 per cent of first-episode, drug-naive schizophrenic patients (Caligiuri, Lohr and Jeste, 1993; Chatterjee et al., 1995), observations that provide a new perspective on the neurology of this condition.

In routine clinical situations, sparrows abound while cockatoos are few, and in the outpatient department one's decisions are rightly more focused on practical than on theoretical considerations. In understanding the intricacies of the issue, such information is nonetheless valuable.

Epidemiology

The commonest cause of parkinsonism is Parkinson's disease, with drugs being the commonest cause of secondary disorder. It has been estimated that, in neurological settings, drug-related disorder accounts for about 4 per cent of cases (Stacy and Jankovic, 1992), although, interestingly, for a much higher proportion (up to 50 per cent) – in those referred to geriatric services (Stephen and Williamson, 1984). When one considers the numbers of patients nowadays exposed to drugs possessing the potential to cause parkinsonism (see Table 2.4), the vast majority of whom are never seen by neurologists, it is likely that drug-related disorder runs idiopathic disease a close second in prevalence.

It is remarkably difficult to come up with clear figures from the literature on the epidemiological characteristics of drug-related parkinsonism. Estimates for prevalence range from 5 per cent to 90 per cent (Gershanik, 1994). It is important to appreciate that the reasons for this diversity reside mainly in the nature of the problem and not in the incompetence of the investigators. Both the prevalence and the incidence of drug-related disorder depend on a particularly wide range of variables which encompass pharmacological, pharmacokinetic, treatment practice, temporal and assessment factors (Table 4.5). It is difficult, if not impossible, to control for all or even most of these in a clinical trial situation.

The first and most obvious set of factors is the recurrent trio of dose, potency and rate of increments. The development of parkinsonism is more likely with high-dose regimes of potent antipsychotics rapidly attained. A further consideration is that the psychopharmacologically

Table 4.5. *Factors influencing the observed prevalence of drug-related parkinsonism*

Pharmacological	Potency (D_2)
	Receptor-binding profile
	Prior exposure history
Practice related	Dose
	Rate of increment
Patient related	Age
	Anatomy of dopaminergic systems
	Coincidental pathology (e.g. Lewy bodies)
Timing	Natural history
	early increase
	subsequent spontaneous resolution
Conceptual	'Symptom'
	Syndrome
Examination	Sensitivity
	Comprehensiveness

experienced patient may be relatively less vulnerable to these influences than the previously drug-naive and, hence, on similar regimes may produce less in the way of neurological adverse effects.

These are not the only determinants of prevalence. It must also be remembered that prevalence increases over time (see below), at least for the first few weeks or months of exposure. Furthermore, it seems that in some patients the symptomatology may plateau, after which a degree of resolution may take place on stable regimes (Simpson et al., 1964; Marsden, Mindham and Mackay, 1986). Hence, the absolute figure attributable to any particular population depends on the mean period of exposure to antipsychotic drugs, all other things being equal. Studies reporting on populations in the initial period of treatment will tend to show lower absolute figures than those whose subjects had been treated longer, while groups studied after periods of treatment stability will once again tend to reduced prevalence figures.

Perhaps the most important determinants of prevalence, however, are the breadth of the concept of disorder one adopts – how wide one sets the boundaries – and the sensitivity of the examination procedure itself. Clearly, where the view of what comprises drug-related parkinsonism is a broad one encompassing a wide range of symptomatology, the prevalence of abnormality will be higher than when only core features are rated globally. Furthermore, where the examination technique is highly sensitive and geared to very mild or equivocal disorder, prevalences will again be higher than when only definite abnormalities are unarguably present. In Ayd's study, for example, mild akinesia was not considered of sufficient import to be recorded (Ayd, 1961), so the prevalence figure here is clearly an underestimate.

The question usually left unaddressed in studies of the prevalence of drug-related parkinsonism is the one relevant to these two issues – namely, whether one is considering disorder at the 'symptom' or the syndromal level. In the former case, the presence of any 'symptom', regardless of type or severity, would be sufficient to determine abnormality (although it will be clear that while conventionally psychiatry has considered this taxonomy as 'symptom' led, signs should also be included, and in the present context are the major consideration). In the latter case, abnormality would be defined in terms of the presence of a constellation of features at a minimum degree of severity.

In practice, the syndromal method gets down to what is considered clinically significant, a judgement that depends on a combination of both examiner and patient perceptions. Firstly, this should involve the examiner in an evaluation of the pattern of signs. A mild, unilateral reduction in arm swing, for example, may be considered of lesser clinical import than an upper limb tremor at a comparable level of severity; or a postural tremor of the dominant hand may be more clinically significant than one of equal severity affecting the non-dominant side. Secondly, a judgement would be required on the severity of any individual feature. Rigidity only evident on reinforcement is likely to be considered of lesser clinical significance than that evident without reinforcement. The third essential is the patient's perception of disability. Symptomatology only considered mild by objective evaluation may exert a disproportionately large impact on the patient's quality of life, or two patients with objectively similar levels of disorder may perceive this in markedly divergent ways.

Thus, there are sound reasons why figures for the prevalence of drug-related parkinsonism vary greatly in the literature and why bald estimates of incidence are probably of little value.

Excluding the less competent extremes represented in the range quoted above, prevalence figures for drug-related parkinsonism in patients on antipsychotic medications range from 15 per cent to 31 per cent. The literature has not as a rule addressed whether this refers to 'symptom' based or syndrome-based data, though the impression is that it is the latter. This certainly seems reasonable – that between one-fifth and one-third of patients exposed to standard antipsychotics have a clinically significant parkinsonian syndrome.

If the author's experience is anything to go by, however, the prevalence of symptom/sign-based disorder is much – very much – higher, and not just for those on potent drugs. The above-quoted figure of 90 per cent refers to gross abnormality with the use of high-potency compounds but, in a radical departure from conventional wisdom, the author is willing to suggest that, with sufficiently detailed and protracted evaluation, it is unlikely many patients adequately treated with standard antipsychotic compounds escape the development of at least some features of the disorder at some time. Whether this means in fact that *all* patients get something at some time is perhaps a bit too radical for even the present volume – but the author is ready to be persuaded!

This, of course, takes us perhaps uncomfortably close to old battle grounds, if not quite on to them. To say that a particular undesired effect of a drug is frequent or even universal is *not*, however, the same as saying that this is a necessary part of the therapeutic package. Many preparations can cause major gastrointestinal upset with regularity, but it would be preposterous to suggest that the therapeutic benefits of such drugs depend on how profusely the patient vomits! Nonetheless, the above statement does raise the question of something that, if not therapeutically necessary, may, with standard drugs at least, have a certain inevitability about it.

Predisposing factors

Apart from the treatment practice variables of dose, potency and rate of increment (duly noting the proviso mentioned in the previous chapter with regard to potency), little is known about the factors predisposing to the development of drug-related parkinsonism (Table 4.6).

Even with these clearly established factors, we must once again raise the 'It ain't necessarily so' qualification. I am reminded of an obstinate schizophrenic woman in her early thirties and her extremely trying husband, who steadfastly resisted my attempts to introduce some degree of logic into her management. They were strong advocates of self-medication and constantly altered recommendations. On one occasion the patient, who was profoundly damaged, presented particularly gratifyingly. She reported feeling relaxed and confident and for the first time in many months had not required her husband to check the garden foliage for agents of the Secret Services. I was pleased at this response to trifluoperazine which, in the recommended dose of 20 mg per day, was a regime I thought could be maintained for some time. As I contemplated this comforting prospect, the husband introduced the words I had been awaiting: 'You're not going to be happy,' he said presciently. 'We've increased to 30 a day.' During my discourse on the advantages of 20 mg a day over 30 mg a day, I was interrupted: 'Oh no,

Table 4.6. *Proposed predisposing factors to drug-related parkinsonism*

Treatment practice	Dose
	Potency
	Rate of increment
	(Prior exposure)
Demographic	Age
	Gender
Individual	Structure
susceptibility	Function

doctor. Not 30 mg – 30 *tablets!'* On 300 mg of trifluoperazine a day the woman could have danced Swan Lake! Apart from a mild and previously evident tremor, there was not a sign of extrapyramidal disturbance.

Similar cases have reached the literature and no doubt many more have not. The above is not presented as an example to be followed but to illustrate the occasionally striking unpredictability of the problem. At one time there was an argument, referred to previously, that as a result of the interplay of non-dopaminergic actions, very high doses of especially high-potency antipsychotics 'broke through' the extrapyramidal barrier and patients who, on lower doses would seize up, melted into motor fluidity once again. As the above case illustrates, some patients do appear inexplicably immune to extrapyramidal adverse effects, but to assume this reflects a parabolic relationship with dosage is to venture a long way beyond the facts *and* therapeutic prudence.

The variable most frequently associated with drug-related parkinsonism is age: the older the patient, the greater the risk (Ayd, 1961; Montastruc et al., 1994; Gershanik, 1994). Indeed, it has been pointed out that the increasing prevalence often reported with advancing age closely parallels the age relationships of Parkinson's disease itself (Marsden et al., 1986). This has been one factor in cementing the idea that antidopaminergic medication may act to promote a tendency to disorder in those constitutionally predisposed to Parkinson's disease. While there is ready information to hand to explain an age association in the fall-off in nigrostriatal neurons that occurs as part of the ageing process, other pathological changes may be important, as noted below.

Gender is a further factor suggested as predisposing. Females have been reported to show abnormality more often than males, with the female:male ratio as high as 2:1 in some studies (Ayd, 1961; Montastruc et al., 1994).

Despite these reported associations, neither age nor gender findings can be taken as establishing direct cause-and-effect relationships. The observations with regard to age could, for example, be complicated by pharmacokinetic factors. A number of pharmacokinetic parameters alter with age, relating to changes in hepatic and renal function, alterations in plasma protein levels, increases in lean body mass etc., with the net effect that blood levels of many drugs, including antipsychotics, tend to rise. While the development of drug-related parkinsonism can be correlated only poorly and inconsistently with plasma levels, a role for pharmacokinetic factors in contributing to the increasing prevalence with age cannot at this stage be ruled out.

Furthermore, the associations with increasing age have not been universally found. Indeed a higher prevalence of disorder has been found in younger patients, independent of prescribing practice (Moleman et al., 1986). This was established in retrospective work but so too was the finding of a positive association with age. Such an observation could have its roots in the dampening effect of chronic exposure that was mentioned in relation to acute dystonias. Younger patients may be subject to fewer of the perturbations associated with long-term antipsychotic exposure and thereby may remain more vulnerable to parkinsonian adverse effects.

Thus, while the balance of the literature favours increasing age as a factor predisposing to drug-related parkinsonism, this is not a unanimous finding nor one that can be taken as necessarily reflecting direct mechanisms.

With regard to gender, an excess in females has also been a frequent but *not* a universal finding. It was most consistently reported in the 1960s and early 1970s in studies mainly involving mental hospital residents. In such populations, females have consistently been shown to be older on average than males (Owens and Johnstone, 1980). If the consensus view of a positive association with age is correct (or even partially correct), this could explain the gender differences in these studies. Furthermore, at that time a number of reports noted that females also tended to receive higher absolute doses of antipsychotic medications than males (Laska et al., 1973; Prien, Haber and Caffey, 1975; Simpson et al., 1978), an interesting observation that has largely gone without comment or explanation. Even today, detectable gender differences may also reflect dosing factors for the same reason that was discussed in relation to one aspect of acute dystonias. Milligram equivalent dose regimes are likely to translate into higher milligram *per kilogram* doses for females relative to males.

The question of individual susceptibility nonetheless remains intriguing. Early studies purporting to show an increase in Parkinson's disease in the families of patients with drug-related disorder were so methodologically flawed as to be unworthy of further consideration, although the general principle is not, and more recent associations with the human leucocyte antigen HLA-B44 require confirmation (Metzer et al., 1989). As with akathisia, the role of intracerebral iron status, of interest in idiopathic disease, is unclear.

However, evidence is emerging of brain abnormality underlying at least some cases of drug-related parkinsonism. Thus, associations have been reported with structural brain change in the form of enlargement of the lateral ventricles using computerised tomography (CT) (Hoffman, Labs and Casey, 1987). More recently, it has been suggested from magnetic resonance imaging (MRI) findings that persistence of symptomatology may depend on different changes depending on the age of the patient, with putamen *hypo*intensity associated with persistence in younger patients and striatal *hyper*intensities in the elderly (Bocola et al., 1996), though this awaits confirmation.

The role of structural change as a predisposing factor is further illustrated in more gross form in the case of a 22-year-old man who presented with a florid, if slowly evolving, psychotic illness of schizophreniform type. At the age of 6, he had developed mumps complicated by meningitis, which resulted in aqueduct stenosis. A shunt was inserted, which in his teens was removed then re-inserted, and had been assessed as competent only two weeks before his first psychiatric presentation. At that time, he had a generalised parkinsonian syndrome of moderate severity. His psychosis demanded treatment but within one week of commencing low then modest doses of chlorpromazine, he became profoundly rigid and bradykinetic, with marked sialorrhoea and postural instability, which represented a severe exacerbation of his prior, organically based symptomatology. On clozapine, his neurological signs eased substantially, though his sialorrhoea worsened, supporting the view that clozapine-induced hypersalivation is not mediated by purely extrapyramidal mechanisms.

Nigral dysfunction has been suggested in some patients with drug-related parkinsonism studied with positron emission tomography (PET). Burn and Brooks (1993) found significantly reduced uptake of ^{18}F-Dopa in the putamen in 4 of 13 elderly patients with drug-related disorder who in fact had levels of uptake that were within the range associated with Parkinson's disease. At follow-up 12–21 months after stopping antidopaminergic medication, three of these patients had persistent clinical signs and continuing abnormal putamen tracer uptake. This raises the prospect that underlying subcortical Lewy body disease could represent the predisposing variable in such patients.

Work of this sort offers an exciting new window on the understanding of drug-related parkinsonism but suggests that different sets of factors may predispose in different patients. Both the structural and functional work thus far has focused on older subjects in whom pre-clinical Parkinson's disease or other organic pathology is likely to be relevant. In addition, age-related cell drop-out not sufficient to alter gross structure may act on individual dopamine 'endowments' that are at the left-hand end of the distribution curve, as possibly in at least one of the 'uni-striatal' men described above. With young individuals earlier in their treatment cycles, however, disorder is more likely to be a relatively pure reflection of practice variables.

There is much yet to learn about factors predisposing to the development of drug-related parkinsonism and much to caution us against treating superficial associations superficially. It is important to be dissuaded from the seductive belief that one can carry around a stereo-typed or composite picture of the 'typical' patient who is likely to develop this type of disorder. There is in reality no such entity, and to assume there is or practice as if there were is the surest route to mighty omissions.

Onset, course and outcome

The onset of drug-related parkinsonism tends to be gradual over days or, more usually, weeks. It is, however, dependent on the practice variables noted previously so will, for example, be more rapid in drug-naive patients exposed to high-doses of high-potency compounds, or in the elderly in the same treatment situation.

The figures of Ayd (1961) remain widely quoted (Fig. 4.6). Ayd found the steepest part of the cumulative onset curve lay between 10 and 30 days, during which time approximately 40 per cent of all cases occurred. Ninety per cent of cases emerged within 72 days of first exposure.

Just how early in exposure symptomatology can commence is impossible to determine from the overwhelmingly sign-based literature. However, if *mild* disorder does indeed have a genuinely subjective component, it is likely that these features precede objective signs and may have a very early onset, after possibly a few days. It is clinical experience that some patients can very soon become aware of an uncomfortable, ponderous slowness about which they often complain bitterly. This is, of course, difficult, if not impossible, to distinguish from the unwanted experience of sedation in patients eager to remain active, but it is likely that part of this phenomenon is extrapyramidal. One should, therefore, be alert to the possibility of symptomatology right from the period of earliest exposure.

The pattern described in Ayd's study of more or less linear onset levelling off in the third month must overwhelmingly refer to syndromal parkinsonism. There is little that the literature can tell us about the

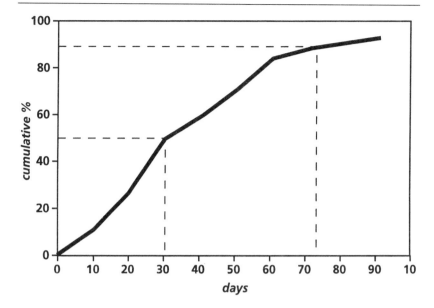

Fig. 4.6. The onset of drug-related parkinsonism. (After Ayd, 1961, with permission.)

pattern with which signs develop individually and in relation to one another – or even about whether predictable patterns exist. The author's impression is that subjective slowness, loss of arm swing, and postural tremor manifest themselves early. Experimental evidence noted above supports this contention with regard to tremor, for which instrumentation has been able to detect changes after only one or two doses of antipsychotic (Arblaster et al., 1993). Gait disturbance, postural flexion, resting tremor and impaired initiation are late or more established signs of disorder. Postural instability is certainly more common than is generally appreciated but where it comes in the scheme of things is unclear. It is probably to be found more towards the later end of the spectrum. As the case described above illustrates, however, in particular patients it may dominate in the presence of relatively unobtrusive additional symptomatology.

Just as the onset of drug-related parkinsonism reflects aspects of treatment practice, so the course will to a large extent be dependent on the pattern of drug administration over time. Indeed, the rising incidence over the first 10 weeks or so of exposure is likely to reflect increasing dose regimes during the acute phase of illness management (see Fig. 4.7). On stable or relatively stable regimes thereafter, the symptomatic picture will also tend to remain stable, at least for a few weeks or months. Pharmacokinetic factors resulting in accumulation of drug over time may be responsible for new cases emerging or some exacerbations, but an interesting and unexplained phenomenon is the tendency noted above for established, stable disorder to remit somewhat after two to three months on stable drug regimes (Simpson et al., 1964; Marsden et al., 1986).

If psychotic patients are managed on an 'acute-to-maintenance' basis (that is, a programme of de-escalating doses from florid phases of illness through to maintenance, as described below), then clearly parkinsonian symptomatology will tend to mirror this in a degree of resolution. In the author's experience, however, it often appears that a threshold effect operates in this situation. As doses come down, parkinsonian symptomatology often changes little until a certain point is reached when patients seem to experience a striking and disproportionately greater improvement than previously – as if they had crossed an invisible threshold. It must be said that this probably relates more to symptoms than to signs, but it could emphasise again the indirect relationship that symptomatology bears to dosage. It might be that such a phenomenon is actually a manifestation of pharmacokinetic factors.

Staehelin's view that was quoted above as reflecting general opinion at the time is still general opinion. Drug-related parkinsonism continues to be seen as invariably resolving on discontinuation of the offending agent. However, this is a view that must be taken with circumspection. It is certainly general psychiatric experience that in affected patients whose drugs are discontinued or who fail to comply, the features of parkinsonism do seem to resolve, with the subjective symptoms going *before* the signs. It is not uncommon, however, for objective symptomatology to remain in evidence for a very long time – in some cases for 12–18 months. This experience has been reflected in the literature by others (Marsden et al., 1986).

What is also clear is that reversibility is not a dictum that can be universally extended, as was suggested above. Sufficient material has now reached the literature to confirm that symptomatic persistence of drug-related parkinsonism *is* a reality (Aronson, 1985; Wilson, Primrose and Smith, 1987; Burn and Brooks, 1993). As was noted, this is likely to be a function of age or underlying latent Parkinson's disease. In one discontinuation study of a geriatric population, drug-related disorder resolved in two-thirds of patients in a mean of seven weeks (range 1 to 36 weeks) following cessation of antidopaminergic medication, but persisted in attenuated form in 11 per cent (Stephen and Williamson, 1984; Table 4.7). The majority of patients in this group had been exposed to prochlorperazine, a relatively weak dopamine antagonist, and it might be argued that these figures represent the most favourable scenario. A longer term follow-up of this group (average 41 months) suggested a high mortality and, in survivors, high levels of dependency (Wilson et

Table 4.7. *Outcome of drug-related parkinsonism (follow-up 1 year: elderly population). (From Stephen & Williamson, 1984.)*

Outcome	Percentage
Resolved	66 (mean 7 weeks; range 1 to 36 weeks)
Attenuated	11
Persistent	6
Resolved (but followed by PD)	11
Died	6
Unknown	2

al., 1987). Furthermore, after showing initial resolution of their drug-related disorder, 25 per cent of the survivors had gone on to develop Parkinson's disease. Thus, in the elderly in particular, drug-related parkinsonism is not necessarily a benign disorder nor one which retains the characteristic of reversibility.

As a general rule, most patients discontinuing or exhibiting major compliance problems with antipsychotics tend to be younger, and thereby a group in whom reversibility would be more likely. It is from this group that the standard view on the reversibility of drug-related parkinsonism has sprung. The fact is, however, that this generally held view is not one that can claim as its justification an unassailable body of good-quality trial data. No such body of information based on discontinuation studies of adequate quality or duration exists, and the belief is essentially supported on the back of clinical wisdom. It would be a mistake to assume that such wisdom, at once both the strongest and the weakest font of knowledge, can be carried to all corners of clinical practice.

This takes us back to the circular world of 'Is it the drugs or is it idiopathic disease?' from which, at the clinical level, there can currently emerge no satisfactory answer, though in future functional imaging may help resolve the dilemma. For the present, the plea is simply for caution in accepting the accepted wisdom.

Treatment

If there is one fact every psychiatric trainee knows it is that the treatment of drug-related parkinsonism is with anticholinergics. This is a lesson instilled early, usually by nursing colleagues, and it is one that is put into practice daily. However, this issue is one that deserves thoughtful consideration rather than an over-learned response.

Modifications of antipsychotic regimes

The emergence of drug-related parkinsonism is *not* necessarily an indication for specific treatment. Whether or not this is deemed appropriate depends on the tests of 'clinical significance' discussed above. If intervention is felt to be indicated, the first step should *always* be a re-appraisal of drug schedules. The potency of the first-choice drug, the absolute dose and, perhaps most importantly of all, the rate of dose increments should all be reviewed.

Managing psychotic disorders requires considerably greater skill than those who do it well are usually credited with. An essential element is structure, though any structure must be pragmatic and somewhat arbitrary. An example of one structure espoused by the author is shown in Figure 4.7. The important point is to establish clear treatment goals, the attainment of which will reflect in medication regimes and help at all times to ensure the minimal antipsychotic exposure commensurate with the maximal likelihood of efficacy in each phase.

Parkinsonism is most likely to emerge during acute phase management. While all those involved with the patient during the acute phase of treatment may be aiming for the same end-point, they may entertain different priorities in getting there, and the responsible physician is frequently in the position of having to balance a number of competing interests: the focus of nursing staff on safety and behavioural control; the realistic anxieties but unrealistic expectations of family; the gulf between patients' and others' perceptions of the situation; the requirements to operate within a legal framework, and many more. All of these must be balanced in the context of treatments whose adverse effects are likely to be manifest before their therapeutic benefits.

Treatment plans are usually determined by what happens in the first week or two after medical contact, yet this is not a time during which the specific goal of management can be achieved. It has been known for many years that there is a built-in delay in the onset of specific antipsychotic effects, though whether this is as long as the two to three weeks usually cited (which may be partly an artefact of methodology and analysis) is unclear. Nonetheless, it is certainly the case that any benefits accruing from antipsychotics within the first week or so are likely to be non-specific (Fig. 4.8a).

Even where out-patient care is espoused, those with more florid psychotic illnesses are still likely to be admitted and the focus of management in the initial acute phase treatment period will be geared as much to avoiding or treating behavioural disturbance as to resolution of

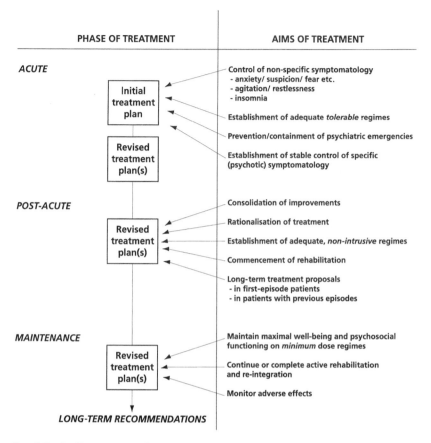

Fig. 4.7. Outline structure for the treatment of schizophrenia.

specific psychotic symptomatology. During this initial period, treatment plans often capitalise on the non-specific effects of early exposure,
in particular sedation. The problem is that the minimum doses required
to ensure safety and behavioural control may be in excess of the
minimum doses required to achieve antipsychotic efficacy, and well
within the ranges liable to produce adverse effects. Escalating doses in
this early period are likely to increase adverse experiences *without*
bringing forward the time scale of therapeutic benefits (Fig. 4.8b).
Protecting patients and staff from the consequences of psychotically
mediated behavioural disturbance is of course a major part of the
doctor's responsibility, but so too is the avoidance, where possible, of
unwanted drug effects which may themselves in the short term contribute to conflict and disturbance and in the long term seriously impede
compliance.

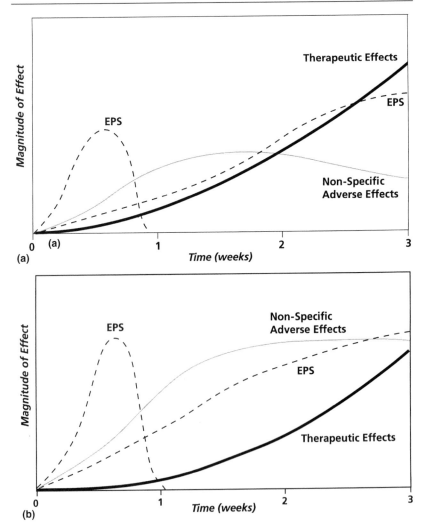

Fig. 4.8. The relationship between adverse and therapeutic effects of antipsychotics in acute phase treatment. (a) Average dose/gradual escalation regimes. (b) High dose/rapid escalation regimes. (EPS, extrapyramidal side-effects.)

The prescribing physician should always keep close tabs not only on the doses being used in acute phase exposure but also on the reasons for them. If rapid escalations have other than antipsychotic efficacy as their goal, the temporary introduction of alternatives, such as benzo-diazepines, should be considered.

The issue is somewhat different for those undertaking community-based management and relates to the difficulty of 'fine tuning' regimes in the absence of continuous and specific monitoring and the consequent difficulty of obviating, as opposed to merely responding to, adverse effects. It may also be legitimate to suggest that the priorities of those supervising such programmes are likely to be much more focused on practical and interpersonal aspects of functioning. It is important in this situation that these considerations do not hijack assessment and relegate extrapyramidal effects to the sidelines. Once again, there is a strong case for extending education on the recognition of EPS to community psychiatric nurses who carry a major burden of responsibility in these situations.

The point therefore is that acute phase or early management needs close monitoring, with a clear focus on the goals of treatment. Only when clinically significant extrapyramidal disorder is evident but alteration of antipsychotic regimes has proved ineffective or is deemed inappropriate should the question of specific additional medication arise (World Health Organisation, 1990).

For most practitioners, the first choice for 'additional' medication is anticholinergics. Whether this ought to have such an axiomatic status, is discussed below, but as the primacy of this option must be accepted, the use of these compounds is considered first.

Anticholinergics

Anticholinergics achieved their introduction as treatments for drug-related parkinsonism via neurology, where they were introduced empirically for the treatment of Parkinson's disease in the 1920s. It must be appreciated, however, that the scientific evidence in support of their efficacy in drug-related states is actually much less than their widespread – indeed, almost universal – use would imply (Mindham, 1976). In fact, in randomised controlled trials it has not always been possible to demonstrate any efficacy that is superior to placebo. This has tended to be particularly the case when more objective, timed manoeuvres have been evaluated. There may be methodological reasons for this in the selection of patients, their prior treatment regimes, the assessment procedures adopted, and so on. However, it is certainly in line with the author's experience that while patients may feel better on anticholinergics, signs of parkinsonism often seem stubbornly to persist. In explaining these findings there is a further factor worth considering.

As already noted, anticholinergics are euphorogenic, a conclusion for which there is ample, if anecdotal, evidence in the literature (Shader and Greenblatt, 1971; Jellinek, 1977; Smith, 1980; Kaminer, Munitz and Wijsenbeek, 1982). As a result of this property, the currency of these drugs amongst some patients is on a par with cigarettes. One student in his early twenties initially tried subterfuge in his efforts to obtain extra doses by simulating acute dystonic episodes. Having little confidence in his own histrionic capacities, which did indeed fall short of Oscar standards, he eventually decided to appeal at a more direct level. On one such occasion he approached the author, sleeve rolled up, antecubital vein bulging, with the pleading request 'Go on, doc, give us a buzz!' Doc didn't, but was provided with a vivid and lasting illustration of this point. To what extent such artificially induced euphoria may act to counter the dysphoric component of bradykinesia, and thereby improve parkinsonian symptomatology by indirect or secondary mental state mechanisms, is unclear, and indeed the proposition is entirely speculative. It is nonetheless one that is worth considering.

Most clinicians operate on the principle that there is nothing to choose between different anticholinergics and prescribe freely from the range available. However, there is evidence that muscarinic cholinergic receptors exist in a number of different forms (at the time of writing, five: M_1–M_5), which have different balances of central versus peripheral distributions (Avissar and Schreiber, 1989). To avoid as far as possible unpleasant and occasionally serious peripheral side-effects, the choice should probably be concentrated on compounds with greater degrees of M_1 selectivity, and hence of central action, rather than what has become simply habit, although there is no trial evidence to support this suggestion. As we have seen, biperiden is the most M_1 selective of the group used widely in psychiatric practice, with procyclidine a relatively selective alternative.

Procyclidine is the one with perhaps the best scientific credentials for efficacy and, by chance, is the one most frequently used in the UK. There is no clear guidance that can be offered with regard to dosages, but ranges of 20–30 mg per day of procyclidine or its equivalent often recommended for Parkinson's disease should be modified downwards.

In psychiatric practice, anticholinergics tend to be used in predictable fixed-dose schedules. Used in this way, they have a rather narrow therapeutic index, with higher dose regimes taking one uncomfortably close to toxicity. In fact, when administered from a low starting point and with slow increments, it appears that very high doses of anticholinergics can be tolerated, at least in the psychiatrically normal. In the treatment of chronic idiopathic dystonias, for example, benzhexol (trihexphenidyl) in doses of up to 130 mg per day has apparently been tolerated without undue adverse effect (Marsden, Marion and Quinn, 1984).

However, common psychiatric practice in the treatment of drug-related parkinsonism is that patients are started on a fixed regime, e.g. procyclidine 5 mg t.i.d. or q.i.d. or its equivalent. This is to be regretted, as not only does this principle increase the risk of adverse effects and frank toxicity, it precludes the identification of the minimum dose requirement.

The potential risks of fixed-dose usage of anticholinergics are exacerbated when, as is common, the co-administered antipsychotic (or other medication) also has significant anticholinergic activity. It is rare for clinicians to stop to consider the combined anticholinergic 'load' such regimes may be asking patients to bear and the consequence of this on mental state, but this is something good practice should demand.

The author recalls being asked to see, for an 'nth' opinion, a young woman who had become the focus of intense interest on the part of a range of specialists because of her '? neuroleptic malignant syndrome' – at the time still a bit of a diagnostic rarity. It was clear that one was at risk of adding to a Tower of Medical Babel, but as the request came from the patient's distressed husband, it was hard to refuse.

The woman, who suffered from a bipolar disorder, did indeed have features compatible with the presumptive diagnosis, including temporal disorientation, frequent but inconsistent misidentifications, extrapyramidal signs and startlingly raised creatine phosphokinase (CPK). However, in the 24 hours prior to my seeing her, some five days after admission she had received 1000 mg of chlorpromazine (including two doses of 100 mg administered i.m.), 200 mg of amitriptyline and 60 mg of procyclidine, two 'stat' doses of which were also administered i.m. In the face of such an anticholinergic tornado, it was hard to go along with exotica, and the author opted for therapeutic overenthusiasm, an opinion which, remarkably, was immediately and universally accepted. Following discontinuation of everything, and sparing use of benzodiazepines, the woman made a full recovery.

The most important reason for avoiding high-dose regimes of anticholinergic is the simple fact that there is *no* conclusive evidence that they are more effective. The author has certainly rarely seen improvements take place with doses above 20 mg procyclidine or its equivalent that were not well established with less.

Because of their relatively short half-lives, administration of anticholinergics should be spread throughout the waking hours, but equally, because of the euphorogenic and stimulant actions noted above, the last dose should not be given within four to six hours of retiring, if possible. Efficacy, at least in subjective terms, accrues fairly rapidly so the benefits of any schedule can be evaluated after three to five days and the schedule modified if required.

An initial regime might involve procyclidine 2.5 mg b.d., which can be increased to 5 mg mane plus 2.5 mg in the evening (6 p.m.) if necessary after a few days, and to 5 mg b.d. and so on with modifications based on *frequent* clinical assessment. Such a gradual and flexible approach to management is much to be preferred over the fixed-dose method.

Table 4.8. *Adverse effects of anticholinergic drugs*

Peripheral	Central
Paralysis of accommodation	Elevation of mood excitement
Precipitation/exacerbation of closed angle glaucoma	Impaired duration of sleep
Impaired salivation stomatitis	Impaired cognition (learning/memory)
Reduced peristalsis constipation paralytic ileus	Toxic confusional state
Impaired sweating/ temperature control	Exacerbation of 'positive' schizophrenic features
Impaired elimination urinary retention	Exacerbation of choreiform manifestations of tardive dyskinesia
Impaired sexual function	

There are a number of reasons for being circumspect in the use of anticholinergics as they do have their own profile of unpleasant and occasionally serious adverse effects (Table 4.8). One of the most serious – a toxic confusional state or anticholinergic psychosis – has already been alluded to. A further mental state issue is the effect of these drugs on psychotic symptomatology. It has been clearly shown that addition of anticholinergics in acutely ill schizophrenics being treated with antipsychotics results in a small but definite exacerbation of the 'positive' or productive features of the condition (Johnstone et al., 1983). This effect, despite some reports to the contrary, does not seem to be a consequence of pharmacokinetic factors such as reduction in antipsychotic blood levels (Johnstone et al., 1983). This phenomenon of productive symptom exacerbation, replicated from several sources, has failed to gain the recognition in routine practice that its potential significance would justify, but it is something clinicians should be aware of, especially in evaluating patients who fail to respond adequately.

A further adverse effect of anticholinergics is on sleep. One study in which the author participated involved the addition of either active or placebo procyclidine three times daily to antipsychotic regimes stabilised over the prior 10 days (Johnstone et al., 1983). Those who started active anticholinergic experienced an immediate and striking reduction in sleep time measured from sleep charts, which could be up to four hours in some cases; this was in a design where the last dose of pro-cyclidine was administered at 6 p.m. Clinicians should be thoroughly familiar with this effect when evaluating the sleep problems of patients receiving combined therapy.

Cholinergic mechanisms are also crucially important in the physiology of learning, processes that can be disrupted by antagonistic medication. This has potentially great theoretical importance in children though impaired learning in children, under treatment for dystonia musculorum deformans has been difficult to detect thus far. However, it is certainly the case that in the elderly, interference with cholinergic mechanisms can produce striking cognitive deterioration, especially in those with incipient dementia. In routine as well as research conditions, such treatment effects may act as a confounding factor in interpreting formal cognitive assessments.

Although the evidence to date does not support the blanket contention that anticholinergics predispose to the development of tardive dyskinesia, this does remain a possibility in some individual cases. What does seem clear, however, is that anticholinergics can exacerbate the choreiform manifestations of tardive disorder.

Peripheral anticholinergic adverse effects are well known to practising psychiatrists. Indeed, it may be that familiarity has bred a degree of contempt. But anticholinergic effects are always unpleasant and can occasionally be serious. Urinary retention is not something we would wish for ourselves, while impaired accommodation can precipitate or exacerbate closed angle glaucoma, and actions on bowel peristalsis may result in problems of greater magnitude than constipation. Paralytic ileus can be fatal in the elderly. Sexual dysfunction is something that is frequently unexplored in psychotic patients and rarely volunteered and, although usually the consequence of a complex interaction of hormonal and neurotransmitter influences, can be associated with cholinergic antagonism, especially in males. By impedance of sweating, anticholinergics can also impair temperature regulation and contribute to hyperthermia. Finally, of course, there is the very practical point that over-prescription provides yet another vehicle for abuse and self-harm. Thus, anticholinergics are to be avoided where possible and administered sparingly when used. But, having started them, what then?

The nineteenth-century British Prime Minister, Lord Palmerston, commenting on one of the great political issues of his day, said 'Only three people understood the Schleswig-Holstein question. One is dead, one went mad, and I'm the third – but I've forgotten!' How often in our careers have we taken over the care of a patient receiving anticholinergics, the reasons for which (assuming there ever were any) are buried in the mists of time? Nurses continue to insist they are written up on each new prescription sheet and junior doctors dutifully continue to comply, without anyone knowing – or the case notes revealing – why. Like any drugs, the use of anticholinergics needs better justification than merely the fact that it has always been so.

Having achieved maximum impact on the target symptomatology, anticholinergics should be held stable for two to three months in patients whose antipsychotic regime is also undergoing no modification. An attempt should then be made to reduce dosage with a view to seeing whether discontinuation is feasible. For someone receiving 15 mg procyclidine per day, an initial reduction of 5 mg could be followed after one to two weeks by decrements of 2.5 mg, also over intervals of one to two weeks.

There is no clear consensus in the literature as to what the likelihood is of symptoms remaining in abeyance once anticholinergics have been stopped. Some reports suggest the majority will not experience a recurrence (Caradoc-Davies et al., 1986; Double et al., 1993), whereas others state that most will (Rifkin et al., 1978; Manos, Gkiouzepas and Logothetis, 1981). Nonetheless, the implication is that *some* will remain symptom free and this in itself would justify an attempt at cessation. Even if complete removal is not possible, the result may still be a lower maintenance dose than previously.

If this initial attempt at cessation is unsuccessful and it proves necessary to return the patient to the original regime, the process should not end there. Further attempts are justified at three-monthly intervals over the next year, although if by then the goal remains elusive, it is unlikely to be attainable.

The essential characteristic of transitional periods between acute and maintenance phases in the management of psychotic disorders (see Fig. 4.7) is antipsychotic dose reduction. As noted, it may take several reductions before the patient experiences an improvement in his or her parkinsonism. If coincidental anticholinergics have been deemed necessary, reductions in these should also be undertaken, but should be delayed for a couple of weeks or so after each reduction in oral antipsychotics in order to avoid unpleasant symptomatic flare-ups. This is because any improvement in neurological tolerability ensuing from dose reduction will be some time in the happening. As a result of their lipid solubility, antipsychotics have large apparent volumes of distribution. Reduction in dose translates into a proportionately lower fall in plasma levels because of leakage back into the systemic circulation of drug that has been reversibly bound in tissue stores. Hence, the unblocking of central receptors takes longer than might logically be expected. This is one likely mechanism underlying the very slow resolution of extrapyramidal symptomatology following discontinuation of antipsychotics mentioned above. Because of the pharmacokinetic properties of depots, anticholinergic reductions in line with reductions in long-acting injectable formulations should be correspondingly slower (e.g. monthly).

At the end of the day, the important message is that reviews of medication must not focus solely on antipsychotics. Coincidentally administered anticholinergic regimes must also be simultaneously reviewed and their long-term administration repeatedly justified.

Dopamine agonists

The now-standard treatment for idiopathic Parkinson's disease is, of course, L-dopa, yet despite three decades of neurological experience, this drug has been largely side-stepped as a treatment of drug-related disorder. Several clinical evaluations have been published with contradictory results, although the volume of work is slim and the quality poor (Bruno and Bruno, 1966; Yaryura-Tobias et al., 1973; Fleming, Makar and Hunter, 1970; Hardie and Lees, 1988). The major reason for this inadequate exploration of the therapeutic potential of L-dopa is in fact largely theoretical, and springs from the inferences of the classical dopamine hypothesis of the pathophysiology of schizophrenia.

There are two versions of this, one of which implicates presynaptic the other post-synaptic mechanisms. Both, however, have the same practical implications: that productive schizophrenic symptomatology results from a hyperdopaminergic state, with the primary pathological locus probably situated in meso-limbic/meso-cortical dopamine systems. Neither of these theories has received substantive experimental support but this has been no bar to the powerful sway they have held over our conceptualisation of schizophrenia. This is largely a consequence of the third plank of the hypothesis, for which there does continue to be support – namely, the dopamine antagonist theory of antipsychotic action.

One area in which the limitations of the dopamine hypothesis can be seen is the clinical effects of dopamine agonists and psychostimulants in psychotic patients. Review of this literature reveals that far from producing a universal symptomatic exacerbation, drugs of this type promote deterioration in only a minority (Lieberman, Kane and Alvir, 1987; Chiarello and Cole, 1987; Table 4.9). It does seem these drugs can cause a florid exacerbation in patients with active 'positive' schizophrenic symptomatology, but this is by no means a predictable phenomenon, especially in those coincidentally receiving antipsychotics. Thus, our caution in the exploration of the therapeutic potential of dopamine agonist drugs may have some basis, but is extreme.

Concerns about the mental state consequences of L-dopa are not, of course, based solely on theory or a culling of the experimental literature. It is common clinical experience that the use of L-dopa in patients with

Table 4.9. *The effects of psychostimulants* in psychotic patients. (After Lieberman et al., 1987.)*

| | Percentage | | |
	Worse	Unchanged	Improved
Schizophrenics (*n* = 459)	40	41	19
Non-schizophrenics (*n* = 480)	18	40	40
	(+ 2)		

*Amphetamine, ephedrine, methylphenidate.

Parkinson's disease can be associated with the precipitation of psychotic symptomatology, although this is more of an organic problem consequent upon the agonist action of the drug on a deficient cellular substrate.

For a number of reasons, therefore, psychiatry has been diffident about the use of specifically L-dopa as a treatment for drug-related parkinsonism, and the evidence to date does not allow for its general advocacy. However, it may be considered for empirical trial in patients who, for whatever reason, are intolerant of more conventional treatments or unresponsive to them. Such evidence as there is at present would suggest that if first-line or second-line approaches have failed, L-dopa is also unlikely to be successful. There is, nonetheless, scope for further investigation of this question in good-quality, controlled trials.

The same might be said for selegiline (L-deprenyl), which has been shown to delay the need for initiation of L-dopa in patients with Parkinson's disease and to reduce their subsequent L-dopa requirements. While there is some evidence of efficacy in drug-related disorder (Gewirtz et al., 1993), the question has not been adequately explored and, at the time of writing, concerns about selegiline's long-term safety remain unresolved.

Neurology now has at its disposal a number of dopamine agonists that are routinely used in the treatment of Parkinson's disease, including bromocriptine, lisuride and pergolide. Again, no systematic evaluation of these in drug-related disorder has been attempted. The reasons for this and the likelihood of success or of creating problems with their empirical trial are probably the same as for L-dopa.

An alternative approach to dopamine agonism is provided by amantadine. The pharmacology of this compound is poorly understood but it is thought to involve dopaminergic enhancement, either by increased release or re-uptake inhibition. Amantadine was originally introduced as an antiviral agent but was reported as effective in alleviating the features of Parkinson's disease, though its benefits appear ill-sustained and

with long-term use it can, like L-dopa, be associated with the development of dyskinesias (see Table 2.4). Although greeted with some optimism in psychiatry also, early controlled trials in drug-related disorder
were not especially encouraging. In one influential study, amantadine
was no better than placebo (Mindham et al., 1972) – but, in this study,
neither was orphenadrine! Nonetheless, especially in the UK, amantadine never gained more than a loose foot-hold in the treatment of drug-
related parkinsonism.

More recent work in psychiatric populations has confirmed an antiparkinson action with amantadine that appears comparable to that of
anticholinergics and, of note, better tolerability particularly in terms of
cognitive function (McEvoy, 1987; Fayen et al., 1988; Silver, Geraisy and
Schwartz, 1995; Silver and Geraisy, 1995). There may, therefore, be a
greater place for the use of amantadine than practice up until now
would suggest, most notably in the elderly, who may have an increased
likelihood of developing exacerbations of cognitive impairment with
anticholinergics, and in the young, in whom these compounds may
impair learning. However, overdose of amantadine can be associated
with fatality (Cook, Dermer and McGurk, 1986; Simpson, Ramos and
Ramirez, 1988) and the potential for planned or impulsive misuse must
be a consideration in recommending its use.

Before leaving the topic of the therapeutic benefits of dopamine
agonism in parkinsonism, it is of interest to return briefly to anticholinergics, for there is evidence that, in addition to the major action
by which they are classified, most, if not all, of these compounds also act
as indirect dopamine agonists through a combination of presynaptic re-
uptake inhibition and enhanced release (Modell, Tandon and Beresford,
1989). Some, in addition, share the property of re-uptake inhibition of
noradrenaline and, to a lesser extent, serotonin. As the antiparkinson
action of these drugs does not correlate well with their antimuscarinic
potency, it may be that some of their therapeutic benefits (and, indeed,
some of their adverse effects) reflect these dopaminergic, and possibly
noradrenergic, actions.

Other strategies

An alternative approach to the management of drug-related
parkinsonism represents a total departure from the above methods
since it is only indirectly targeted on dopaminergic systems. This
involves blockade of serotonergic mechanisms, specifically the 5-HT_{2A}
receptor subtype.

There is, as already noted, experimental evidence that striatal 5-HT
neurons interact with dopaminergic systems, and so it could be hypothesised that 5-HT antagonism might enhance certain aspects of striatal dopamine function. Theories equating acute extrapyramidal

dysfunction with disruption in the balance between serotonergic and dopaminergic mechanisms in the striatum remain crude, and no single theory is as yet all embracing, but at a clinical level the actions of SSRIs empirically validate such a link.

A number of standard antipsychotic compounds have 5-HT antagonist properties, although no evidence has ever accrued that standard drugs with differing affinities for 5-HT sites differ accordingly in neurological tolerability – or, for that matter, in their efficacy. Potent 5-HT_{2A} antagonism is nonetheless a feature of the pharmacology of clozapine and was spot-lighted early as the possible basis for both the drug's better neurological tolerability and its enhanced efficacy (Huttunen, 1995)).

Serotonergic systems are now very much a focus of antipsychotic psychopharmacology and, while taking this as *the* element of clozapine's complex pharmacology that explains enhanced efficacy may be speculating beyond the evidence, with regard to better tolerability it may not. The relatively selective 5-HT_2 antagonist ritanserin, for example, was shown to be an effective treatment of parkinsonism (Bersani et al., 1990), and, as discussed later, of akathisia also. Had this drug not been rather suddenly deleted in 1995, we might well have been discussing it as a reasonable and interestingly alternative therapeutic approach to drug-related parkinsonism. Nonetheless, the efficacy of ritanserin in this situation would support the view that 5-HT_2 antagonism is a potentially useful strategy to explore in the search for therapeutic innovation at the 'acute' end of the drug-related extrapyramidal spectrum, and new selective tools for further appraisal of this question are awaited with interest.

There is now available or in late-stage development a new generation of antipsychotics that put this idea to the test, at least in the combined format of a single agent. All of the first wave of these compounds – represented by risperidone, sertindole, olanzapine, quetiapine and ziprasidone – are embodiments of the idea that better tolerability and, it is to be hoped, enhanced efficacy will result from compounds with greater affinities for 5-HT_{2A} relative to D_2 receptors.

Early results from clinical trials of these new drugs are encouraging and do indeed point to better neurological tolerability, as assessed in a number of ways such as patient subjective complaints, objective examination-elicited signs and requirements for additional anti-parkinsonian medication (Fig. 4.9). The question of enhanced efficacy on productive symptomatology remains open, but presently seems to this author doubtful, and reported benefits on 'negative' states may reflect the better neurological tolerability rather than efficacy effects.

Risperidone provides an interesting test of the serotonin–dopamine antagonist (SDA) hypothesis in that the prediction should be that

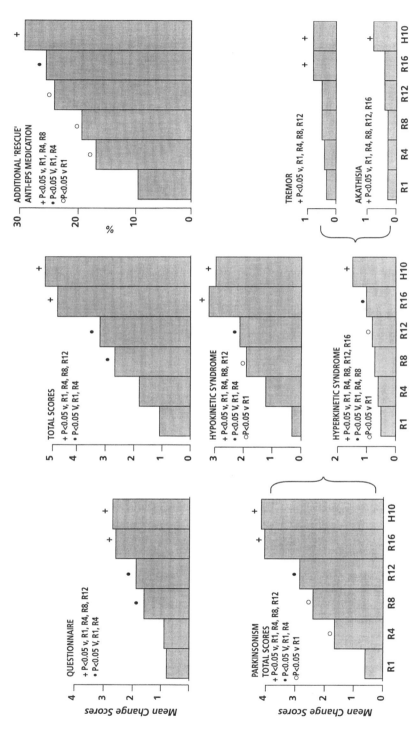

Fig. 4.9. Risperidone multinational study: neurological tolerability measured on ESRS plus requirements for additional anti-EPS medication.

improved extrapyramidal tolerability should follow proportionately from an increasing ratio of 5-HT$_{2A}$ to dopamine D$_2$ antagonism. Risperidone has one of the highest 5-HT$_{2A}$:D$_2$ binding ratios of any drug available or in the immediate pipeline and hence it might be reasonable to predict that it would be especially well tolerated neurologically.

In fact, viewed from this perspective, its advantages appear modest, at least in relation to haloperidol, the major comparitor against which it has thus far been most rigorously tested. A clear dose–response relationship exists, with increasing doses associated with increasing predilection to the development of EPS (Peuskins and Risperidone Study Group, 1995). However, within the recommended (and restricted) dose range, risperidone does seem to possess better tolerability than haloperidol in terms of subjective complaints, objective signs and requirements for additional antiparkinsonian medication (Owens, 1994). This reflects in rating scale scores that cover parkinsonism (amongst other things) but it is a concept of parkinsonism that incorporates akathisia. As shall be seen, the particular advantages of risperidone (and possibly the other newer drugs also) appear to be targeted on akathisia and tremor (see Chapter 5).

However, an overview of the risperidone data to date does not provide a ringing endorsement of the 'balanced' antagonism theory, and while 5-HT antagonism may be one factor in modulating the liability to neurological adverse experiences, the net effect of other receptor interactions known to produce a similar result must not be relegated to obscurity. The profile of extrapyramidal tolerability for any antipsychotic agent is likely to remain dependent on the 'algebraic sum' of *all* its receptor interactions rather than on something reducible to a single combination.

At the time of writing, the new-generation compounds would appear to offer a way of minimising liability to the extrapyramidal neurological adverse effects so frequently encountered with standard antipsychotics, and, by extrapolation, may provide an alternative management strategy in those who develop these disorders with standard compounds. However, it will be some time before adequate comparative data produce a clear picture of their absolute and relative merits.

Finally, we must not forget clozapine. Currently one of the two licensed indications for clozapine is EPS intolerance to standard compounds, and in this regard the drug scores across the board. With regard to parkinsonism, clozapine does not appear to be completely free from liability, but it has been estimated that the prevalence of disorder is approximately half that of patients on standard drugs (Casey, 1989). As with parkinsonism associated with standard antipsychotics, bradykinesia appears to predominate in clozapine-related disorder, although tremor has been reported as less frequent (Gerlach and Peacock, 1994), a finding which has echoes in the risperidone data and may reflect one of the major clinical effects of potent 5-HT$_{2A}$ antagonism.

Although this brief advocacy of clozapine began with 'finally', this should not be taken to imply that one has to be at therapeutic rock bottom before it can or should be considered. Indeed, it might be argued that clinicians are perhaps unduly conservative in using clozapine in the situation of neurological intolerance as opposed to treatment resistance. The issue is that a recommendation for this cumbersome, costly and potentially dangerous treatment should *always* be preceded by clear and logical attempts to manage the problem along lines that demonstrate both diagnostic and therapeutic acumen, of which the use of clozapine is but an example.

An outline proposal for the management of drug-related parkinsonism is presented in Figure 4.10.

Pathophysiology

The pathophysiology of parkinsonism is at one level the most straightforward of that of any of the drug-related neurological syndromes. The analogy is with Parkinson's disease, a condition long known to be associated with impaired dopaminergic transmission in the basal ganglia. This was an insight that was itself originally contributed to greatly by an understanding of drug-related disorder.

Recent in-vivo functional imaging studies using both PET and SPET have found that patients with 'acute' EPS (i.e. parkinsonism rated on the Simpson–Angus Scale and akathisia rated on the Barnes Scale) have higher levels of dopamine D$_2$ receptor occupancy in the striatum than patients free from these neurological signs, confirming the basic premise (Farde et al., 1992; Scherer et al., 1994). Furthermore, in an echo of older claims, these groups suggest that for standard drugs a threshold exists for the development of these features. With PET, the therapeutic threshold is proposed to lie between D$_2$ occupancy levels of 74 per cent and 82 per cent, with higher levels associated with the development of EPS (Fig. 4.11). This is resonant with the reductions in dopaminergic fibres associated with symptomatic Parkinson's disease.

The implication, therefore, is that there exists a therapeutic dose range above which extrapyramidal adverse effects become manifest and below which the degree of dopamine antagonism attainable is insufficient to bring about clinical benefit. The inference also is that this range is rather narrow. Enhanced neurological tolerability associated with combined 5-HT antagonism may be the result of either a widening of the therapeutic threshold with lower levels of D$_2$ occupancy producing clinical benefit, or a simple widening of the therapeutic dose range

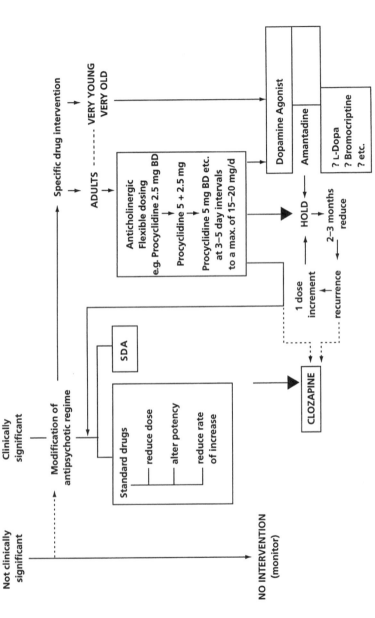

Fig. 4.10. Outline management of antipsychotic drug-related parkinsonism. (SDA, serotonin–dopamine antagonist.)

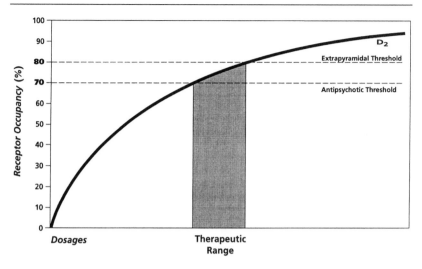

Fig. 4.11. The concept of thresholds: standard drugs.

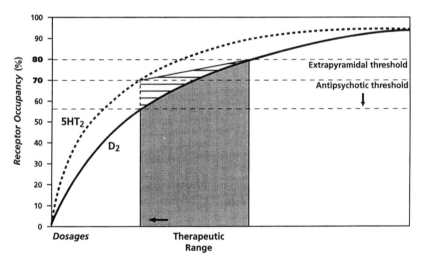

Fig. 4.12. The concept of thresholds: serotonin–dopamine antagonists.

within which antipsychotic efficacy can be achieved (Fig. 4.12). The former scenario may pertain for clozapine but, of the new generation compounds, the evidence to date does not support the view that this is the case for risperidone at least (Farde et al., 1995).

The implications of discrete therapeutic versus extrapyramidal thresholds are considerable, not least in providing a powerful justification for the present volume, but whether these data can be translated into something of clinical utility any more easily now than 40 years ago remains to be seen.

While great strides have been made in understanding the functional anatomy of the basal ganglia and the pathophysiology of Parkinson's disease, our knowledge in both these areas remains superficial. With regard to drug-related parkinsonism, we have very little appreciation of the detailed mechanisms whereby antipsychotic drugs produce their adverse effects. In-vivo imaging has thus far only confirmed our general impressions, not unravelled the nuts and bolts. The following brief overview (Fig. 4.13) is presented only to orientate the reader to the terrain wherein the problem germinates and to provide a small canvas for some speculations.

The corpus striatum is the largest of several subcortical grey matter nuclei involved in the control of motor function and anatomically comprises the caudate, the putamen, the globus pallidus (the latter two sometimes referred to as the lenticular or lentiform nucleus), and the amygdaloid nuclear complex. As opposed to this strict anatomical classification, the term 'basal ganglia' is more frequently applied to those motor nuclei that are, in clinicopathological terms, closely linked functionally, and comprises in addition to the caudate, putamen and globus pallidus, the substantia nigra and the subthalamic nucleus.

The cells of the basal ganglia are 'compartmentalised' into functional domains subserving skeletomotor, oculomotor, associative and limbic functions. The system can be seen as a series of re-entrant loops arranged in parallel, each originating from its own specific cortical fields and returning to cortical areas via specific regions of the dorsal thalamus, thereby forming cortico-basal ganglia-thalamo-cortical circuits. Virtually all areas of cortex feed into this system, progression through the layers of which is associated with very high levels of convergence, in the order of at least several hundred to one. Despite this, these loops are largely closed, with little cross-communication between circuitry subserving different domains.

Cortical inputs to the basal ganglia are largely focused on the putamen although there are also topographic projections directly to the subthalamic nucleus. Both these cortico-striatal and cortico-subthalamic projections are excitatory and probably glutaminergically mediated. The two main projections from the putamen are via gamma aminobutyric acid (GABA-ergic) medium spiny neurons to the external globus pallidus and to either the internal globus pallidus or the pars reticulata of the substantia nigra. The putamen also contains large aspiny interneurons which appear to be cholinergic and may possibly inhibit the spiny neurons. Projections from the respective parts of the internal globus pallidus and the pars reticulata constitute the major

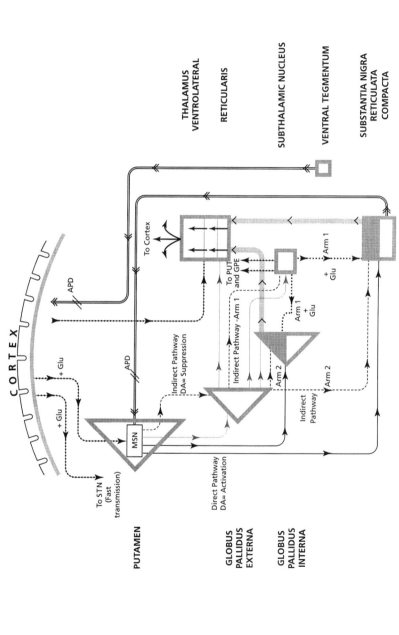

Fig. 4.13. Schematic representation of the functional anatomy of the basal ganglia. (APD, antipsychotic drugs: MSN, medium spiny neurons; STN, subthalamic nucleus; broken lines, indirect pathways; dots, excitatory (glutaminergic) pathways. All other pathways GABA-ergic (and inhibitory) except ▭▭▭ which are dopaminergic. Shaded areas, sensorimotor output nuclei.

sensorimotor outflow of the basal ganglia to centromedian nucleus and ventrolateral thalamus. These two pathways, which are also GABA-ergic, appear to form a functionally integral unit. Fibres from the external globus pallidus to thalamus appear to have comparable characteristics.

Connections from putamen to the outflow nuclei of the internal pallidum/pars reticulata comprise what is known as the direct input pathway. In addition, an indirect input also exists via the subthalamic nucleus. These fibres originate in the GABA-ergic neurons of the external globus pallidus and project to the subthalamic nucleus, which in turn sends excitatory glutaminergic feed-forward connections to the internal pallidum/pars reticulata. Recently, a second arm of the indirect pathway has been described whereby fibres project from the external to the internal pallidum/pars reticularis.

In line with its pervasive distribution, the role of dopamine within this system is complex and poorly understood, as, therefore, are the consequences of its blockade. The most predictive theory, based on primate models, relates hypokinetic movement disorders to thalamic disinhibition. The major striatal dopaminergic input is to the putamen from nigrostriatal fibres originating in the pars compacta of the substantia nigra. There is also input to the nucleus accumbens, olfactory tubercle and ventral striatum from dopaminergic neurons arising in the ventral tegmentum. Functionally, dopamine appears to have reciprocal effects on direct and indirect pathways, with activation of medium spiny neurons that comprise the direct pathway to internal pallidum/pars reticularis and suppression of those projecting to the external pallidum and the indirect pathway.

One net consequence of disruption to this balance from striatal dopamine deficiency is excessive basal ganglia outflow and thalamic disinhibition. This results from impaired activation of the GABA-mediated direct pathway and also from impaired suppression of the indirect pathway resulting in excessive discharging of excitatory neurons in the subthalamic nucleus.

A single mechanism cannot account for all the symptomatology of parkinsonism, but the results of targeted surgical lesioning in patients with Parkinson's disease have provided insights into possible localisations of the pathophysiological disturbances underlying some of the clinical abnormalities. The first surgical intervention was pallidotomy, which was effective in alleviating rigidity and what has been referred to as the 'secondary' bradykinesia associated with this. Surgical attention later shifted to the ventrolateral thalamus as lesioning here seemed to offer more practical advantages by, to some extent, alleviating tremor as well as rigidity. Subsequently, tremor has been reported to be abolished by lesions of the ventral intermediate nucleus but not of the ventrolateral nucleus per se. Pallidotomy and ventrolateral thalamotomy can also be effective in appeasing dopa-induced dyskinesias, which may thus share a common final pathway with rigidity.

Elucidation of the mechanisms underlying the component symptomatology of drug-related parkinsonism has hitherto not been a priority. In view of the frequency of the condition and its potentially serious consequences, this must change and is likely to be aided by new techniques such as functional brain imaging. While for the present we can indeed say that the pathophysiology of drug-related parkinsonism is based on striatal dopamine blockade, this covers the fact that at a functional level it is as yet not possible to specify precisely what this means.

5

Akathisia

Introduction

The concept of akathisia had a long history in the shadows prior to and following the introduction of antipsychotics. It has become customary for authors approaching this topic to begin by explaining its origins, and the present author will maintain the tradition.

The term literally means 'not sitting' or an absence of the ability to sit (still). It was coined by Lad Haskovic in 1902 to describe the 'compulsive' standing and sitting of two male patients he thought – in tune with the times – to be suffering from 'hysteria'. However, there were earlier descriptions of a similar, if not identical, phenomenon going back to Willis in the seventeenth century, and the American George Beard included a recognisable description as part of his 'syndrome' of neurasthenia (Sachdev, 1995a).

It was with the advent of epidemic encephalitis that the concept caught the wider attention of neurology, with a number of reports describing what Wilson referred to as a 'paradoxical' restlessness in association with post-encephalitic parkinsonism. Although the neurological basis of this symptomatology was established early, it would be some time before even neurologists could be clear about whether the features were of independent origins or merely secondary to core parkinsonian symptomatology such as the 'stiffness' of rigidity. This process was facilitated by the eponymous Dr Ekbom, who made his first appearance in 1944 with his accounts of the Restless Legs Syndrome, which was subsequently established as being a neurological condition that could occur in the *absence* of parkinsonism.

For the first account of this phenomenon in a pharmacological context we are once again indebted to Sigwald and colleagues, who reported restlessness in a patient with Parkinson's disease treated with promethazine, (Sachdev, 1995c) which, as already mentioned, was one of

the major early clinical indications for antihistamines. With the introduction of antipsychotics, the association was quickly acknowledged,
though some psychiatrists, as is so often the case, preferred to tread old
dynamic waters rather than accept a purely neurological basis. The
impairment of autonomy over bodily functions was seen as bringing
'closer to the surface their fears of retribution for "sins" and guilt in
terms of bodily disease, as though it is expressed in a living tableau
before their very eyes' (Sarwer-Foner, 1960), which is of course inventive, poetic – and totally fanciful. It is not advised that such a tack be
tried in one's defence against charges of negligence before a court of law
nowadays!

Despite the early recognition of restlessness associated with antipsychotic drug use and the general acceptance of the pharmacological
basis of this, akathisia remained one of the two 'poor relations' of drug-
related extrapyramidal disorders in terms of dedicated research. It is
only comparatively recently that this unjustified omission has been cor-
rected.

Terminology and concepts

The English language is blessed with a rich and subtle vocabu-
lary which plays into the hands of psychiatry's tendency to use terminology imprecisely. The language is possessed of a number of similar
concepts, the meanings of which are usually not considered with their
interchangeable applications. This question of the varied manifestations
or qualities of aimless, affect-driven behaviours has been discussed by
Sachdev (1995a), to whom the reader is referred for a more detailed
exposition.

Restlessness and agitation are especially accustomed to synonymous
usage, even in dictionary definitions. Personally, the author could live
with Kraepelin's definition of agitation as 'anxious restlessness',
emphasising the role of affective arousal from whatever source in
fuelling the motor overactivity. Restlessness would then assume a more
generic role, with less of an implication regarding the underlying affect
and more of an emphasis on the objective motor component.

Related terms include fidgetiness, hyperactivity and jitteriness. To
some extent, these are overlapping concepts, although several have
found rather specific homes in clinical psychiatric practice. An example
is hyperactivity, which tends to be restricted in use to children with
what is now characterised as a particular disorder. Fidgetiness also has
a specific usage implying manipulation of body parts or objects in the
environment but is applied to general as well as to psychiatric contexts;
while jitteriness, which has been applied to the restless lack of ease

described in some patients receiving tricyclic antidepressants (Pohl et al., 1986), would seem to serve little specific purpose.

Having said this, the predominant terminology applied in the literature to the symptomatology of akathisia is *restlessness*. Thus, two essential characteristics are described: the first is an unpleasant, distressing inner restlessness, and the second is a drive to move, either the whole body or an affected part, in an attempt, (usually vain or only partially or periodically successful) to appease the subjective discomfort.

Viewed in this context, therefore, akathisia is *not* strictly a disorder of movement per se, and is probably best considered as essentially an unpleasant or dysphoric affective state. Motor activity may be inappropriate, purposeless or semi-purposeful and non-goal directed, but it is not abnormal in the way it clearly is in the other extrapyramidal syndromes associated with antidopaminergic drug exposure. By this, what is essentially meant is that movement does not appear disrupted by *involuntary* mechanisms.

The distinction between what is voluntary and what is involuntary in motor behaviours is, one has to admit, sometimes more gut reaction than keen observation. It certainly does not spring from the application of specific rules. For example, the fact that sufferers from akathisia can, at will, temporarily suppress or abandon their aimless overactivity helps us little, for the same is true of those with tardive dyskinesia, a syndrome comprising features universally – and, indeed, by definition – considered *in*voluntary. By the same token, no-one suggests that the motor activity of those with depression or generalised anxiety is involuntary, yet in some such cases one would have to tie the patient to a chair to prevent him or her moving.

It is the patients themselves who usually acknowledge that their aimless akathisic activities are willed and voluntary. They continue to feel that such movement is under their own control – potentially at least – in a way that the movements of tardive disorders are not, and certainly such movements do retain the sophistication and integration of willed behaviours. Having said this, motor activity in this situation is 'willed' rather in the sense of someone with a pistol to their head. The patient can exert will but *not* choice. This gives the motor activity of those with akathisia the driven quality. It is not a case of 'I will', but rather 'I must'.

There is one important omission from the above which requires correcting for, left as it stands, the implication is that the term akathisia refers to a single concept. This is not the case. Just how many concepts can legitimately be considered under this heading is not entirely clear, but there are certainly more than one.

There is an arcane quality to writings in this area, which seem to represent the speculations of the bewildered. For our purposes we need not explore the various proposals in depth and will adopt a simple approach.

Table 5.1. *Operational diagnostic criteria for akathisia. (After Sachdev, 1995a.)*

A. Prerequisites
1. Presence of characteristic subjective and/or objective features of restlessness
2. History of exposure to a provoking drug
3. Absence of a primary medical cause

B. Subtyping

i. Acute	Starting within 6 weeks of initiation or increase in dose or change of regime, involving *any* provoking agent
	No decrease/discontinuation of any drug with anti-akathisic properties in the previous 2 weeks
ii. Tardive	Commencement after a minimum of 3 months' exposure to an *antipsychotic* agent
	No increase in dose or alteration in type of antipsychotic in the previous 6 weeks
	No decrease/discontinuation of any drug with anti-akathisic properties in the previous 2 weeks
iii. Withdrawal	Exposure to an antipsychotic agent for a minimum of 3 months
	Onset within 6 weeks of discontinuation or substantial dose reduction
	No decrease/discontinuation of any drug with anti-akathisic properties in the previous 2 weeks

In line with terminology in the field of drug-related movement disorders in general, those forms of akathisia that are not 'acute'- that is, early in onset – are de facto delayed in onset and hence represent 'tardive akathisia'. The literature in general recommends that delayed onset in this context should be considered to mean after a minimum of three months' continuous treatment with stable dose regimes. Within this rubric of 'tardive' – and, again, in line with convention – two main subtypes can be identified: one in which disorder is treatment emergent and the other in which it is withdrawal emergent. These definitions have been operationalised by Sachdev (1995a; Table 5.1), and although they are clearly aimed at the research market, there may be merit in encouraging those in routine practice to consider acquiring familiarity with them also in order to enforce a greater awareness and a more considered recognition.

The problem with such paper exercises in classification is that in practice it is often difficult to be sure precisely when akathisia emerged in the course of treatment. This is particularly the case when psychiatrists seem disinclined to undertake regular, systematic monitoring or practices increasingly act against the practicality of this by encouraging earlier and more complete transfer of 'at-risk' patients to the care of non-medical agencies. Cross-sectionally, therefore, in view of the similarity of features, it may be extremely difficult to tell if akathisia is acute or treatment-emergent tardive, as early-onset disorder can persist for many months and certainly well into the arbitrarily defined time scale for onset of the tardive type.

A possibly useful point, that is raised as a general rule in Chapter 2 and that has been used as the basis for more detailed classifications, is that the symptomatology of acute akathisia should continue to maintain an intimate relationship to pharmacological interventions, particularly to alterations in antipsychotic dose, no matter how long it persists, while in tardive disorder these associations should be tenuous, indirect or absent.

Classification has also been confounded by a more basic conceptual question. As will be evident, in the terms we have been discussing it, akathisia comprises two elements: a subjective one (the predominantly affective symptoms) and an objective one (the observable behaviours or signs). The question then arises as to whether you can have either of these on its own and still have akathisia.

Akathisia is not, of course, the sole condition that can never occur in mild form, and it is certainly clinical experience that some patients develop inner discomfort shortly after starting relevant medication that does not reflect outwardly in behaviour. These patients say they feel 'twitchy', ill-at-ease or 'anxious inside' when asked, but do not necessarily complain spontaneously or show untoward motor activity. Whether this represents mild akathisia is unclear, although during phases of (usually) acute psychotic exacerbation, such non-specific symptomatology is weak evidence on which to base a firm neurological diagnosis. It has been suggested that this state of affairs be referred to simply as 'possible' akathisia (Sachdev, 1995a). This is certainly reasonable but, particularly in routine clinical situations, it must not be seen as a static state of affairs. 'Possible akathisia' would be a presumptive diagnosis, with the implication that the true situation would be clarified by regular monitoring.

The second scenario – signs depleted of symptoms – has been more controversial. Validation of the observation takes no greater effort than an amble around any facility where chronically treated patients are to be seen, combined with the briefest of enquiry. It is what to make of it taxonomically that has been the focus of debate. As shall be seen, the symptomatology of akathisia in those with prolonged exposure histories does modify over time, particularly in terms of the intensity of the subjective component. As a rule, patients seem to lose that distressing edge so characteristic of the early exposure or acute variety. Whether this reflects a primary amelioration of the affective distress or merely a numbing of the mechanisms of conveying distress is unclear, though the latter would seem unlikely to account entirely for this phenomenon. Carried to its extreme, patients may exhibit *only* the motor behaviours.

The issue in this situation has been much to do with whether such movements are voluntary or involuntary, though this approach may not address the realities. A further issue is where purely objective disorder lies in relation to tardive dyskinesia in general.

No definitive answers are possible on these points, though to this clinician's eye the bulk of the abnormality comprising the 'sign' component of tardive akathisia does *not* have the characteristics of involuntary disorder. In fact, what patients seem to demonstrate in this situation is once again not movements per se but complex, integrated behaviours. Relative to involuntary movement types, motor activity retains an element of sophistication and variability in terms of both its form and its content. The impression conveyed is of disorder that is more 'automatic', not necessarily initiated or maintained by conscious will, but amenable to it. In this respect, such behaviours may be more akin to mannerisms.

Research into motor activities of this sort has long been the preserve of ethologists, who have largely espoused behavioural and social/environmental explanations which may be valid for some contexts. Biological models rooted in disrupted neural mechanisms have largely gone by default. It remains unclear as to where stereotyped/manneristic disorders lie in relation to normal, willed activity on the one hand and classical involuntary movements on the other, but this is an area that could do with further scientific exploration.

Thus, in patients with tardive akathisia it may be extremely difficult to categorise movements as to type. There is a further and totally practical issue, however. Even if one possesses the expertise to be clear that a particular pattern of 'restless' behaviours is involuntary, with what confidence can one distinguish this from other involuntary motor disorders that make the patient look restless without restlessness actually being – or ever having been – a component feature? This situation can arise with some presentations of tardive dyskinesia comprising especially dystonia of the lower axial, pelvic and upper thigh musculature. Such patients can certainly look 'on the go', but this is only an *appearance* of restlessness.

Terminology in this field reflects the confusion of concepts it represents. The term 'pseudoakathisia' has been applied by some authors to tardive disorder depleted of symptoms. But if akathisia is conceived of as a syndrome of component parts that may differ in emphasis, this is illogical. No-one would suggest that when schizophrenia wears a coat of a different colour and presents with predominantly negative symptomatology, it thereafter becomes 'pseudoschizophrenia'. Tardive akathisia without evident symptoms is perhaps best referred to quite simply as 'symptomless tardive akathisia', which leaves 'pseudoakathisia' with logic and value, not as a synonym, but as a useful descriptive term for a pattern of clearly involuntary – and especially dystonic – movements that create the appearance of restlessness but from which the inference is of tardive dyskinesia and *not* akathisia.

Clinical features

The core characteristics enshrined in the definition of the disorder discussed above provide an obvious lead-in to the clinical symptomatology (Table 5.2). The features of classical, acute akathisia are focused on first, followed by discussion of the modifications imparted by the tardive state.

Before launching into abstracted detail, however, it might be useful to present highlights of the experience by someone who has been there. Kenneth Kendler, who has subsequently gone on to a distinguished research career in psychiatry, began his professional authorship with a lucid and compelling account of his own experiences of akathisia, which he developed as a medical student after – students take note! – volunteering for a research project. Kendler (1976) wrote:

> 'At 9.00 pm I received 1mg of haloperidol intra-muscularly. I felt drowsy by 9.20. By 9.30 the drowsiness had dissipated and was replaced by a diffuse, slowly increasing anxiety. My uneasiness soon began to focus on the idea that I could not possibly sit still for the rest of the experiment. I imagined walking outside: the idea of walking was particularly attractive. I could not concentrate on what I had been reading ... As soon as I could move, I found myself pacing up and down the lab, shaking and wringing my hands. Whenever I stopped moving the anxiety increased ... The reaction peaked at 10.30 pm ... At home, I walked rapidly several times around the apartment complex ... I did a little jig, moving my arms and legs quickly. By midnight the intensity of the reaction was decreasing ... the intensity of the dysphoria was striking ... (and) the sense of a foreign influence forcing me to move was dramatic.

This superb account encapsulates the essential elements of the disorder and, although more graphic, contains echoes of the experience of Dr Quatri a quarter of a century earlier with chlorpromazine, referred to previously. The insistent and distressing nature of the symptomatology in these descriptions must not be lost.

Table 5.2. *Summary of the major features of akathisia*

Symptoms	Signs
'Dis-ease' (psychological)	'Troubled' facies
Dysphoria	Shifting weight sitting
Apprehension	Straightening trunk movements
Anxiety (psychic and/or somatic)	Crossing/uncrossing legs
Tension (psychic and/or somatic)	Swinging crossed legs
Impatience	Abduction/adduction
Irritability	Writhing/rotational ankle movements
Impaired attention	Fidgeting fingers/hands
Impaired concentration	Fidgeting objects
Discomfort (physical)	'Picking'
Inner restlessness (especially lower body)	Folding/unfolding arms
Fidgetiness	Body caressing
Inability to remain still	Rubbing thighs/knees
Compelled to move	Rubbing chair
'On the go'	Massaging body/face/hair
Dysaesthesiae	Rocking
Jerks	Sudden standing
	Walking on the spot
	Pacing

Symptoms

As a general rule, the balance of signs versus symptoms remains more harmonious in acute akathisia than in other drug-related extrapyramidal syndromes, so the identification of a particular level of objective behavioural disturbance permits the inference of a proportionate degree of subjective symptomatology, and vice versa (Fig. 5.1).

The subjective features (i.e. the symptoms particularly associated with acute disorder) are built around the feeling of inner restlessness. Patients become increasingly ill-at-ease, anxious, apprehensive – victims of a peculiarly unnerving disquietude. They feel 'keyed up', 'tense' or 'fidgety' in a way that is singularly self-absorbing and consequently become increasingly preoccupied with the motion they are more and more drawn to. They are often to be seen intently focused on their 'rituals' of appeasement to the exclusion of all around them. In this situation they can become readily intolerant of the intrusions of the

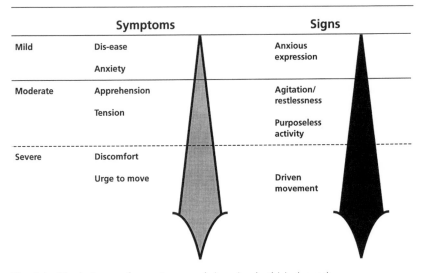

	Symptoms	**Signs**
Mild	Dis-ease Anxiety	Anxious expression
Moderate	Apprehension Tension	Agitation/ restlessness Purposeless activity
Severe	Discomfort Urge to move	Driven movement

Fig. 5.1. The balance of symptoms and signs in akathisia (acute).

environment and may show flashes of irritability and even anger at perceived encroachments.

This sense of restlessness can be experienced as a psychic (i.e. 'in the mind') phenomenon, a primarily somatic (i.e. 'in the body') one, or something emanating from both sources. For the majority of patients, however, the unusual and dominating characteristic is of a state of 'dis-ease' that is peculiarly somatic. Of particular note is the frequent tendency for patients themselves to localise the restlessness to the legs, a fact encapsulated in their account of being 'on the go', or, as one of van Putten's patients put it, being the victim of her 'hurry up feelings' (van Putten, 1975). This lower limb localisation can be of potential use diagnostically. In addition, patients may also experience uncomfortable and often bizarre sensations in the legs, sometimes described as 'stretching', 'cramping' or 'creepy-crawly' feelings.

In keeping with a state that might be construed descriptively as one of 'hyperarousal', sufferers may appreciate impairment in attributes of cognition such as concentration and attention. The normal pattern of sleep may be strikingly disrupted, both by initial insomnia and by an inability to sustain sleep in the face of an exacerbation of symptomatology associated with lying.

The inability of victims to hold to uninterrupted sitting, standing or lying, something of which they are all too painfully aware, has sometimes been referred to as an inability to maintain a particular position. One must be careful about the implications of this terminology as this is, strictly speaking, the literal translation of 'athetosis' as we have seen. No primary disturbance of postural mechanisms has been identified in akathisia and, as has been discussed, the movements are *not* involuntary in the sense that those of athetosis are.

Signs

The first observation relates to expression and demeanour (see Table 5.2). Writing on the subject often fails to point out that, unsurprisingly, patients with acute akathisia often *look* tense, anxious and to varying degrees, distressed. It must be remembered, however, that akathisia frequently occurs in the presence of coincidental parkinsonism, which can modify this aspect of the presentation. Nonetheless, it is often striking how the appearance of discomfort and unease can emerge through the 'masking' effect of bradykinesia.

To some extent, the symptomatology varies with whether the patient is sitting, lying or standing. When sitting, the trunk is stiff and upright, but in frequent motion. Patients shift from side to side in their seat, alternating their weight from one buttock to the other or repeatedly straightening themselves up. They may rock back and forward with the regularity of a metronome. Often they fidget with their fingers or a handkerchief or other object in their hands, and engage in rubbing or 'massaging' behaviours. Thus, they may wring their hands, rub their forearms or face, stroke their hair or massage their thighs repeatedly.

The legs are constantly shifting in position. A characteristic action is crossing and uncrossing the legs, either fully at the knees or at the ankles with the legs outstretched. These movements are striking for their lack of grace and fluidity. They do not emanate as part of a graded sequence of action, but invariably appear without 'build up' either in terms of postural change or expressive gesture. They are suddenly, unpredictably and coarsely executed, to be as suddenly and crudely reversed. Equally characteristic is swinging of the crossed leg backwards and forwards, which is reminiscent of the aimless antics of the bored and indignant, if slightly apprehensive, airline passenger delayed yet again for 'operational reasons'.

All other manner of complex motor activity may be seen, such as rotational or inversion/eversion movements of the ankles, abduction/adduction of the thighs, folding and unfolding of the arms and rapid jerks of whole limbs, any or all of which may be accompanied by sighs and moans of despair.

As the problem progresses, the stage will be reached when the patients may not only be unable to sit still, they may be quite unable to sit at all for other than the briefest of moments. Some patients who find themselves in this awkward position during an interview may retain sufficient social presence and, with regard to their level of symptomatology, may still have sufficient time to seek leave to stand, or at least announce their intention. However, both these prerequisites of acceptable behaviour may have departed, leaving them no choice but to stand suddenly, often in mid-sentence. Even in the face of significant bradykinesia, it is remarkable how swiftly this action can be effected. It can be disconcerting for the novice examiner to have his or her efforts interrupted in this way, but it is essential to acknowledge the reasons.

When standing, the inability to hold to a still and sustained attitude is again evident. Characteristically, patients shift weight from side to side, though to describe this as moving from 'foot to foot' does not convey the essence of the disorder. The movement actually appears to mimic walking, with elevation of the heel followed by lift off from the ball of the foot. Hence, the idea of 'walking on the spot' is probably more accurate, though in fact the appearance has as much of a dancing as a walking quality. At the level of crude symbolism, the over-imbibed football supporter in urgent need of vesicular relief provides a fairly comparable image. Restless, aimless activity in other body parts, as noted above, will usually also be evident.

The major mechanism utilised by the patient in an attempt to alleviate the distress is pacing. This 'need' to walk in the face of an inability to stand still was referred to by Jean Sicard as tasikinesia, (Sachdev, 1995c), though the distinction between this and akathisia is probably only quantitative rather than qualitative. Those afflicted by the condition take more and more to purposeless walking up and down. This pacing is clearly not purposeless in the literal sense of 'serving no purpose' – it ameliorates their discomfort and that is 'purpose' enough – but it is so in the behavioural sense of not being directed towards any defined external goal. To begin with, this may be something resorted to only intermittently, but as symptomatology builds up, patients resort to it more and more. The 'driven' quality then becomes most evident. Patients feel compelled and, to the observer, have the look of someone approaching the task with the greatest of commitment. They appear highly focused, watching not the view before them but, with eyes downcast, only their immediate path. It is interesting that not any path would seem to suffice; patients appear to map out a very specific one for themselves – usually the longest straight line in the ward – and can often be quite intolerant of obstructions to it. The day becomes more and more devoted to pursuance of such an increasingly impoverished repertoire of behaviours.

Lying down may ease the subjective distress and its accompanying signs somewhat, but even in this position symptomatology similar to that noted above may intrude into relaxation. This may seriously impede the induction of sleep. A potentially disturbing feature that may be especially evident in bed is myoclonus. This is similar to myoclonus occurring in other situations and is characterised by spontaneous but ultra-brief, jerky muscular contractions that are quite definitely involuntary. The contractions are typically described as 'shock-like' in their effects. Myoclonic jerks may be a relatively frequent occurrence, especially in those who are profoundly akathisic, although the evidence is somewhat contradictory. It does seem, however, that they are themselves only infrequently severe.

There is one further issue in connection with the presentation of acute akathisia that, although it relates more to a possible adverse consequence rather than a primary feature, is of sufficient importance to merit emphasis. This is the issue of aggressive behaviour. As has already been seen, irritability can result from akathisia, but in rare instances this has been reported as ending in violence, both suicidal and homicidal in nature (van Putten, Mutalipassi and Malkin, 1974; van Putten, 1975; Shear, Frances and Weiden, 1983; Schulte, 1985; Drake and Erlich, 1985). In view of the prominence of akathisia in general, reports of such an outcome are very few and may, of course, represent merely chance associations. However, while we might justly assume this is at most an uncommon association, in view of the potentially devastating consequences, it is one that should *always* be borne in mind.

Tardive akathisia

Clinically, the manifestations of akathisia in tardive form are not, on the face of it, qualitatively different from those of acute disorder just considered. The major difference lies in a shift in the balance between the subjective and the objective symptomatology. In the acute state there is a harmonious and often proportionate relationship between the two (see Fig. 5.1). Tardive states tend to be characterised by a decline in prominence of the subjective. Patients may still complain of restlessness – indeed, the single most common complaint is inability to keep the legs still – and such complaints may at times be bitter. Behaviours clearly ameliorating in their intentions can still be identified. But in general the inner restlessness so distressing to the acutely afflicted patient seems to subtract itself from the symptomatology, the anguish to blunten. It also seems that the purely sensory component of acute disorder, i.e. the 'creeping', 'pulling' type of symptoms, becomes less evident.

As noted before, these sorts of changes are unlikely to be merely a reflection of illness-related changes in the experience or expression of affect, but are more likely to represent fundamental shifts in pathophysiological mechanisms.

This decline in emphasis of the subjective symptomatology is mirrored by behavioural changes. Aimless activity – and, in particular, the 'driven' quality of the motor response – usually abates and patients seem more able to exhibit the greater part of their abnormality while sitting, often somewhat vacantly, in a chair. Pacing, when evident, is less hectic, more ritualistic. Shifting, squirming, straightening movements of whole body/trunk may continue along with, perhaps most character-istically, constant leg activity – crossing/uncrossing, swinging back and forth and, strikingly, abduction/adduction, all executed with the same ill-refined and graceless quality noted with acute disorder. Myoclonic jerks infrequently occur.

It must again be emphasised that the more the subjective wanes, the greater the difficulties – both practical and conceptual – of establishing a firm distinction between akathisia of tardive onset and those features that comprise the syndrome of tardive dyskinesia.

One question that has bubbled under the surface of antipsychotic psychopharmacology for some years relates to whether or not these drugs promote tolerance and therefore are associated with a with-drawal syndrome on rapid discontinuation. The bulk of the evidence does *not* support the development of withdrawal as a general phenom-enon, except perhaps in those suddenly removed from treatment with compounds of relatively high anticholinergic activity, especially thiori-dazine (Luchins, Freed and Wyatt, 1980). It has been proposed that 'withdrawal' is a misattribution and that the anxiety/restlessness/ insomnia etc. of such cases actually represents a withdrawal-emergent akathisia (Sachdev, 1995a). This is an interesting proposition to bear in mind from a routine clinical point of view, although it is unlikely to account for all such cases and has as yet received no research confirma-tion.

Modifying factors

When it comes to evaluating akathisia, it is important to bear in mind that it shares a number of characteristics common to all the drug-related extrapyramidal disorders. Thus, its features relate to the mental state so that those 'aroused' by virtue of their psychiatric disorder will show more prominent abnormality, while states of tranquillity or seda-tion will diminish it. Symptomatology disappears during sleep, although the poor-quality sleep patients often complain of in associa-tion with akathisia may cause them to rouse in the night, with motor restlessness keeping them awake thereafter. Myoclonus may, when prominent, cause its greatest disruption at this time. The clinical presentation will also vary over time in any individual and, although no clear diurnal pattern has been established, it would seem sensible, as with other disorders, to undertake serial evaluations at the same time each day.

As shall be seen, instigation of voluntary motor activity in an unre-lated body part has been repeatedly reported as being associated with the emergence or exacerbation of latent or minimal involuntary movements in a part under examination. The procedures to demonstrate this are referred to as 'activation' procedures and are an integral part of the standard extrapyramidal examination technique (see Chapter 10). As shall also be seen, the author has long been rather troubled by this blanket assertion as it has not always seemed consonant with his own experience.

With regard to akathisia, 'activation' tasks have met with contradictory responses, – some reports confirming worsening, others supporting improvement or abolition. In a detailed study, Sachdev and colleagues could not demonstrate the 'activating' effects of an 'activating' motor task – rather, the opposite. In their studies, disorder diminished or disappeared altogether (Sachdev, 1995a). They have suggested that this is an attribute distinguishing akathisia from tardive dyskinesia, but in the author's view this conclusion is hardly justified because of the issue surrounding the precise task chosen to address this question, and in particular how much it requires the exercise of mental functions, especially concentration. In the author's experience, the more any such task demands a sophisticated level of cognitive input, the more likely it is to result in suppression rather than activation. With regard to akathisia, this alas does not appear to be the experience of others. Fleischhacker et al. (1993) found reduction with a motor task but exacerbation with a mental one! The only certainty at present would seem to be that the choice of 'activating' task is crucial, but no matter what, the response is likely to be unpredictable.

Diagnosis

The picture of apparently aimless, fidgety restlessness is common in everyday life as in general psychiatric practice. Such behaviours are a universal response in situations of boredom, frustration, confrontation and apprehension. As an organiser of the MRCPsych examination for some years, the author can vouch for the veracity of this observation, at least in relation to exam candidates! However, these behaviours are circumscribed and time limited. They nonetheless do offer an invaluable platform for the diligent clinician to learn the foundation to his or her trade, for what represents inappropriate behaviours of this sort are best understood via what may be extreme but appropriate. It is not merely the degree of the distress that sets akathisia apart, but the absence of appropriate context. Of his experience, Kendler noted that 'with the possible exception of going on stage on an opening night (*appropriate*), I cannot remember any feeling of anxiety so intense' (*inappropriate*).

Table 5.3. *Distinguishing akathisia from psychomotor agitation: 'a high index of suspicion'*

Temporal association with antipsychotic introduction or alteration
Patient's graphic descriptive language
'Almost' alien/imposed nature of symptomatology
Resistance to distraction or amelioration by engagement
The 'driven' quality of the motor response
Localisation to lower body, especially legs
Abnormal sensations, especially in legs
Myoclonic jerks, especially nocturnal
Response to a specific therapeutic intervention

In general psychiatric practice, this sort of picture is also a frequent occurrence and is to be found in any state of 'arousal'. Restlessness of this sort is not, of course, the sole preserve of psychotic disorders, but it is in these conditions that antipsychotics will be most used, so the focus is appropriately there.

The major diagnostic issue is the separation of akathisia from psychomotor agitation (Table 5.3), for the phenomenology of the two can be indistinguishable. A particular source of confusion is that acute akathisia is most likely to develop at an early stage of active illness when agitation is also likely to be a prominent feature anyway. Furthermore, a tense, 'coiled-up' restlessness may be the patient's response to the experience of admission to hospital and the relative confinements that that imposes. Suspicion or bewilderment and brooding resentment feeding off one another can, therefore, result not only in escalating behavioural disturbance but also in increasingly florid psychotic symptomatology. Thus, the introduction of medication that may promote akathisia is taking place at a time when a crescendo of agitation and aimless, disorganised activity is most likely.

A further issue to bear in mind is that the over-stimulation of akathisia may itself exacerbate the productive features of the psychotic illness. It is well known that states of high emotional arousal or anxiety can have an adverse effect on schizophrenic symptomatology. It is perhaps less considered that the dysphoric affect comprising the subjective component of akathisia and other extrapyramidal syndromes may also fire positive symptomatology (van Putten et al., 1974; van Putten and Marder, 1987). One woman, relieved at the easing of her akathisia, described its effect as like 'giving them (the voices) whiskey – they went berserk'. This relationship is much neglected in routine practice but is of potentially great importance in evaluating the comparative benefits of the new antipsychotics.

The elderly present specific problems, especially those suffering from dementia. Akathisia can all too readily be mistaken for the increasing loss of composure caused by the substitution of the familiar with the unfamiliar, or for the worsening of confusion that may be a consequence of hypotension or other drug effects. It is a moot point just how beneficial antipsychotics are in the restlessness not infrequently found in dementing patients, but accepting that they are still commonly used in this situation, particular alertness is called for.

The clinician has, therefore, to bear in mind a complex interplay of circumstances. There are several areas that may help in delineating akathisia. The first is the temporal sequence. With any exacerbation of these affects and behaviours following within a few days of starting treatment, changing to a compound of higher potency, or increasing dose schedules, akathisia must be considered. Secondly, it is (as always) worth listening to what the patients themselves say, because many will be able to state quite categorically that what they experience is *different* from agitation. Thirdly, even with profound degrees of agitation, it is still often possible to engage patients sufficiently to distract them away from their purposeless behaviours, whereas with akathisia even relatively modest levels of disorder usually continue to intrude through engagement that appears of good quality. Fourthly, the 'driven' quality of akathisia has been repeatedly emphasised and is characteristic. Patients acknowledge the willed nature of their actions but often tell of the *almost* alien desire that is compelling them (see Kendler's quote above). Finally, and perhaps most importantly, is the localisation the patients frequently give to the source of their discomfiture, which for the majority is to the lower limbs.

At the end of the day, none of these points may be of any use, and the most important element in diagnosis is a high index of suspicion. Resolution of the diagnostic issue may only be possible by utilising one of the surest characteristics of acute akathisia and that is the intimate relationship between symptomatology and treatment regimes. Increases in dose, potency and speed of exposure will all result in swift exacerbation; decreases, in more gradual amelioration. Hence, gauging response to some therapeutic intervention may be the soundest way of enlightening the dilemma. However, this is not a strategy that will be of practical worth with tardive akathisia.

A wide range of neurological and medical disorders can feature restlessness (Table 5.4). Mostly, these do not present a diagnostic dilemma. The position of *Parkinson's disease,* however, is worth mentioning. Although acknowledging akathisia early, neurology has been remarkably leaden in incorporating this into the symptomatology of one of its major constituent disorders. One would hesitate to suggest that this might be a result of generations of neurologists seeing the

Table 5.4. *Differential diagnosis of akathisia*

Psychiatric	Psychomotor agitation (causes of)
Neurological	Parkinson's disease
	Restless legs (Ekbom's) syndrome
	Subthalamic lesions
	Peripheral neuropathies
	Myelopathies
	Myopathies
	Tardive dyskinesia
Deficiency states	Iron
	Folate
Metabolic states	Hyperthyroidism
	Hypoparathyroidism
	Chronic renal failure (dialysis)
	Hypoglycaemia
Other	Pregnancy
	Vascular (including venous) disease

features as psychogenic – hesitate perhaps, but not refrain! What scant formal research has been undertaken would point to definable akathisia at some time afflicting between 25 per cent and 44 per cent of those with idiopathic Parkinson's disease and to this not being directly related to treatment (Lang and Johnson, 1987; Comella and Goetz, 1994). It is, perhaps, ironical that it should, in this one small area at least, be psychiatrists urging neurologists towards a more organic viewpoint!

One specific neurological differential to be kept in mind is the restless legs (or Ekbom's) syndrome already referred to. The precise prevalence of this condition is unknown but even if the minimum figure of 1.2 per cent of the population is accepted (Sachdev, 1995a), this speaks of a far from esoteric disorder.

The author must plead a certain culpability on this issue, as most of the cases of this disorder he can recall have been recognised in retrospect with the knowledge of protracted hindsight and sometimes spectacular therapeutic infertility. In defence, however, it could be argued that others have pointed out the relative absence of such cases from medical clinics, one small justification for lack of familiarity and recognition. It may be that this is a condition patients rarely bring to medical attention unless specifically asked, either because it is usually mild or considered too 'weird', or because it most often lies buried beneath other more pressing concerns.

It certainly does appear that much higher prevalences of more striking disorder are to be found in special situations. A particular association is with iron-deficiency anaemia, with rates of 25–40 per cent reported, while 11–27 per cent of pregnant women have been reported to experience the problem, especially in late pregnancy (Sachdev, 1995a). A similar set of features has been found in about one-fifth of those receiving renal dialysis. Isolated reports have also concerned patients with a range of neurological disorders, including peripheral neuropathies, and a few who had vascular disorders, especially on the venous side. The condition may occasionally be familial.

Ekbom's syndrome also has both a subjective and an objective side to its symptomatology. The subjective features comprise an element of distress commensurate with the severity of the condition, and occasionally extreme, and a relief of symptomatology with movement. However, perusal of published accounts strongly suggests that the symptomatology being relieved is of a much more primarily sensory nature than that of akathisia – more dysaesthesia than dysphoria per se. Thus, patients are reported as describing this in terms of an internal itching or pulling or creeping 'sensation', with much use of entomological similes, 'like ants' or worms or other undesirables crawling through their bones or sinews. The impression is also of a more conclusive localisation than with akathisia, so patients seem clear that the problem is internal and most frequently seems to reside in the region of the shin. Worsening on lying is characteristic, and this condition is usually associated with profound disturbance to, especially, the early phase of the sleep period.

Patients with Ekbom's syndrome also exhibit behavioural ploys aimed at symptom relief, which include purposeless movement such as walking, although from the published literature they do appear somewhat more inventive than the average victim of akathisia. Thus, they may massage their site of localisation, dance or do a little yoga before retiring, swing their legs over the bed or even steep them in cold water (beware the patient who cannot stand the 'heat' of the blankets!). Unlike akathisia, myoclonic jerks are a prominent feature of the restless legs syndrome and may occur in the day but are characteristically nocturnal (beware the patient who cannot stand the 'heat' of the blankets and whose partner has had to retreat to the spare bedroom to avoid the bumps!).

The author has learned of Dr Ekbom the slow way, and although our paths have only occasionally crossed, his story is a useful one to know for those in general psychiatric practice.

While Ekbom's syndrome may only infrequently test one's diagnostic powers, the symptomatology of tardive dyskinesia may commonly do so. As has been mentioned, there is an inherent assumption in the concept of tardive akathisia that the features of this can in all circumstances be distinguished from those of other tardive disorders conventionally considered separately. This is by no means the case. Particular problems arise with some segmental or generalised manifestations of chronic dystonia, which can impart to the patients exactly the objective appearance of fidgety restlessness considered characteristic of akathisia. Examples include axial hyperkinesis, a kinetic dystonia of the lower back and pelvic muscles sometimes referred to accurately, if rather insensitively, as 'copulatory' movements, and dystonias of the anterior or adductor/abductor thigh muscles. One elderly man had such a profound dystonia of the hip flexors that he could not wear slippers for fear of projecting them onto an unsuspecting public. He would frequently cross and uncross his legs when sitting, which made him look profoundly ill-at-ease, but this was a willed and voluntary action which he had discovered aborted full-blown dystonic spasms (see Chapter 7). Not all that *looks* restless, is.

Epidemiology

As has been noted, akathisia has been neglected in the literature to a degree that is out of all proportion to its clinical importance. No-one can come up with a satisfactory explanation as to why this should have been the case, though 'tramlining' is unlikely to have been entirely innocent of some blame. In acute settings, parkinsonism was more clearly known as neurological and hence a less easy victim of psychodynamic 'explanation'. With tardive hyperkinetic disorders, the priority was to define the boundaries – the classification of subsyndromes could wait. However, perhaps when we look back to the study of Weiden and colleagues (1987) mentioned earlier, we should be grateful for small akathisic mercies!

As with the other drug-related syndromes discussed here, the literature on akathisia has not been too careful in distinguishing prevalence from incidence. While this certainly reflects a sloppy approach to epidemiological investigation, it is not quite as terminal as it seems because, as has been mentioned in other contexts, it is unlikely there is a single figure or tight range of meaning that can be provided for either of these. Rates of occurrence depend on the same range of individual, pharmacological, treatment practice and other variables which were discussed in connection with parkinsonism and which somewhat blur the value of the distinction between these two concepts.

The two other problems in evaluating epidemiological information on akathisia are that, firstly, researchers have not always consistently considered both objective and subjective components of symptomatology

Table 5.5. *Some prevalence studies of akathisia*

Study	Prevalence	Comment
Freyhan (1959)	13.0	No standardised assessment Slightly different rates for different drugs but no dose equivalences
Ayd (1961)	21.2	Those with akathisia only and no other EPS
Kennedy et al. (1971)	38.5	Evaluation unstandardised
Braude et al. (1983)	25.0	
Barnes and Braude (1985)	48.0	Acute 7% Chronic 28% Pseudo 12%
Curson et al. (1985)	19.6	Evaluation unstandardised
Gibb and Lees (1986)	3.0	Inpatients – 'definite' only Outpatients 41% movement 55% body restlessness 46% psychic restlessness
McCreadie et al. (1992b)	30.0	Questionable 10% Definite 18% Pseudo 5%
Halstead et al. (1994)	42.0	Chronic 24% Pseudo 18%
Sachdev (1995a)	33.0	24% with stricter criteria

and, secondly, disorder has usually not been categorised in terms of acute as opposed to other forms of akathisia noted above. The published figures (Table 5.5) are therefore influenced by several other interposing factors in addition to the usual ones of sample selection and evaluation methodology. They must at present be taken only as a rough reflection of probability and not as absolute figures.

Ayd's open retrospective study of over 3500 patients remains the largest, and found akathisia to afflict 21.2 per cent (Ayd, 1961). For the reasons noted before, this must represent an underestimate, but not as much of one as was the case for acute dystonias. In general, the literature would suggest that between 20 per cent and 45 per cent of those exposed will develop akathisia – that is, disorder comprising both subjective and objective symptomatology (Sachdev, 1995b).

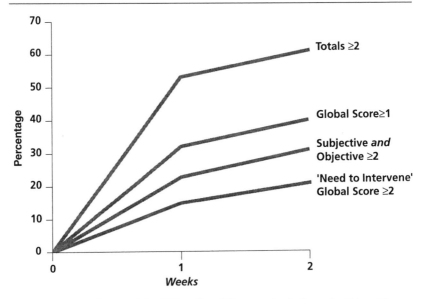

Fig. 5.2. The incidence of akathisia using different criteria from the Prince Henry Hospital Scale. (Data from Sachdev and Kruk, 1994.)

With regard specifically to the incidence of acute disorder, the study of Sachdev and Kruk (1994) is the most informative so far. These authors assessed 100 consecutive patients admitted for non-organic psychoses and who had been medication free for a minimum period (two weeks for those on orals: six weeks for those on depots) and who had no evidence of akathisia. The patients were examined at baseline prior to starting antipsychotics and at one and two weeks, or sooner if akathisia developed.

The incidence depended on the cut-offs adopted on the scale used (the Prince Henry Hospital Scale, see Chapter 11). With a global score, it was found that over a two-week period 40 per cent of patients were rated as having akathisia (Fig. 5.2). However, as the authors pointed out, this did not correspond to clinically significant disorder, which they defined in terms of 'a need to intervene' (i.e. of at least 'moderate' severity). Using this criterion, they found a 21 per cent incidence figure over two weeks. By applying the more satisfactory method of summing the subjective *and* objective items of the scale and applying the more stringent criterion, they calculated incidence figures that they suggest as being suitable for research purposes but that are perhaps more clinically relevant than those based on global ratings – namely, 23 per cent by day seven, with an overall incidence figure over two weeks of 31 per cent.

Figures for the frequency of other than the acute form of akathisia are based on even flimsier evidence because of the differentiation problems relating both to the classification of established disorders in any clinical population and to the separation of tardive akathisia from tardive dyskinesias in general. Barnes and Braude (1985) reported a prevalence of 28 per cent for what they defined as chronic akathisia in long-standing schizophrenic patients attending depot clinics, while the same group more recently reported a comparable figure of 24 per cent in long-stay hospital residents (Halstead, Barnes and Speller, 1994).

Gibb and Lees (1986), in an interesting study of long-stay mixed diagnosis hospital inpatients, found a prevalence of only 3.2 per cent for definite akathisia (i.e. 17 per cent of those with motor disorder). They did find a group of patients (50 per cent) who had orofacial dyskinesia and restless motor activity, but this lacked both the subjective and the objective features of akathisia. A further third of the sample demonstrated restlessness but without subjective features or orofacial dyskinesia.

We also found an extremely low figure for 'akathisia' (1.2 per cent objective symptomatology only) in a severe long-stay schizophrenic population. However, this was using a scale (the Simpson or Rockland Scale) that is conceptually confused in the akathisia department (see Chapter 11). Thus, in addition, we found that around 3–5 per cent of the sample rated on items for 'restless legs', body 'rocking', 'stamping' and 'rubbing' movements.

The Sydney group has also provided data on the prevalence of tardive disorder. Sachdev (1995a) has reported figures from 100 chronic schizophrenic patients attending community health centres and whose medication had been kept stable. Using a global criterion (from the Barnes Scale, see Chapter 11), a figure of 33 per cent was found for disorder concluded to be a mixture of chronic and tardive. However, the figure shrank to 13 per cent for those with no signs of coincidental tardive dyskinesia.

The range of figures for the prevalence of non-acute forms of akathisia is as wide as for tardive dyskinesia, and the average in the studies reviewed by Sachdev (1995d), at 23 per cent, is also comparable. It is probable that sample and conceptual – and consequently rating – differences account in some part for such wide discrepancies.

Overall, the literature on the epidemiology of akathisia is weak and there is a pressing need for long-term prospective investigation of the extent of the problem. From what we know so far, around one-third of those exposed to standard antipsychotics will develop features of acute akathisia, and somewhere in the region of one-quarter will continue to demonstrate on-going symptomatology, a situation that for many is bound up in the web of tardive motor disorders discussed in the next section.

Predisposing factors

Once again, those obvious factors that predispose to the development of acute akathisia are predominantly pharmacological and practice related. These are what we have already seen with parkinsonism – namely, the type of drug in terms of its potency, the dosage and the rate of dose increments (Sachdev and Kruk, 1994).

It is certainly possible for patients suddenly exposed to high doses of potent antipsychotic to develop a rapid-onset hypokinetic-rigid syndrome and become, as it were, suddenly 'locked in'. This is most likely to occur in the drug naive, or when patients in relapse have excessive additions made to their baseline regimes, or when similar follies afflict the elderly. It is, however, a fortunately infrequent occurrence. It seems that with regard to signs at least, the great majority of individuals have a sufficient functional reserve in the relevant dopaminergic pathways to allow for a more gradual onset of parkinsonian symptomatology following the implementation of treatment decisions.

The same may not be the case with acute akathisia. There is evidence, for example, that a significant proportion of normal volunteers may experience identical symptomatology within a very short time of receiving even a single dose of antipsychotics (King, Burke and Lucas, 1995). The usual 'culprit' in these studies has been haloperidol. It seems that akathisia, especially when associated with the use of potent medication, may have very early origins – even as early as after a single dose. In this situation, a further predisposing factor closely related to those above is mode of administration – with a greater likelihood of symptomatology associated with intravenous than with oral administration. In support of this, Magliozzi and colleagues (1985) found that while one-third of those (healthy volunteers) given haloperidol orally developed akathisia, the problem was evident in two-thirds of those who received it intravenously. Thus, particular care should be exercised in the use of high-potency antipsychotics given intravenously, and particular vigilance exerted in the monitoring for adverse experiences that may ensue.

Once again, with the above associations accounted for, there is no evidence of any demographic or other variables that predispose to the development of acute akathisia, including age, gender, race etc. (Sachdev, 1995b). By analogy with Ekbom's syndrome, it has been proposed that patients with iron deficiency may be at greater risk. Investigations on blood-based parameters have been inconclusive (Sachdev, 1995b) and resolution of the question will probably need to await wider application of techniques that provide more representative evaluations of iron status in the brain itself, such as, for example, MRI. The author's experience of working in a multi-ethnic environment, and in a hospital where the 'normal' haemoglobin for Hindu vegetarian women was set lower than that for Western carnivores, did not lead him to observe strikingly greater rates in such women.

It has been suggested that, as with tardive dyskinesia, those with affective disorders (specifically depression) are at greater risk of developing acute akathisia (Gardos et al., 1992), but this remains an isolated observation and not one that, even if replicable, can be taken to imply a primary relationship.

What might be encompassed under the rubric of 'individual susceptibility' is unclear, although experience would point to the fact that this is an important part of the equation. However, the precise neurochemical or other components that comprise it are a distance away from the elucidating.

There are no clearly established factors predisposing to the development of other varieties of akathisia – tardive, chronic etc. At the level of common sense, acute abnormality would be likely to represent a predisposition, but even this requires to be established with clarity. An association has been reported between tardive disorder in schizophrenic patients and the presence of 'negative' features and cognitive impairment (Brown and White, 1991). This finding with regard to negative features has not been replicated (Halstead et al., 1994) but, as shall be seen, is of considerable interest with relation to similar observations in tardive dyskinesia.

Onset, course and outcome

As far as the literature is concerned, the onset of acute akathisia has tended to be seen as a somewhat leisurely affair, measured in days to weeks with a cumulative development roughly, if not exactly, paralleling parkinsonism. Again, Ayd's large retrospective study from 1961 has been influential. In this study, development over time appeared gradual, with 90 per cent of the cases of akathisia evident within 90 days of exposure (Fig. 5.3). These data certainly seem to be reflected in clinicians' attitudes towards akathisia – that this is something that may come on 'after a while'.

There is increasing evidence that this approach is too laid back by far. Indeed, a closer look at Ayd's data should have raised warnings: although 90 per cent of cases were evident in the first two to three months, 60 per cent had developed within a month. This represents a slightly earlier pattern of onset than that found with drug-related parkinsonism.

Prospective studies have suggested that clinicians would do well to shorten their time scale of risk. Braude, Barnes and Gore (1983) found that 85 per cent of their cases developed within one week, while, as has

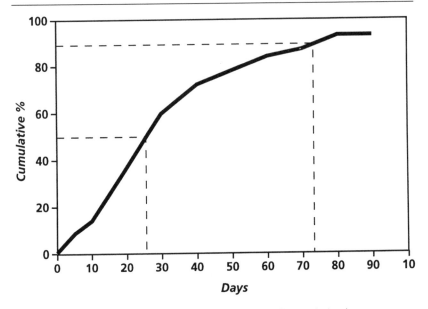

Fig. 5.3. The onset of akathisia. (After Ayd, 1961, with permission.)

been seen, about three-quarters of Sachdev and Kruk's patients had symptomatology within the same period. This latter group, whose patients, like those of Braude et al., were receiving oral medication, found that the diagnosis was 'usually' first made on day three of treatment (Sachdev, 1995a). This would clearly suggest that clinicians must be alert to the possibility from a very early stage of exposure to even oral antipsychotics. The question then is whether vigilance ought routinely to be extended back as far as the first dosage.

As mentioned above, there is a small but consistent body of evidence to suggest that a significant proportion of normal volunteers receiving antipsychotics experience dysphoric restlessness with accompanying urgent, non-goal-directed movement within a short time of receiving antidopaminergic medication. King et al. (1995) found that, with a high index of suspicion, 16 per cent of volunteers could be identified as exhibiting mainly subjective restlessness within three hours of taking haloperidol 5 mg orally, although in addition 40 per cent complained of dysphoric mood that was separate from sedation. Van Putten, May and Marder (1984) reported that 40 per cent of subjects given a single i.v. dose of 5 mg haloperidol developed features within six hours.

However, there is evidence that with parenteral administration, onset may be very rapid indeed: Kendler's graphic account above referred to symptomatology experienced within 30 minutes of receiving 1 mg of haloperidol i.m. Nor, incidentally, does the problem appear to be limited to antipsychotics. A similar rapid onset, in 15–30 minutes, has been reported to occur after a single i.v. dose of 10 mg metoclopramide (Jungmann and Schoffling, 1982).

This has not always been acknowledged as akathisia per se, though phenomenologically it seems to be very similar, if not indistinguishable, and does appear rateable on scales for akathisia developed from patient experiences. Why this very early symptomatology is rarely if ever detected in patients, even in prospective incidence studies, is unclear. It has been suggested that perhaps patients and volunteers may differ in their reaction to medication, based, most obviously, on their levels of 'arousal' and hence tolerability. This has not been systematically investigated, but experience would suggest it is not the case. Alternatively, it may simply be that this early drug-related disturbance is 'buried' in the existing psychopathology and thereby mistaken for it until it reaches a certain level of prominence. It might also be worth considering, however, that this early restlessness is indeed in some way different and may fade, to be replaced subsequently by the clinical syndrome of akathisia, though, again, such prospective work as has been done is generally unsupportive of this hypothesis.

There is clearly a need for further detailed investigation of the patterns of drug-related restlessness in both patients and non-patients, including the profile of its evolution over ultra-short time intervals. In the meantime, clinicians would be well advised to view akathisia as a *possible* development from the very first implementation of treatment plans that involve either initiation or increase of antipsychotic drugs, particularly when management has included emergency intravenous use of a high-potency compound.

It seems that this aspect of very early onset is something that must also be borne in mind with depots – at least those of fluphenazine. Ayd found that 90 per cent of the acute akathisia associated with the use of fluphenazine enanthate and decanoate became evident within four days of administration (Ayd, 1974). As far as the decanoate is concerned, this may be related to the unusual pharmacokinetics noted above, namely its unique and rapid post-injection peak.

The omissions in the research literature on akathisia are particularly evident in those forms other than the acute. Almost all data have been derived retrospectively, a study methodology unsuited to address the problem, and where there have been blanks to be filled in (and that is often), analogies have been drawn from observations on tardive dyskinesia. By operationalised definitions, treatment-emergent tardive akathisia shows itself only after a minimum of three months' exposure, with regimes held stable for at least half that time. Burke and colleagues (1989) found a curvilinear pattern of development for tardive akathisia, with about one-third of cases becoming affected in the first year and around half by the end of the second year. However, this study was conducted retrospectively on patients attending a tertiary referral centre.

Withdrawal-emergent disorder is that which emerges within six weeks of drug cessation or substantial dose reduction. This again emphasises the tenuous relationship that tardive disorders bear to treatment regimes. One possible exception to this is a phenomenon reported in patients on depots, some of whom describe a few days of restless discomfort in the latter phase of their inter-injection interval, immediately prior to their next injection. The author has certainly not infrequently come across statements by patients or their relatives to the effect that by the pre-injection period they feel they 'need' the next injection, or that the beneficial effects are 'wearing off' because they feel more tense or ill-at-ease. Although drug levels for most depots peak at about four to seven days post-injection, the decline thereafter is gradual, and whether such reports always, or indeed often, represent the evolution of mild withdrawal-emergent akathisia must depend on individual pharmacokinetics and the duration of the inter-injection interval. However, it is a possibility to bear in mind.

Symptomatology developing early in treatment and conforming to the concept of acute akathisia can be durable. This, therefore, maintains an intimate association with alterations in drug regimes and has been referred to as 'acute persistent akathisia'. Such disorder would tend to remain stable on stable treatment regimes, which could, of course, mean that it may endure for many years. Thus, although the onset of akathisia and its relationship to treatment may, for classificatory purposes, characterise disorder as 'acute', one cannot allow the inference that it is therefore of short or limited duration. However, the resolute continuation of such symptomatology would be a legitimate justification for vigorous and imaginative review(s) of medication.

Like other tardive syndromes, tardive akathisia can persist for weeks or years or ease over time. Unfortunately, the relationships between course and time and the eventual outcome are highly variable and none of these elements can be predicted in the individual case. In what proportion of sufferers the disorder may endure, perhaps permanently, remains a mystery, but the possibility of this as an outcome in itself again emphasises the need for close long-term monitoring.

Treatment

As with parkinsonism, the presence of akathisic symptomatology is *not* in itself a sufficient requirement for the instigation of treatment. As always, the decision to treat will be based on a consideration of the clinical impact of the adverse experiences. With acute akathisia, it has to be said that the implications for the patients' well-being and their compliance – both immediate and long-term – are such that some form of active intervention will usually be demanded. In tardive situations, a more considered judgement may be required.

The bulk of the following concerns acute akathisia, for this is what clinical experience and the literature provides most information on. Issues in the treatment of tardive disorder will be touched on latterly.

Modifications of antipsychotic regimes

The first consideration in the management of acute akathisia is not what drug to add. As with parkinsonism, clinicians all too often seem moved to intervene by addition of yet another drug rather than considering in what ways antipsychotic regimes may be modified to achieve the desired effect. To some extent, this is understandable, as having implemented a specific antipsychotic regime – especially one that may be appearing to work – no-one is keen to rock the boat. However, akathisia, once present, will of itself produce big waves that may readily swamp one's little therapeutic vessel!

The first thought should be towards modifying the antipsychotic regime. This may be by means of dose reduction (and there are few patients in whom this is not a possibility) or, slightly more radically, by a change to a drug with a lesser liability – which in practice usually means a less potent compound. In less 'critical' situations, simply holding dose schedules steady for a period of a week or two and then increasing only slowly may sometimes be sufficient. However, the author has never been particularly impressed by the effectiveness of either of the latter two.

These interventions all require a degree of time for benefits to filter through – a week or two at least – and hence will not be the best approach for those with highly symptomatic disorder. But if cautious therapeutic decisions and close monitoring have allowed early detection of mild or early features, they should represent one's initial efforts.

Specific additional medication: first-line approaches

When a specific additional drug is required, *anticholinergics* remain the first choice of most clinicians in the UK at least, although these have become a less popular option in the USA. They were certainly the initial recommendation – often enthusiastically endorsed – in the 1960s, when the question of specific treatment was first raised. Their introduction in this context, however, was on a more empirical basis than their use in the other extrapyramidal syndromes, and their continued widespread use in acute akathisia is even less justified by the scientific evidence than is their use in parkinsonism. At time of writing, only four controlled studies have investigated the efficacy of anticholinergics in acute akathisia (DiMascio et al., 1976; Friis, Christensen and Gerlach, 1983; Adler et al., 1993a; Sachdev and Loneragan, 1993) and only three of these included a placebo condition. To the present time, the widespread use of anticholinergics in acute akathisia is based on controlled data from some 39 patients – and six of these were investigated in a single challenge study! To say that this hardly represents a solid body of scientific evidence is stating the obvious.

It is, of course, also stating the obvious to point out that the sample size on which a scientific finding rests need not be large if the effect is substantial and unequivocal. But this is not the case in relation to the present issue. Overall response rates vary from 21 per cent to 73 per cent, with an average in the region of 45 per cent in all studies and 55 per cent in the controlled ones.

This whole saga illustrates an important issue: namely, that much of what we do in psychiatric practice is a left-over from the days when things were 'done this way because this is the way they're done'. No licensing authority nowadays would sanction the use of anticholinergics for the treatment of acute akathisia on the basis of the available scientific evidence. Yet, because their use is so entrenched, the area is not an obvious one for young researchers to devote their energies to or for funding bodies to support. Few reputations are made out of 'We knew that already' research. In these days of evidence-based medicine, however, such attitudes may not be tenable for long. There is little point in us taking justifiable pride in the firm foundations of some modern psychopharmacological methodologies when such basic practice issues continue to stand on hills of sand.

The above figures may be interpreted as justifying a persistent state of investigative inertia. After all, 50 per cent or so of patients improve. But, of course, 50 per cent do not! The response is not a uniform one, and its predictors and correlates are unknown. One interesting suggestion is that those who do respond to anticholinergics are the patients who also have coincidental parkinsonism (Braude et al., 1983), though this requires confirmation. At a practical level, however, it may provide a rough guide to formulating treatment plans based on the findings of one's assessment examination.

The relative merits of different anticholinergics with particular affinities for subtypes of the muscarinic receptor are also unknown in the treatment of akathisia. However, the principles expounded in relation to parkinsonism are valid here, too.

While British psychiatrists have been impressed by the 50 per cent improvement rate with anticholinergics, colleagues in the USA have been more taken with the 50 per cent failure rate, and exploration of an alternative strategy has been more vigorous there.

In 1983, two reports suggested the possible value of propranolol. The first was a single case report by Wilbur and Kulik (1983), and the second an open study of 12 patients by Lipinski and colleagues (1983). Since then, the efficacy of propranolol has been the focus of a number of studies both open and controlled (Fleischhacker, Roth and Kane, 1990; Sachdev, 1995a), and the impression of many is that this should now be the drug of choice. Relatively low doses, in the range of 20–60 mg per day, seem to be adequate, most appropriately given in a twice-daily regime in view of the drug's short half-life, although a sustained release preparation may achieve the same effect. There is agreement that, if effective, propranolol's benefits show themselves soon after introduction – usually within 48 hours.

A practical schedule, therefore, might be 20 mg b.d., increasing to 40 mg b.d. after 24 hours if no benefit is evident. If after three to five days significant symptomatology persists, a limited trial of three to five days on 120–160 mg per day would be justified. If, however, no clinical improvement can be detected at this stage, the evidence suggests that little will be gained by further dose increments, which, of course, are likely to run into increasing difficulties with side-effects, some of which can be major.

The author has for the last few years been of the American persuasion in the treatment of acute akathisia, favouring the use of propranolol as a first option, particularly in cases without coincidental parkinsonism. However, experience certainly does not suggest miraculous powers. Indeed, reports would not indicate improvement rates much different from those with anticholinergics. In a comprehensive review, Sachdev (1995a) has pointed out the weakness of the literature supportive of the efficacy of beta-blockers. Studies have utilised varying methodologies, making comparisons difficult, and while he acknowledges that the trend of the literature suggests that propranolol may be a useful therapeutic tool, he concludes that 'its earlier promise is unlikely to be borne out '.

A related question is whether or not any benefits are confined to propranolol or may be shared by other beta-blockers. It does appear that any therapeutic effect is centrally mediated (Adler et al., 1991). This conclusion comes from the generally negative effects reported for the less lipophilic compounds nadolol and sotalol and the hydrophilic atenolol. Indeed, there is a suggestion of symptom exacerbation with atenolol. The question of whether benefits are mediated via a particular receptor subtype (i.e. beta-1 versus beta-2) is unclear at this stage, although it does seem that compounds with intrinsic sympathomimetic activity, such as pindolol, are not especially helpful.

Thus, as far as the *evidence* is concerned, there seems little to choose between anticholinergics or propranolol as first-line specific interventions for acute akathisia. The former perhaps have familiarity on their side as well as the possibility of alleviating coincidental parkinsonism, while propranolol is likely to be better tolerated in itself. Whatever one's first choice, the alternative can be held in reserve as a second-line approach in the case of treatment failure.

Other strategies

An alternative approach that has 'face validity' with some clinicians is the use of a benzodiazepine. The rationale is not hard to deduce from what has been said about symptomatology, although whether there is any more specific benefit deriving from the action of benzodiazepines in facilitating GABA inhibition is unclear. The evidence that there is to support the efficacy of benzodiazepines in acute akathisia – specifically diazepam, lorazepam and clonazepam – is largely anecdotal or derived from open studies, so although these compounds may represent a safe and familiar treatment modality, the justification for their use must continue to rest on the basis of clinical practice rather than clinical science. Some practitioners – and patients – may be wary of benzodiazepines because of the unfortunately bad press they have attracted in recent years, but their prescription in this specific situation is an indication for *supervised* use and such concerns should be easily assuaged.

The suggested merits of amantadine in the treatment of drug-related parkinsonism have already been seen, and although its use in akathisia has been even less extensively investigated, there is some evidence supportive of efficacy (DiMascio et al., 1976). However, this is certainly not such that the drug could be recommended for anything other than a third-line trial.

The most radical recent approach to the treatment of drug-related parkinsonism is also pertinent to akathisia – and that is 5-HT$_2$ antagonism. Once again, pursuit of this line has to some extent been hindered by the discontinuation of the best specific probe, ritanserin. However, there is evidence in the literature that ritanserin was an effective and well-tolerated treatment for akathisia, including a small number of cases who had been resistant to conventional approaches (Miller et al., 1990). A less satisfactory antiserotonergic tool, cyproheptadine, has been reported on favourably (Weiss et al., 1995), but in view of potential problems with its use, this should only be considered in exceptional cases.

This returns us once again to the possible role of the new generation antipsychotics. At time of writing, the most detailed data relate to risperidone. Phase III evaluation of this was undertaken on approximately 2000 patients world-wide who were entered into one of three main studies comparing risperidone to haloperidol and a control condition, which in two of the investigations was placebo and in the third an ultra-low dose of the trial agent assumed to be subtherapeutic. As noted in Chapter 4, benefits were evident by a number of methods of assessing extrapyramidal tolerability. Improvements in total scores on the ESRS (see Chapter 11) largely reflected benefits on the 'Parkinsonism–Hyperkinesia Subscore' of the scale which comprises tremor and akathisia. The advantage remained significant for akathisia considered separately (Owens, 1994) and was evident across the dose range (see Fig. 4.9). Thus, it may be that the particular benefits of the new-generation drugs lies in a advantage targeted largely on akathisia.

This apparently focused advantage of risperidone – and presumably the other new-generation drugs modelled on the same principles – needs to be proven against milligram equivalent dose regimes of haloperidol and a range of other standard compounds. The populations in which lower rates of akathisia have been found comprise for the most part patients with established illness and prolonged antipsychotic exposure, so advantage is, strictly speaking, valid only for such patients who switch treatments. Furthermore, it is not possible to say to what type of akathisia the finding best applies. If it stands, however, and can be shown to generalise to other new compounds utilising the combined $5\text{-HT}_{2A}/D_2$ strategy, it will be a practical endorsement of the model and will endow these compounds with particular clinical advantage, which is likely to extend to all forms of akathisia.

The recommendation for clozapine is now firm. Initial reports in patients with established akathisia who were transferred to clozapine were not encouraging, with the suggestion that it may not be associated with any advantage over standard drugs. However, its benefit has now been clearly established. The original confusion undoubtedly arose from inadequate follow-ups (Owens, 1996), which were usually only of one month, so that the assessments were, in fact, including hang-over effects from previous standard antipsychotic medication (an observation which could to some extent vitiate the interpretation of the risperidone data presented above). Longer-term follow-up has shown that, after transfer, features of akathisia do fade, improvements that are evident over about a 12-week period. This literature has not been careful in categorising what variety of akathisia is benefited most by clozapine, although it is likely that the reduced liability extends to both acute and tardive forms.

With regard to the development of akathisia, Kurz et al. (1995) have shown that the cumulative incidence of disorder over a 12-week trial period was 31.7 per cent for patients on haloperidol and 5.6 per cent for those on clozapine.

In view of the profoundly distressing nature of, especially, acute akathisia, clozapine must now be readily considered as an effective treatment option.

The imperative to treat in cases of tardive akathisia may be somewhat diminished in comparison with the acute situation, and the considerations somewhat different. Thus, for example, in the relative absence of distressing subjective symptomatology, one may instead have to take into account the socially embarrassing nature of constant and inappropriate objective behaviours and how these might impede rehabilitation.

It is perhaps as well that the imperative is less pressing, for the options are limited. As shall be seen in relation to tardive dyskinesia, the emphasis is on primary prevention, which is a reflection of the unsatisfactory nature of treatments so far available. Primary prevention accentuates the minimum utilisation of antipsychotics and the constant justification of their use in *all* clinical situations (see Chapter 6) and, although the rightful advocate of sound practice, is a poor substitute for specific therapeutic interventions effective against established disorder.

Where downward antipsychotic dose titration has gone as far as it can and achieved as much as it will for tardive akathisia, each of the measures described for acute akathisia is worthy of systematic evaluation, as are those mentioned for tardive dyskinesia. 'Systematic' does not, of course, mean indefinite, and in tardive akathisia, where the evidence for and likelihood of efficacy are less, the move to a new-generation antipsychotic or clozapine should be a ready one.

An outline proposal for the systematic management of akathisia is shown in Figure 5.4.

Pathophysiology

The pathophysiology of akathisia, acute or otherwise, is unknown. As with the other syndromes described here, the range of drugs, with their varied pharmacologies, that are capable of producing disorder points to either a range of mechanisms or a series of possible inputs into a final common mechanism. In view of the integrated arrangement of brain circuitry, some version of the latter theory is the more likely, but the details remain obscure.

The drugs most frequently implicated in the production of akathisia are once again those which either directly or indirectly interfere with dopaminergic functions, and it is reasonable to conclude that this is a fundamental mechanism underlying development of the disorder. However, a paradox immediately becomes evident: how is it that drugs so regularly associated with the development of motor poverty can also, and within the same dose ranges, cause motor overactivity? The most obvious explanation is probably also the correct one: a different localisation for the different pathophysiological processes (Marsden and Jenner, 1980).

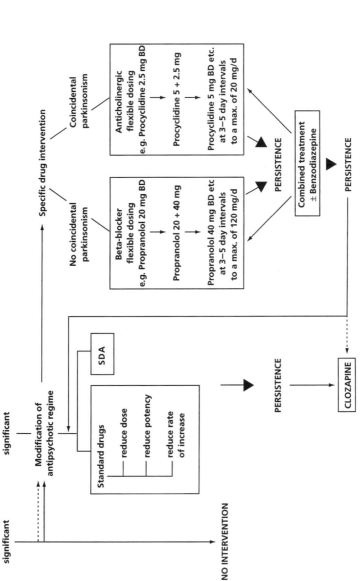

Fig. 5.4. Outline management of akathisia. (SDA, serotonin–dopamine antagonist.)

It has already been seen that parkinsonian symptomatology emanates from blockade focused on nigrostriatal basal ganglia inputs. It is unlikely, however, that a variant of this can explain akathisia (Sachdev, 1995a). While the two disorders can and do occur simultaneously, the correlation for their co-occurrence is rather poor, and the treatment response of one does not necessarily predict a similar response in the other. Furthermore, a substantial body of animal work consistently points to inhibition of motor function as the consequence of disruption to nigrostriatal dopaminergic mechanisms, and although the question of varied symptomatologies dependent on varied affinities for different subtypes of the dopamine receptor within the striatum has not been explored, this does not seem a likely explanation.

The other major dopaminergic pathway has been of interest to psychiatry for a number of years. The mesolimbic/mesocortical system arises mainly from area A10 of the ventral tegmentum and passes rostrally to limbic areas, including nucleus accumbens, septum, olfactory tubercle and amygdaloid complex, as well as areas of limbic cortex, including medial prefrontal, cingulate and entorhinal. Dopaminergic projections within this system are extensive to motor, premotor and supplementary motor regions.

Support for this system as a site for the primary pathophysiological events underlying akathisia is scant, but includes the fact that mesocortical dopamine neurons appear to exert a tonic inhibitory action on aspects of locomotion. Thus, in rats, lesioning of these pathways results in an increase in purposeless motor activity. Such lesions also appear to impede learning on certain cognitive strategies. In addition, Penfield and colleagues, as part of their cortical stimulation studies, noted that a restless urge to move was reported with stimulation of the supplementary motor area, while isolated case reports of accidental injury associated with akathisia have concerned lesions of the prefrontal cortex.

A loss of cortical (especially prefrontal) dopaminergic input from antagonism of mesocortical systems might result in a loss of inhibition at these sites, with a consequent increase in glutaminergic drive to the striatum. This would then be expected to result in an increase of GABA-mediated inhibition of the internal globus pallidus and pars reticulata of the substantia nigra, with the effect of disinhibiting thalamocortical fibres. A more sophisticated model incorporating the effects of several other transmitters has been presented by Sachdev (1995a), to which the carnivorous reader is referred for more meat.

Interest in mesolimbic/mesocortical pathways has to date centred largely on their relevance to the pathophysiology of schizophrenia and as the possible site of antipsychotic drug action. They have not traditionally been considered as a focus of adverse motor events, which is no doubt part of the somewhat naive perception that nigrostriatal systems subserve solely motor and mesolimbic systems solely mental events. This view, so much a bastion of new drug development, is certainly in need of revision (Lidsky, 1995).

The evidence in favour of a mesolimbic/mesocortical site for the pathophysiology of akathisia may be weak but is less damning to this hypothesis than the evidence against a nigrostriatal one. Nonetheless, it is clear that much remains to be understood about the mechanisms underlying this common problem and even commoner, and possibly related, clinical phenomena.

6

Tardive dyskinesia

Introduction

Few topics have so dominated the psychopharmacological literature as has tardive dyskinesia. By any appraisal, however, it was not a topic that psychiatry came to with alacrity or enthusiasm. What, by the 1980s had become a torrent of publications, started life as a little trickle and built only gradually, reflecting the profession's reticence in acknowledging the potential deluge to come.

In the field of tardive dyskinesia, aficionados demonstrate their 'aficionado-dom' by debating on whom priority should be bestowed for publication in the field. The candidate favoured by some is the German psychiatrist Schonecker. In 1957, he described a syndrome of abnormal movements in three elderly chronic psychiatric patients with cerebral arteriosclerosis. The abnormalities consisted of 'automatisms with licking and smacking movements of the lips' (Schonecker, 1957). They were, therefore, orofacial in distribution and complex and recurrent in nature, and occurred in subjects who had all been on chlorpromazine. However, these disorders were reported in patients whose duration of exposure ranged from 'the first days of treatment' to a maximum of only eight weeks. It, therefore, seems likely that Schonecker's patients had acute or initial dyskinesias and not tardive dyskinesia, as this subsequently came to be conceived.

On the basis of conceptual purity it is probably once again Dr Sigwald and his colleagues who should be credited with priority. In 1959, they published a report of four cases of orofacial movement disorder which had remained persistent for up to 27 months after stopping antipsychotic medication. The patients, all of whom were female, were aged from 54 to 69 and none was psychotic. One had an anxiety state, another an obsessional disorder, while the other two had been treated for postherpetic and trigeminal pain syndromes. They had been exposed for only relatively brief periods (8–18 months) and to doses that by modern standards were extremely low (Sigwald et al., 1959).

An increasing number of reports appeared in the Continental literature around this time, perhaps the most influential of which was that of the Danes, Uhrbrand and Faurbye (1960), who, in the first English language publication, provided descriptions that would be recognisable by modern accounts. Their paper was even famously illustrated by images that would become all too common to clinicians in the years to come. They described involuntary movements, which they believed in some instances to be irreversible, occurring in 33 mainly psychotic, long-stay patients. These authors emphasised the 'bucco-linguo-masticatory' predominance in signs, although they did mention, almost in passing, movements in all body parts. The patients had been treated by a variety of physical means, including electroconvulsive therapy (ECT), but despite this Uhrbrand and Faurbye concluded that the outstanding factor amongst their patients was prolonged exposure to what they referred to as 'psychopharmaca'. In fact, although some patients had been exposed to reserpine, what Uhrbrand and Faurbye were unequivocally proposing was the concept of 'antipsychotic-caused' involuntary movement disorder that was durable and possibly irreversible.

The term 'tardive dyskinesia' first appeared in a paper by Faurbye et al. in 1964. The paper comprised a series of descriptions of neurological features associated with antipsychotic drug use. The authors began by describing dyskinetic movements as 'co-ordinated, involuntary, stereotyped, rhythmic' movements and stated that tardive dyskinesia was 'first and foremost characterised by the occurrence of dyskinetic movements'. However, they did have a wider understanding of the boundaries of the disorder than would be acceptable now, stating that '(in addition) tremor and autonomic symptoms may occur'.

Their comments on facial dyskinesia are easily recognisable, but as far as whole-body disorder is concerned, they once again clearly had a wider concept in mind than what today's tighter boundaries would permit. Thus:

> Dyskinesia of the body appears when the patient is standing as swaying to and fro, in some cases with torsions of the body, [with] in [the] sitting position rocking movements and in pronounced cases nodding of the head in the opposite direction of the body movements.

The controversies over the taxonomic position of tardive akathisia were to be for later years.

The authors emphasised the orofacial predominance embodied in the term 'bucco-linguo-masticatory triad' and anticipated the debate on the associational or mutually exclusive relationship with parkinsonism.

They described the variable onset, the fact that features could emerge after many years symptom free, and the associations with high-potency compounds and increasing age. They also pointed out that signs could first emerge in the period immediately following cessation of treatment.

In fact, this early work from Denmark could be read as a summary of the first 25 years in the research life of tardive dyskinesia rather than the announcement of its birth. Perhaps, in a world of scientific censorship, official sanctioning of this paper might have spared us many of the meandering excursions through the back-waters of clinical psychiatric research that characterised so much of the published literature in this field – excursions that on many issues merely ended in us returning to the point of our departure. However, psychiatry being as it is, have theme, will travel!

It is interesting to note the differing trends in perception in the UK and the USA that, in retrospect, the literature on tardive dyskinesia demonstrates. In the UK the topic never fired the research community, despite some important individual contributions. Indeed, it was from the UK that some of the most trenchant attacks on the scientific foundations of the concept were launched. In the USA however, the subject went on to occupy a dominant position in the research litany, in no small part due to the dogged influence of Dr George Crane, who, in an extensive series of publications from 1967 (Crane and Paulson, 1967) in mainly, though not exclusively, the American literature, did more than most to bring the issue to the attention of the wider profession. Indeed, it might be argued that by the mid-1980s the response of some sections of American psychiatry was something approaching professional hysteria!

This mood of pessimism and worry seems to have been as much fuelled by medicolegal as by purely clinical fears, and although the medicolegal issues (to which reference will be made later) remain largely unresolved in most jurisdictions, the mood has changed somewhat. This probably reflects partly the demonstration that the prognosis for tardive dyskinesia is less relentlessly negative than was at one time thought, and partly the perception of progress in the development of new compounds that may conceivably deflate the magnitude of the problem.

The meanderings of the literature over the first couple of decades resulted in modification of the concept of tardive dyskinesia in more or less all of its essentials (Table 6.1). It might, therefore, be of some interest to explore the nature of the concept in the context of the literature over these early years. This may, in addition, provide some awareness of why, at one point, it was possible – and, indeed, necessary – to challenge its scientific foundations and why epistemologically it may still have its limitations.

Table 6.1. *Early modifications to the concept of tardive dyskinesia*

Criterion	Constituent movements	Distribution	Implicated drugs	Duration of exposure
Initial proposal	'Any abnormal (hyper-)kinesis Choreiform Athetosis/dystonia Tics Ballism Myokymia Tremor	Whole body	Antipsychotics (reserpine)	6 months–2 years
Modification	Removal of tremor	'Orofacial' and 'tardive' become synonymous	Widening of classes: tricyclic antidepressants antihistamines anticonvulsants antiemetics benzodiazepines BUT NOT L-dopa	Elasticity: weeks–indeterminate time

The concept of tardive dyskinesia

A useful starting point in the investigation of any concept might be the literal meaning of the name given to it. We might, therefore, begin by asking what 'dyskinesia' and 'tardive' actually mean.

Prior to its incarnation in the present context, 'dyskinesia' did not have much of a existence within neurology. Some years ago, the author undertook a search of the published literature for the meaning of 'dyskinesia', in order to embellish with a morsel of precision an otherwise somewhat factually barren review. As it turned out, it might have been a more productive use of time to have searched out the meaning of life! The term was infrequently and then variably applied without specific definition, a practice that psychiatry seemed simply to have adopted. 'Dyskinesias' were the sorts of disorders that were called 'dyskinesias'! The author then submitted to one of the world's leading experts a six-line definition, carefully honed from both the literature and, by then, some degree of clinical experience. The response was tactful but devastating. Forget my efforts at precision. 'Dyskinesia' in its generic sense, one was informed, meant 'any abnormal kinesis'- no more, no less! The author's own wit told him that this (with due deference) could not be entirely acceptable, as the bradykinesia of parkinsonism – the opposite from the current focus – would also be covered by such a definition. The implication would have to be more specific to have clinical utility. In fact, usage seemed to be restricted to '*hyper*kinesis', which implied that the disorder of movement was characterised by motor activity that was additional to the norm in either type or degree (i.e. a sort of 'positive' motor pathology) and unequivocally *involuntary* in nature.

It was certainly the case that, according to the literature, most clinical varieties of involuntary movements – tics, chorea, athetosis/dystonia, myoclonus, ballism, myokymia – were to be found as part of tardive dyskinesia. However, there was a notable exception. Marsden and colleagues (1975) wrote: 'Tremor, however, does not occur as a part of this syndrome'. Presumably, although it was unstated, tremor was ex-communicated on the grounds that its presence in such patients represented coincidental parkinsonism. Be that as it may, the most common hyperkinetic disorder of all was out, to the detriment of our modified generic definition.

The roots of 'tardive' are straightforward enough. It comes from the French 'tardif', meaning 'late' or 'late in the day'. In the present context this was, of course, meant to delineate the disorder from those other extrapyramidal disorders that came on soon after exposure. It is important to appreciate that the idea of 'lateness' of onset was significant as a defining characteristic because the early literature used very similar terminology to describe what we now call acute dyskinetic, especially dystonic, abnormality as it did for tardive disorder. Indeed, the idea of a 'bucco-linguo-masticatory triad' originally applied to reversible signs of sudden onset in the first two or three days of exposure.

Just when 'early' became 'late' was never clear and always arbitrary. Faurbye et al. suggested a minimum of six months' continuous exposure, although the bulk of the literature favoured something more in the region of a year or two (Ayd, 1967). However, it was not long before movements were being called 'tardive' after only a few weeks – occasionally days – of exposure (Chouinard and Jones, 1979).

A further change that took place was that authors increasingly forgot Uhrbrand and Faurbye's account of disorder in all body parts and focused more on the most obvious manifestations, that is, the orofacial. Crane and Naranjo (1971) provided a series of neurological definitions pertinent to the issue of adverse effects of antipsychotics, in which they stated: 'Complex dyskinesias are the most common disorders observed in long-term patients and are often referred to as tardive dyskinesias'. They did mention that peripheral movements could be found in psychiatric patients, but their description gave clear emphasis to slow, 'complex' repetitive orofacial activity. In particular, they separately defined and described chorea, athetosis, tics etc. from 'complex' or 'tardive' dyskinesias.

Thus, the topographically descriptive term 'orofacial' and the aetiological one 'tardive' became confusingly confused. Much of the early descriptive literature continued this trend of concentrating on the lower third of the face, a tendency that was only really reversed by the widespread introduction of standardised rating scales that incorporated whole-body evaluations.

Perhaps the most fundamental assault on the original concept came with a widening of the classes of compound that became implicated as putative aetiological agents (see Chapter 2). Although 17 of Uhrbrand and Faurbye's patients had been treated at some time with reserpine, only one patient had received this alone, all the others having also had conventional antipsychotics. These data emphasised the original idea of antipsychotics as being the essential causative agent, but reports began to appear implicating other classes of drug also. These included tricyclic antidepressants, anticonvulsants, antihistamines, antiemetics – and even benzodiazepines (Kaplan and Murkovsky, 1978).

It was becoming increasingly difficult to see in what pharmacological way these diverse compounds could be accommodated in a unified aetiological theory, although dopaminergic antagonism still seemed the most obvious. It had been clear for some time, however, that other drugs with psychotropic properties and that altered dopaminergic function could cause a similar clinical problem. These were the dopamine agonist psychostimulants and L-dopa. Although involuntary movements associated with L-dopa use tend in general to have a

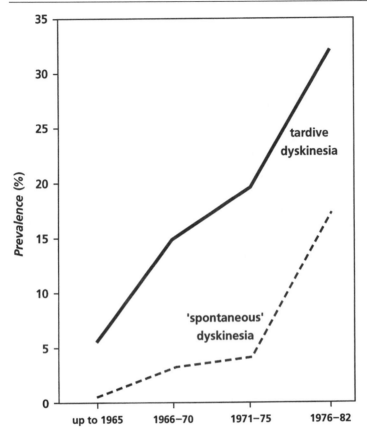

Fig. 6.1. The mean prevalence of 'tardive dyskinesia' in antipsychotic-treated patients, and 'spontaneous' dyskinesias in antipsychotic-free patients over time.

more peripheral distribution than those of tardive dyskinesia, at a clinical level the two can be indistinguishable.

Thus, dopamine antagonist drugs with central (psychotropic) actions were not necessary for the pharmacological production of disorders of this type. In fact, there was an increasing recognition that drugs themselves were not necessary, as similar involuntary movements were to be found in a variety of clinical situations in which drugs could *not* be implicated (Brandon, McClelland and Protheroe, 1971). Awareness of these so-called 'spontaneous dyskinesias' was, by the early 1980s, resulting in prevalence figures for these that were comparable to figures from some studies inferring drug-related pathology and the rates of increase over time were comparable (Fig. 6.1). Spontaneous disorder probably accounted for some of the reported associations, especially with tricyclics and benzodiazepines, where the drugs themselves were probably coincidental and played no aetiological role.

It was, and indeed is, difficult to accommodate these elastic components within a single conceptual definition. Nonetheless, these were 'the facts' as the foundation literature told us. Therefore, a definition based on this literature might be along the following lines:

> Tardive dyskinesia is a syndrome comprising most, but not all, types of involuntary movement developing more or less anywhere in the body, which have been caused by exposure to many, but not all, types of psychotropic medication (and a few other classes of drugs besides), from a period of at least 6 to 24 months but in fact from several weeks to a indeterminate number of years.

This is clearly somewhat cumbersome to commit to memory, especially for the pre-exam trainee engaged in the task of assimilating a host of facts. It might, therefore, be simplified thus: 'Tardive dyskinesia is what authors of papers on tardive dyskinesia believe it to be'.

The point is not as flippant as the mode of expounding it. Tardive dyskinesia is an *epidemiological* concept whose validity rests on a statistical association – namely, that between the development of specified involuntary movement disorders on the one hand and exposure to certain pharmacological agents (antidopaminergics and in particular antipsychotics) on the other. There are, as shall be seen, sound data of a *statistical* type to justify the validity of the concept at the correlational level. If we really wish to advance our understanding of the nature of the problem, however, we need to be more ready to acknowledge the limitations of the concept and not simply its strengths. This is a point expounded in more detail in Chapter 8.

Clinical features

Tardive dyskinesia is different from the other syndromes discussed above in that, unlike them, it appears to have no elusive or easily over-looked or misattributable subjective symptomatology (Fig. 6.2). Indeed, while patients may complain bitterly and understandably about their motor disorder, what is often striking is how *little* they complain about abnormality that for most of us would be intrusive, unnerving, and profoundly socially embarrassing (Alexopoulos, 1979; McPherson and Collis, 1992). The reason why this should be is unknown, though it has often been pointed out that this phenomenon of insouciance is most frequently observed in chronic schizophrenic patients. Possible reasons why the subjective symptomatology of tardive akathisia might diminish are noted above, and any of these

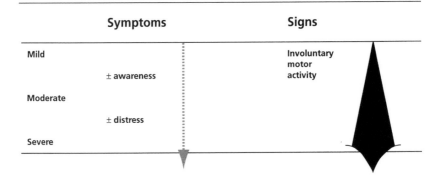

Fig. 6.2. The balance of symptoms and signs in tardive dyskinesia.

might be pertinent to tardive dyskinesia in general. In addition, however, there is evidence that such lack of awareness in tardive dyskinesia may correlate with cognitive impairment (McPherson and Collis, 1992).

The author has not infrequently come across indifference amounting to total lack of awareness in institutionalised patients, who, even on prompting, quite regularly seem to remain oblivious to gross disorder, but is less sure that the phenomenon occurs to the same degree in the non-institutionalised. These patients may, indeed, not offer any spontaneous complaint, but seem more ready to acknowledge their signs when specifically asked, even if they express less than expected concern.

No data have been generated to address the issue of subjective awareness in institutionalised versus non-institutionalised schizophrenic patients as such, though there is evidence that the presence of tardive dyskinesia may be associated with reduced likelihood of discharge from long-term care (Kucharski, Smith and Dunn, 1980), which, rather than reflecting social factors, may again be associated with deficits in cognition. It would be of interest to evaluate the question of whether awareness can be seen to emerge with developing re-socialisation.

In assimilating the following, summarised in Table 6.2, the reader is advised that it is to some extent a caricature – or, perhaps more accurately, a composite. The impression of a systematic progression in the development of signs is misleading. Symptomatology may progress logically or unpredictably, slowly or with alarming speed, or may never extend beyond an initial target area. In reality, no written account can do justice to the variety and bizarreness of the permutations possible, and the reader is heartily advised to use those presented here as no more than a scaffolding on which to rest his or her own observations.

Conventionally, texts present the tongue signs first, with the statement that it is here that disorder starts or can be detected in its mildest

Table 6.2. *Summary of the major clinical features of tardive dyskinesia*

Tongue	'Vermicular' movements (no displacement)
	Displacement on one or more axes (rotation, lateral movement, 'tromboning')
	Extension beyond dental margin
	Irregular sweeping of buccal surface ('bon-bon' sign)
	Irregular non-recurrent protrusion ('fly-catcher' sign)
Jaw	Mouth opening
	Lateral deviation
	Anterior protrusion
	Chewing
	Grinding
Lips	Pursing
	Puckering
	Sucking
	Smacking
	Retraction of lateral angles ('bridling')
Expression	Blepharoclonus
	Blepharospasm (partial/complete – sustained/spasmodic)
	Elevation/depression of eyebrows
	Furrowing of forehead
	Grimacing
	Conjugate eye deviation (tardive oculogyrus)
Head/neck/trunk	Torti-/antero-/retro-/latero-collis
	(Tics)
	Lateral/anteroposterior displacement ('Pisa syndrome')
	Shoulder elevation/shrugging
	Axial hyperkinesis ('copulatory' movements)
Upper limbs	Hyperpronation
	Wrist/elbow flexion/extension
	Metacarpo-pharyngeal flexion/extension ('piano playing')
	Finger filliping
	Lateral outsplaying
	Exaggerated arm swing

Table 6.2. (*cont.*)

Lower limbs	Adduction/abduction
	Flexion/extension hips/knees/ankles
	Ankle rotation
	Inversion/eversion
	Lateral 'outsplaying' of toes
	Flexion/extension of toes
Internal musculature	Dysphagia
	Irregular/audible respirations
	'Dyspnoea'
	Spontaneous vocalisations
	grunting
	moaning
	Speech disorders
	dysarthria
	'nasal' speech
	irregular phrasing
	'staccatto speech' (adductor spasm)
	'breathless whisper' (abductor spasm)

or earliest manifestations. As a general statement, this has some merit in that abnormalities of the lower third of the face (including the tongue) are the commonest. In addition, it has been shown that ratings of questionable abnormality are more frequent in the tongue and that such ratings more often than not turn up as 'definite' abnormality within six months (Kane et al., 1980). However, the above caveat applies and the primary justification for starting with the tongue in descriptive accounts is order.

Worm-like or vermicular movements *in* the tongue are reported as the earliest signs of pathological change. These distort the shape of the tongue, and impart to its surface a low-grade writhing or 'infested' appearance resembling a 'bag of worms'- albeit a small one! The contours seem to ripple or expand and contract with irregularly episodic or more constant small-amplitude movements, but the structure remains bedded on the floor of the mouth and its axes are not displaced. This occurs as choreoathetoid disorder becomes established, when unpredictable displacement can be seen in all three axes – vertical, longitudinal and lateral – though the tongue at this stage remains within the dental margin. This displacement does not substitute for the vermicular movement, but is superimposed on it. The tongue may irregularly curl either backwards on the shaft or under it, or laterally at the margins.

These movements are not restricted to the periphery and the shaft itself may arch independently. The whole structure may twist on its longitudinal axis, or be jerkily displaced laterally, or develop forward/backward movement. This latter action, which may be best observed in the active state of voluntary protrusion, is sometimes called 'tromboning'. Such constant or erratic movement is often perceived as distressing by the patient and may be the focus of spontaneous complaint, though whether this is because of the nature and the site of the disorder or the fact that it tends to occur early in the evolution of the syndrome is unclear.

Progression leads to extension of involuntary activity beyond the dental margin. Thus, the tongue may irregularly abut on the inner surface of the lips, especially the lower lip, in either a repetitive motion to the same point below the mouth or in a sweeping motion upwards from the gingival space towards the mouth. This gives the picture so often reproduced by ham actors attempting to emulate the behaviours of the edentulous elderly. Characteristically, the tongue balloons the cheek on one side or the other and sweeps the inner buccal surface. This can make patients look as if they are manipulating solid material in their mouth and, for the early descriptive writers, the analogy of a sweet seemed the most obvious. This is, therefore, sometimes referred to as the 'bon-bon' sign.

Subsequently, involuntary activity is extended out of the mouth, with the tongue forcibly extruded, sometimes in the mid-line, though more commonly to one side or the other. These movements are invariably associated with some degree of rotation and may be slow and writhing (i.e. dystonic) in nature or jerky and irregular (i.e. choreiform). Rapid, darting tongue protrusions, repetitive but forever changing, were frequently described in the era of encephalitis lethargica, when they were referred to as the 'fly catcher' sign, an apposite term which, to anyone with a passing knowledge of natural history, conveys the essence of the disorder. The term has also been used for the phenomenon in tardive dyskinesia.

Constant involuntary activity of this sort has the effect of a regular lingual work-out, so the tongue, over time, may assume a corrugated appearance from development of individual muscle groups. Eventually, it may become generally hypertrophied and appear to have outgrown the oral cavity. When not engaged in their relentless cycle of activity, such large, beefy tongues are often to be seen hanging limply from the corners of passively open mouths.

Jaw movements take the form mainly of chewing, or grinding movements, so they usually combine elements of involuntary opening and closure of the mouth. The lower jaw, where the disorder resides, may show activity that is restricted to upwards and downwards movement of varying speeds, although frequently there is in addition a component of lateral deviation which, when present, is invariably slow. Alternatively, the mouth may be maintained forcibly open in a grotesque and petrified 'yawn'. Anterior protrusion may also occur, which is again usually a slow and sustained action. Grinding movements resembling bruxism can result in profound damage to the teeth, especially the molars. The author recalls with regret a middle-aged woman whose perfect back teeth were reduced to hideous, painful stumps in only six months. It is of interest, however, that patients with rapid opening/closing movements do not seem to 'chatter'. Such movements appear to be executed on a partially open mouth. It is furthermore interesting to note that jaw movements rarely inflict trauma on the tongue, which, as already mentioned, may itself be abnormally enlarged. This illustrates both the relative slowness and especially the co-ordinated nature of these movements.

The other area to be involved in this complex is the perioral musculature. The lips may purse and/or pucker into sucking movements or the lower lip may be curled outwards, and the lateral angles of the mouth may be irregularly retracted in unison. These angular movements resemble the effects of the bridle on a horse's mouth and are accordingly sometimes referred to as 'bridling'. Occasionally, perioral and other facial involvement may have audible consequences in the form of clicks, smacks and puffing sounds, though such noises often result from dyskinesias affecting internal muscles.

This, then, is a descriptive 'skeleton' of the bucco-linguo-masticatory triad. It will be clear, however, that the 'buccal' component is largely a passive effect of involuntary activity elsewhere, especially in the tongue. The cheeks hardly deserve inclusion to the exclusion of the lips, and the 'triad' could perhaps more accurately be re-christened 'labio-linguo-masticatory'.

This complex of movements is conventionally referred to descriptively as comprising disorder that is 'choreoathetoid' in type. Choreiform movements have the characteristics of being rudimentary, non-co-ordinated and repetitive but non-recurrent (that is, they do not as a rule repeat in the same place over and over). This is clearly quite the opposite of what we see in the bucco-linguo-masticatory triad. The movements here are complex, co-ordinated and almost predictably recurrent – in the undisturbed state, the same cycle often repeating itself ad infinitum.

What one seems to get in the orofacial component of tardive dyskinesia and some other dyskinetic states is something subtly different, something resembling a 'package' of disorder in which severity is gauged more by the extent of involvement than by how bad each individual part is. Furthermore, the whole appearance has a somewhat 'passive' quality to it. This may seem a bizarre statement in view of the above descriptions and the reference to the potential for distress. However, the situations in which tardive movements provoke little or no awareness are usually those in which orofacial disorder predominates (Rosen et al., 1982). Peripheral abnormalities are, as a rule, far more poorly tolerated. The 'passive' nature of the disorder is highlighted when compared to those suffering from primary facial dystonias. To witness someone in this situation is a distressing experience all round; one can almost 'feel' the forces distorting the face into its hideous, anguished expressions.

There may be merit in being pedantic on this point because phenomenologically there is, in fact, nothing 'abnormal' about the orofacial movements of tardive dyskinesia. In another context and voluntarily instigated, as for example during eating, they would be perfectly normal. What is abnormal is their expression in inappropriate circumstances and without willed execution. The impression conveyed by tardive orofacial movement disorder – and it is nothing more than an impression – is that the involuntary movements represent a 'release' phenomenon, in which the entire template for a complex pattern of motor activities of common phylogenetic origins is laid vulnerable to release from tonic inhibition, a process whose progression is mirrored in the extension of symptomatology.

The phenomenological distinction between this sort of disorder and what is conventionally seen in the context of neurological disease has recently been highlighted, though in a way that, from a psychiatric perspective, draws us back into the maze. Stacy, Cardoso and Jankovic, (1993) have described the commonest movement type in tardive motor disorders as 'tardive stereotypies', present in 78 per cent of patients. This takes us back to Rogers' 'conflict of paradigms' argument (Rogers, 1985), that what is seen by psychiatrists and neurologists is essentially the same, but with a different interpretation placed on it via the different paradigms our separate traditions foster (i.e. 'tramlining'). The interesting twist to the tale now is that, at a time when psychiatry is espousing more of the neurological paradigm, certain strands of neurological opinion are donning the conceptual clothing we have discarded! While the quality of 'difference' in many of these drug-related movement types is important, dressing up old terms in reject clothing has, in the author's opinion, only the potential to confuse.

The point on the nature of the movements comprising especially the orofacial component of tardive dyskinesia is of more than theoretical interest, however, because it raises questions about the validity of highly detailed multi-item approaches to recording disorder and the rules that must be adopted to enhance this. Clearly, in order for the tongue to extend beyond the dental margin, the jaw must part, and for it to be protruded out of the mouth altogether, the same must apply to the lips. Should, then, these integral movements also be rated along with those of the tongue, or should ratings concerning the mouth and lips be restricted to the sort of grinding or puckering etc. described above – activity that is clearly qualitatively different? These matters have not been addressed in the literature as yet, but could perhaps do with some ventilation.

The other musculature of the face to be affected is that of expression. This involves elevation and/or depression of the eyebrows, furrowing and wrinkling of the forehead, blepharoclonus and blepharospasm, each in isolation or all in harmony. Oculogyric spasms occurring as part of a tardive syndrome have already been mentioned, although this is rare.

The effect of involvement of the muscles of facial expression can be highly disfiguring, with a composed expression rapidly and unpredictably transformed into surprise, disapproval or an intimidating bared-teeth grimace. Movements of this sort produce socially inappropriate signals, which can be readily misinterpreted. One of the author's young male patients made nursing colleagues very nervous indeed because of his frankly intimidating demeanour. At interview, an air of imminent and indiscriminate homicide sat ill with sweet replies and accommodating behaviour. The young man had, in fact, a partial blepharospasm with sustained partial spasm of orbicularis oculi and leaden eyebrows correspondingly depressed, which accounted for his lowering appearance of menace. Beneath this neurological exterior of intimidation dwelt a psychological pussy cat!

Abnormalities may also involve the axial/truncal muscles and the limbs. Movements evident from involvement of the large antigravity postural muscles of neck and trunk are overwhelmingly dystonic in type and more often sustained, as opposed to intermittent or spasmodic (see below). Thus, distortions of posture are common and easily overlooked or misattributed. All varieties of disturbance in normal head/trunk relationships can be found (torti-/retro-/antero-/latero-collis), with compensatory postural change where appropriate.

Axial dystonia – the so-called Pisa syndrome – has already been mentioned. This may take the form of unilateral disorder (or disorder with a unilateral predominance) with a truncal lean to one side associated with a degree of rotation that advances the shoulder on the opposite side. Bilateral disorder results in an accentuated lumbar lordosis and a backwards lean. Both these situations displace the centre of gravity and can seriously interfere with gait. This is especially so with bilateral disorder, which gives the patient a most bizarre appearance that once again is easily mistaken for 'mickey-taking'. The major problem it presents for patients is the instability it introduces into walking, which has to be compensated for by increasing the length of step. Instability is most marked in situations in which the patient is unable to increase step length, such as in going down stairs. One of the author's patients had to be transferred to a ground-floor ward as he became reluctant to use the stairs after keeling over backwards once too often.

Limb girdle involvement can result in dystonic abnormalities but in the upper girdle, in addition to sustained disorder or shoulder shrugging, tic-like movements can sometimes be seen affecting shoulder, neck and up into expressive facial muscles. In the pelvis, dystonia predominates and may in this location be spasmodic. The rhythmic, thrusting and sometimes rotatory pelvic movements of axial hyperkinesis have already been mentioned, as has their passing descriptive resemblance to copulation. Patients with this unpleasant disorder can frequently be seen with their arms folded tightly over their abdomen or with one arm held thus, resting the elbow of the other arm in that hand while the hand caresses the face. Far from conjuring images of copulation, the demeanor of such patients brings more to mind Tam o' Shanter's wife in Burns' poem, who sat at home 'nursing her wrath to keep it warm'. These arm positions seem to be used as symptom-relieving 'antagonistic gestures', of which more in Chapter 7.

The limbs can fall victim to an almost infinite range of involuntary motor activity, some of which is readily recognisable in terms of the descriptive type of movement, some of which defies rational description, far less classification. The arms may hyperpronate statically or in spasmodic bursts and may flail unpredictably in typical ballistic movements. Alternatively, they may be held in bizarre, statuesque poses. One man maintained his right arm in a perfect 90-degree flexion when he walked, with a clawed hand extending before him.

Shock-like myoclonic jerks may also unpredictably displace arms (or legs). Dystonia of the whole limb may produce a constant writhing, twisting motion, exhausting to watch. Flexion/extension and rotations at the wrist, finger filliping, extension and lateral separation of the fingers (so-called 'outsplaying'), non-harmonious flexion/extension of the fingers ('piano-playing' movements) and many, many more can be found in isolation or combination. Rudimentary choreiform jerks may also be seen.

The legs may similarly demonstrate every permutation of involuntary motor disorder, some examples of which have already been alluded to. These include flexion/extension and abduction/adduction movements at the hip, lower leg movement from activity around the knee, and especially distal disorder such as squirming ankle rotations, inversion/eversion, dorsiflexion/plantarflexion and flexion/extension and 'outsplaying' movements of the toes comparable to those that can also affect the fingers.

Finally, it is important to remember that internal groups may be affected, including oropharyngeal and laryngeal muscles as well as intercostals and diaphragm. Involvement of these muscles can give rise to some of the most dramatic, and indeed sinister, symptomatology of tardive dyskinesia. Dysphagia can result from a disconnection between the voluntarily instigated component of swallowing and the automatic, or from the establishment of an action dystonia in oropharyngeal muscles (Gregory, Smith and Rudge, 1992). Choking, with the very serious risk of inhalation, can occur (Feve et al., 1993) and death may occasionally ensue.

Laryngeal adductor spasm distorts speech into a shrill, strident screech, while involvement of the abductors gives rise to 'breathless' whispering. One middle-aged woman who was a patient of the author was admitted with a mass of tardive movements, including adductor spasm, which convinced a fellow patient that she was a witch and the nurses that she was 'at it'. The author was never quite convinced that his efforts at education overcame the view of the former that her dramatic improvement subsequently was due to 'magic' or of the latter that it was because she had 'pulled herself together'.

Speech may be less obviously affected at a number of levels, with the evident disorder dependent upon the pattern of oropharyngeal, laryngeal and diaphragmatic/intercostal involvement. Random involuntary intrusions can result in irregular articulatory breakdowns similar to so-called hyperkinetic dysarthria, and temporal disorganisation showing in an erratic rhythm (Gerratt, Goetz and Fisher, 1984). Vocalisations may, in addition, appear dull, lacking intonation and 'nasal'.

These functional consequences of motor disorder have been relatively little investigated in comparison to the vast number of descriptive topographical studies, but clinicians ought to be aware of the major impedance they can present to communication and re-socialisation.

Once again, though, a little care in challenging the obvious can sometimes be fruitful. Communication between nursing staff and one elderly woman the author encountered on a long-stay ward had ceased for some time. The woman had a gross orofacial dyskinesia with a massive and constantly protruded tongue, whose ceaseless movement apparently rendered her highly nasal speech incomprehensible. 'She might as well be speaking a foreign language', the Charge Nurse told me. In fact, she was! The lady hailed from the Isle of Lewis in the Outer Hebrides and at some point and for some reason had reverted to her native Gaelic. Her diction in English, which she could speak fluently but chose not to, was not of the best, but certainly rendered her more understandable to Londoners than her mother tongue.

Diaphragmatic and/or intercostal involvement can give rise to loud respirations, hyperventilation and dyspnoea (Weiner et al., 1978;

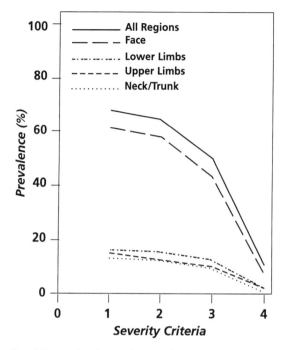

Fig. 6.3. Regional prevalences of involuntary movements at different criteria on AIMS. (From Owens et al., 1982, with permission.)

Greenberg and Murray, 1981)) with irregular rhythm and grunts, groans, sighs and other rudimentary vocalisations. Respiratory dyskinesias have been estimated to affect about 16 per cent of patients with tardive dyskinesia and may be the cause of significant alkalosis (Rich and Radwany, 1994).

Orofacial signs are characteristic in tardive dyskinesia but by no means universal. However, approximately 60–80 per cent of sufferers will show orofacial symptomatology (Fig. 6.3). The above account might have seemed to suggest some differences in the descriptive types of movement comprising orofacial disorder and those of an alternative distribution, differences that could point to a lack of homogeneity within the syndrome. There is, indeed, evidence that this may be the case. Multivariate statistical techniques applied to rating data have consistently shown that orofacial and limb/trunk items cluster separately, suggesting that the syndrome comprises at least two components (Kidger et al., 1980; Glazer et al., 1988; Gureje, 1989; Inada et al., 1990; Brown and White, 1992; Bergen, Kitchin and Berry, 1992). The orofacial component appears to be more strongly correlated with advancing age or illness factors, whereas limb/trunk abnormalities seem to relate more to treatment variables. It may be, therefore, that peripheral disorder represents more of a primary drug phenomenon, while the role of drugs in the former is more a promotional one in the context of other predisposing factors. This is something that will be returned to later.

As with parkinsonism, the movements of tardive dyskinesia can be predominantly or exclusively unilateral in their distribution (Waziri, 1980). Clearly this is more likely with appendicular movements, although it can be relevant to some manifestations of facial disorder as well. This has been the focus of some interest in that a predominance of right-sided disorder may point to biological predisposition in the dominant hemisphere (Wilson et al., 1984). However, it seems that the 'predominant' side for movement disorder is not fixed but can be found to alter with serial evaluations (Egan et al., 1992b). At present, it seems unlikely that any specific extrapolations from a poorly understood clinical observation can help us much.

The totality of tardive dyskinesia can never be fully captured on the written page. The diversity of movements to be found in this syndrome and the distorted appearances they impart to the normal control and flow of movement are infinite and literally indescribable – or so it seems to this practitioner. Indeed, the author has attended 'expert' round tables which took the form of a sort of quiz in which consensus was attempted on video presentations – with limited result! The 'amateur' need feel no diffidence in an awkward inability to categorise particular disorder precisely. At a clinical level, this may not matter too much. To some extent, the imperative for the clinician is to acquire the ability to see that *something* is there to be seen, and to appreciate its implications, rather than to possess the descriptive power to be confident of exactly what it is that has been seen!

Operationalised criteria for tardive dyskinesia

In the context of akathisia, the fact that tardive symptomatology can be either treatment emergent or withdrawal emergent was referred to. These concepts are particularly pertinent to tardive dyskinesia. Involuntary movements diagnosed as 'tardive dyskinesia' may either emerge during a period of continuous antipsychotic exposure or in the immediate period following discontinuation or dose reduction. Alternatively, established (treatment–emergent) disorder may exacerbate in intensity after dose reduction or cessation. However, the precise relationship between these two presentations is unclear.

It is logical to assume that involuntary movements that only emerge on discontinuation of antipsychotic (or antidopaminergic) medication probably reflect a milder or less immutable pathophysiology, and in line with this is the fact that withdrawal-emergent dyskinesias more readily resolve and are the predominant abnormalities found in children, in whom they seem inevitably to remit in the absence of re-exposure (see Chapter 9). It may be, therefore, that dyskinesias that become evident on drug withdrawal represent simply a milder or early form of what, with perseverance, becomes emergent on persistent exposure.

However, the situation may be more complex, as illustrated, for example, by the fact that movements emerging first on discontinuation of drugs may occasionally persist and remain unamenable. The author was referred a 32-year-old woman with mild learning disability whose drugs had been reduced following the observation of slight hyper-pronation of the right arm. Within a month, she had developed a pro-found and disabling dystonia with ballism affecting the entire arm, which was unaffected by a return to her original regime.

Reference has already been made to the variable and inconclusive time criteria that have been used to characterise movement disorder as 'tardive', something which creates a major hurdle to the exposition of standardised criteria for disorder. The most widely utilised operation-alised criteria for tardive dyskinesia are those of Schooler and Kane (1982), which do incorporate a minimum time criterion for exposure of three months, a figure that is essentially empirically derived (Table 6.3). The use of such criteria is nonetheless valuable in imposing some degree of standardisation, which permits more reliable cross-study compari-sons. As was mentioned in the context of similar criteria for akathisia, they can also be commended for imposing a more rigorous standard to routine practice.

Modifying factors

At various places in this volume, emphasis is put on the inti-mate relationship between extrapyramidal symptomatology and the mental state. This point is again made here, not only because it is rele-vant to all syndromes, but because it has particular relevance to tardive dyskinesia. Considerable variations in the severity of disorder can be evident, depending on the psychological climate at the time, and, indeed, movements otherwise latent may emerge only during times of alteration in mental status.

In effect, the determining factor is the degree of 'arousal' the patient is experiencing at the time. The psychological concept of 'arousal' is somewhat more technical than what is necessary for our purposes, but the more alert or anxious patients are, the greater they perceive others' expectations of them to be; the more pressurised or generally 'stressed' they are – the higher their 'octane' levels – the more evident

Table 6.3. *The Schooler and Kane criteria for tardive dyskinesia*

Prerequisites	1. At least three months cumulative antipsychotic exposure (continuous or discontinuous)
	2. Abnormal movements of at least 'moderate' severity in one or more body parts *or* of 'mild' severity in two or more body parts on any standardised recording instrument
	3. Absence of another potentially causative disorder
Diagnoses	
(a) Probable	Fulfills 1.–3. above on a single examination
(b) Masked probable	Fulfills 1.–3. above at first examination but fails to fulfill 2. above at a second examination within 2 weeks of dose increment or re-introduction of drug
(c) Transient	Fulfills 1.–3. above at first examination but fails to fulfill 2. above at second examination within 3 months with no increase or re-introduction of drug (dose reduction permissible)
(d) Withdrawal	Does not fulfill 2. above while on medication but fulfills 1.–3. above within 2 weeks of stopping drugs of average half-life or 5 weeks with long half-life preparations (depots, diphenylbutylpiperidines)
(e) Persistent	Fulfills 1.–3. above at first examination and over at least a 3-month period.
(f) Masked persistent	As in (e) Fails to fulfill 2. above within 3 weeks of dose increase or re-introduction of drug

any disorder will be. By the same token, if the subject is relaxed and composed, involuntary motor activity will be less evident and, if drowsy, whether naturally or via sedation, will be at its lowest ebb. All the movements with which we are concerned here disappear during sleep.

This inherent variability is a crucial element to bear in mind, especially in making serial evaluations. A vulnerable patient sitting quietly in a chair may be considerably discomforted by the simple event of a stranger walking into the room; an interview with an unknown doctor may precipitate the patient into emotional overdrive. In other words, the incidental that may seem trivial to you, may not seem so to a patient, and this must be taken into account in systematic ratings. This emphasises the importance of a period of unobtrusive assessment as an integral part of the examination procedure (something mentioned again in Chapter 10).

It may be that psychological factors underlie the observation that there is a definable diurnal variation to the movements of tardive dyskinesia, with disorder, especially limb–truncal, greater in the afternoon than in the morning (Hyde et al., 1995), though this may, of course, reflect other factors. It is clear, however, that the value of serial ratings as a true representation of the measurable disorder is greatly enhanced if examinations take place at the same time each day. Because of severity fluctuations that occur in relation to changing blood levels throughout the depot cycle, it has further been advised that serial ratings in those on long-acting injectables should be conducted at a standard time in the inter-injection interval (Barnes and Wiles, 1983).

The whole question of the impact of will and willed actions on dyskinetic movements is complex, as has been alluded to. Even at quite advanced levels of severity, patients can usually exert willed control over their involuntary movements when asked to do so, though only for limited periods. The duration of time for which they can do this does not seem to relate simply to the degree of severity. Similar, often total, control can be seen during the initial engagement of active attention when concentration is maximal. Thus, patients may show considerable disorder in the course of a routine conversation, which disappears when they ask for and listen to the repeat of a point they did not catch or when they are temporarily distracted by an event external to the interview, only for disorder to return fully formed with return of the routine. Descriptive accounts of tardive dyskinesia often note this negating action of will almost as a blanket effect, but it seems to the author that it is with the complex, co-ordinated orofacial dyskinesias that this phenomenon is seen most predictably and in most complete form.

The conventional wisdom is that specific intentional action in a distant muscle group will bring out or 'activate' involuntary movements in another body part, and a range of so-called 'activation' procedures has been described which form an important component of the standard examination technique (see Chapter 10). As a general rule, this is no doubt valid, but the facilitation and suppression of involuntary movements are more complex than this simple rule would imply. It is probably only a valid rule with 'activating' tasks that are as rudimentary as possible – in other words, that involve minimal cognitive input. The more active attention and concentration require to be recruited in their execution, the more unpredictable the response is likely to be. In particular, any action involving a degree of concentration is likely to have a marked suppressant effect on movements of dystonic type. Indeed, it has frequently been commented on that patients with dystonias can be seen to exhibit gross disorder in the waiting room that melts away in the consulting room, simply because of the attention the patient is paying to the interview. Activation techniques are, as shall be seen, important to perform, but not without care in their choice or with immutable preconceptions as to the result.

Those 'youngsters' using the Abnormal Involuntary Movement Scale (AIMS; see Chapter 11) might nowadays be somewhat bemused to note its section on the patient's dental status. This is a throw-back to an issue of some debate at the time when the scale was devised and which may not yet have entirely run out of steam. There is little doubt that the edentulous state can of itself be associated with the development of complex, involuntary orofacial movements of the type described above (Sutcher et al., 1971). It has been postulated that this results from a loss of mandibular proprioception following disruption of position sense fibres located around the the root apices.

Many chronic schizophrenic patients have long since parted company with their natural teeth and there was at one time quite a discussion concening the extent to which this fact could account for their orofacial dyskinesias. Schizophrenics are not, of course, the only ones nowadays who bid farewell to their teeth at an early age – the majority of people, in the West at least, do too. Yet one is not aware of hordes of aimlessly gnashing jaws within the populace in general. One must reasonably conclude that, in the absence of other factors, the edentulous state of itself is not a major aetiological contributant to our present problem. However, there is evidence that it may contribute by way of modification (Woerner et al., 1991; Bergen et al., 1992). In one of our studies, females were, somewhat surprisingly, less likely to have their own teeth than males, a factor that correlated with severity of their disorder. Thus, it could be that the widely replicated finding of more severe disorder in older females than in older males (see below) could be partly influenced by such an incidental factor. For those interested in trying to unravel the many remaining mysteries surrounding drug-related (orofacial) movement disorders, attention to dental status may not be an entirely foolish waste of time.

There was also at one time an argument, based largely on theoretical considerations, that the relationship between tardive dyskinesia and drug-related parkinsonism was one of mutual exclusion. This is clearly not the case, though there is evidence of reciprosity. Increasing antipsychotic doses have the potential to suppress the movements of established tardive dyskinesia, and the likelihood of an antipsychotic achieving this may relate to its liability to produce parkinsonism – lower symptomatology in the former being at the price of higher symptomatology in the latter (Nordic Dyskinesia Study Group, 1986). Whether what is in effect symptom 'masking' provides a complete explanation for the suppression phenomenon is unclear, but it does shout loud for the requirement that all evaluations of extrapyramidal status be comprehensive and emphasises the need for current and recent drug regimes to be taken into account in interpreting data on tardive dyskinesia.

Diagnosis

There is no specific laboratory or other investigation into which the clinician can retreat to make the diagnosis of tardive dyskinesia on his or her behalf. As has been noted, the concept is an epidemiological one and the diagnosis in the individual case therefore rests on the exercise of probabilities. On balance, is it probable that antidopaminergic (and specifically antipsychotic) medication has contributed to the clinical presentation and, if so, are you sufficiently confident to convey that opinion to the world via the inference of your diagnosis? The important point is the diagnostic inference, for the term 'tardive dyskinesia' carries *specifically* the implication of a role for these drugs in causation. It follows, therefore, that one cannot talk of 'spontaneous tardive dyskinesia'. This is simply a nonsense, which betrays either an alarming level of conceptual ignorance or a cavalier disregard for the importance of terminology that is equally disquieting.

The major step in establishing a reasonable level of probability is a review of the psychiatric diagnosis. It has been known for the best part of a century that a range of organic disorders can present with schizophreniform symptomatology, often years in advance of physical signs, and that a number of these are disorders in which involuntary movements form an integral part. Huntington's disease is probably the most frequently encountered in a psychiatric context. Carriers may present to psychiatric services with a range of mental state disorders, especially paranoid ideation, many years before the emergence of movement and other neurological disorders. In this situation, the prior use of antipsychotics may, as a consequence of a suppressant action of the drugs, actually delay the appearance of involuntary movements, while the development or exacerbation of these signs following reduction or withdrawal of medication may cement the opinion that the emergent movements are drug related. This is an uncommon scenario, but is one that is nonetheless worthy of remembering.

Some of the major conditions that might be associated with involuntary movements are listed in Table 6.4.

Invoking once again the principle of sparrows and cockatoos, these conditions are to the jobbing psychiatrist very much of the cockatoo – if not the bird of paradise – variety. Once in a while, however, the exotic may fly past your window. During the course of a survey of a long-stay schizophrenic population (the Shenley Study, see Chapter 8) of a large psychiatric institution, the author came across a middle-aged woman frequently and variously used for teaching purposes to demonstrate mannerisms *or* tardive dyskinesia. The woman did, indeed, present a bizarre appearance. She walked in a remarkable mimic of a chicken, weight-bearing on the balls of her feet, with a left-sided lean and buttocks protruded hindwards, steatopygia–like. She had long been noted to be 'unsteady' and stabilised herself with a stick. On closer examination, however, she had a clumsy, broad-based gait, coarse nystagmus, bilateral pes cavus and markedly diminished jerks in the lower limbs. Mannerisms she most definitely did *not* demonstrate – but tardive dyskinesia? Buried in 30 years of case records was the history that her father had died of 'spino-cerebellar degeneration'. Although conforming to operational criteria for schizophrenia and believed by some to demonstrate neurological consequences of its treatment, a hereditary neurodegenerative disorder of the Friedreich's type was a much more likely explanation of her physical signs.

A thorough physical re-appraisal is important in psychotic patients who develop involuntary movements on specific medications, but this can be undertaken in the reasonble expectation that the findings are likely to be non-contributory.

Epidemiology

Figures on the prevalence of tardive dyskinesia originally crystallised out of those epidemiological studies that also sought to establish the validity of the concept. The technique used was the retrospective 'pooled data' method, a sort of elementary precursor to the more sophisticated metanalysis. Essentially, frequency figures were extracted from all those studies conforming to basic predetermined criteria in which patients had and had not been treated with antipsychotics, and a simple mean was calculated for each group. The 'pooled' average from the drug-treated sample gave the prevalence, and a statistically significant increase over the figure for drug-naive samples supported the validity.

The technique was a valuable but crude investigative method, with a number of inherent weaknesses. The first is that it was largely applied

Table 6.4. *Major conditions associated with involuntary movements (excluding tremor)*

Hereditary	Huntington's disease
	Wilson's disease
	Benign hereditary chorea
	Dystonia musculorum deformans
	Tuberous sclerosis
	Familial calcification of the basal ganglia
	Hallervorden–Spatz disease
	Neuroacanthocytosis
Infective	Sydenham's chorea
	Encephalitis lethargica
	HIV
	Spongiform encephalopathies
	Viral encephalitides
	Abscess
	Tuberculoma
Metabolic	Hyperthyroidism
	Hypoparathyroidism
	Electrolyte disturbance
	hyper/hyponatraemia
	hypocalcaemia
	hypomagnesaemia
	Hypoglycaemia
	Hyperglycaemia (including non-ketotic hyperosmolar states)
	Porphyria
	Neurometabolic disorders
	Lesch–Nyhan syndrome
	lysosomal storage disorders
	amino acid disorders
	Leigh's disease
	other inborn errors of metabolism
Immune	Systemic lupus erythematosus
	Sarcoid
	Behcet's disease
	Polyarteritis nodosa
Toxic	Alcohol withdrawal
	Carbon monoxide poisoning
	Heavy metal poisoning

Table 6.4. (*cont.*)

Vascular	Infarction (including transient ischaemic attack)
	Haemorrhage
	Arteriovenous malformation
	Migraine
Neoplasm	Primary
	Metastatic
Trauma	Closed head injury
	Subdural/extradural haematoma
Miscellaneous	Senile chorea
	Multiple sclerosis
	Parkinson's disease
	Progressive supranuclear palsy
	Multisystem atrophy
	Idiopathic torsion dystonia
	Tic disorders (including Gilles de la Tourette syndrome)
	L-dopa responsive dystonia
	Post-thalamotomy
	Edentulous oromandibular dyskinesias
	Mannerisms/stereotypes
	Pregnancy (chorea gravidarum)

to data from strikingly heterogeneous populations that varied in terms of gender composition, residential status, diagnosis and treatment characteristics, amongst others. Indeed, some studies did not even concern patients as such, but elderly nursing home residents. Furthermore, as the boundaries of the condition were unknown, or at least not agreed upon, exactly what different authors had understood by the concept was open to wide interpretation. Finally, even if a modicum of validity could be allowed for, the lack of standardised recording methodology left reliability in the lap of the Gods.

Notwithstanding these very major problems, Kane and Smith (1982) undertook a comprehensive review of the published literature and calculated that the mean prevalence of involuntary movements from samples exposed to antipsychotics was significantly greater than the prevalence of spontaneous movement disorders in drug-naive samples (Table 6.5). These figures were comparable to those of other studies around the time that used a similar methodology (e.g. Jeste and Wyatt, 1981a), and became widely accepted.

From the early 1980s, prevalence figures for presumptive tardive

Table 6.5. *Prevalence of involuntary movement disorders in antipsychotic treated and untreated patients (pooled data method). (After Kane & Smith, 1982.)*

	Sets of data	n (approximate)	Prevalence (%)
Antipsychotic treated	56	35 000	20 ($\pm$ 14)
Antipsychotic untreated	19	11 000	5 ($\pm$ 9)

$p < 1 \times 10^{-5}$.

dyskinesia began to rise strikingly, with figures frequently reported in the range of 40–50 per cent, and occasionally higher. There were several reasons for this. Firstly, these data comprised an element of disorder that was cumulative within the 'at-risk' population. In other words, a baseline of chronic disorder present early in the history of the condition was 'added to' by new cases developing over time. Furthermore, the 'at-risk' population was itself expanding. Some studies, on the other hand, restricted their focus of interest to particular high-risk groups, such as the elderly, and hence understandably found higher prevalences.

Most importantly of all, however, was the fact that from the early 1980s, the published work increasingly utilised standardised recording schedules. These had two effects. The first was to force investigators to consider mild degrees of disorder equally with the more obvious, and the second was to ensure a comprehensive, whole-body evaluation. In some of the author's own work, the prevalence of involuntary movements increased by about 50 per cent from an initial examination, which used a simple dichotomised present/absent recording method, to follow-up of the same sample, in which a standardised recording scale was used. This increase was largely attributable to greater awareness of mild and largely peripheral disorder.

This illustrates once again an important lesson of life: namely, that learning by rote 'the' prevalence figure for tardive dyskinesia is in reality a bit of a waste of time, for no such figure exists, and any single figure without qualification is not only meaningless but potentially misleading. The prevalence of tardive dyskinesia is crucially dependent on both the sensitivity and the comprehensiveness of one's assessment procedure (plus a number of population variables considered later). The 'raw' prevalence figure may be useful as an aid to free communication, but its limitations *must* be appreciated.

Clearly, the ideal way to establish the prevalence of tardive dyskinesia would be to undertake evaluation of defined populations with different treatment histories using standardised techniques and operationally agreed criteria for abnormality. Two such large-scale studies were published in the early 1990s (Table 6.6) and, notwithstanding the concerns about the validity of data derived by the 'pooled' method, they came up with strikingly similar figures. They found in drug-treated patients an overall prevalence for tardive dyskinesia in the range of 20–25 per cent (Woerner et al., 1991; Muscettola et al., 1993).

The study of Woerner et al. (1991) resuscitated some interesting questions. Within their large group of schizophrenic patients, the authors found an effect of site (Fig. 6.4). Those treated in voluntary facilities had a prevalence of 13.3 per cent, while for those in state hospital care the figure was 36 per cent. The obvious interpretation of this is differing treatment patterns, with those in state facilities in the USA simply being more aggressively managed. But an alternative worth bearing in mind is that those who end up in such settings may have more 'severe' or 'different' forms of illness that in some way render them more vulnerable to neurological adverse effects.

In relation to groups *not* exposed to antipsychotics, the authors also made an interesting observation. Overall, they found the prevalence for spontaneous dyskinesias to be only about half that reported with the 'pooled data' method – i.e. 2.6 per cent. The group that did have a prevalence of around 5 per cent was that comprising geriatric inpatients. The conclusion here was that the involuntary movements in these physically ill patients were developing on some sort of 'neuromedical' template – some physical change that predisposed them to movement disorder. The questions of predisposition in relation to features of the illnesses for which antipsychotic drugs are given are returned to in Chapter 8.

These and other point prevalence studies in recent years have reported in terms of percentages conforming to operational criteria. This, of course, does mean that with inclusion of mild or equivocal disorder, the total percentage of any patient group evidencing any signs at any one time will be higher, such as was the case in studies from the 1980s noted above.

While prevalence is an important figure to bear in mind, what is perhaps of greater interest is incidence. This is necessary for attributing the risk to any individual over time, all other factors being equal (in reality an impossible requirement). Although several groups have addressed the issue of incidence (Gibson, 1981; Kane et al., 1982; Yassa and Nair, 1984; Chouinard et al., 1986; Gardos et al., 1988b; Waddington, Youssef and Kinsella, 1990; Table 6.7), figures have varied, no doubt on the basis of heterogeneous sampling and methodology, small sample sizes and relatively short follow-up intervals. It is only in recent years that large-scale, good-quality incidence studies have been published.

Table 6.6. *Prevalence of tardive dyskinesia: summary of two large point prevalence studies*

Study	Sample	Recording method	Criteria	Prevalence (%)	Comment
Woerner et al. (1991)	2250 mixed diagnoses + non-psychiatric and normal elderly	Modified (28 item) Simpson + AIMS	Schooler & Kane single assessment (severity confirmed by second rater) 'presumptive' in 95%	23.4 ($n = 1441$) (c.f. 'spontaneous' 2.6%, $n = 809$)	OFD only: 43% psychiatric patients 85% geriatric patients Correlates: age gender age/gender interaction duration of exposure site
Muscettola et al. (1993)	1651 mixed psychiatric older patients (78% > 40 years)	AIMS	Schooler & Kane + ve patients re-examined after 3 months 'persistent'	19.1	OFD: 13%, only 11% on high doses Correlates: age age/gender interaction high doses longer duration combined antipsychotic and anticholinergics

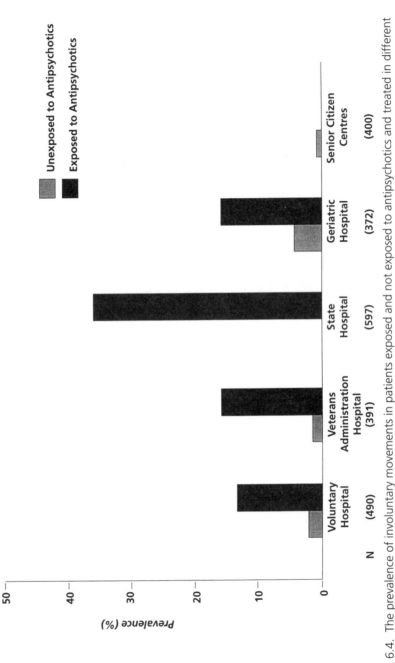

Fig. 6.4. The prevalence of involuntary movements in patients exposed and not exposed to antipsychotics and treated in different settings. (Reproduced with permission from Woerner et al., 1991.)

Table 6.7. *Studies of the incidence of tardive dyskinesia*

Study	n	Follow-up (years)	5-year risk (%)
Gibson (1981)	343	3	⩾ 24.4
Kane et al. (1982)	554	7	17.8
Yassa & Nair (1984)	108	2	17.5
Chouinard et al. (1986)	131	5	35.1
Gardos et al. (1988b)	15	7	28.3
Waddington et al. (1990)	38	5	42.1

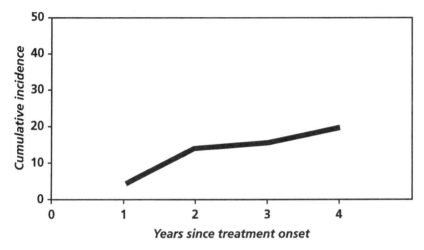

Fig. 6.5. Incidence of tardive dyskinesia in first-episode schizophrenia patients. (From Chakos et al., 1996.)

Two groups, one at Yale and the other at Hillside Hospital, New York, have produced comparable figures. They suggest that the annual incidence figure for tardive dyskinesia is in the region of 5 per cent from populations predominantly but not exclusively comprising patients with schizophrenia (Morgenstern and Glazer, 1993). Although movement disorder was operationally defined by both these groups, the majority of such disorder appears mild and apparently non-progressive.

However, such populations are not only diagnostically heterogeneous, they also comprise patients at different stages of illness and hence of treatment. Of greater interest clinically would be the incidence in first-episode patients. Data bearing on this question have recently been provided from a four-year follow-up of the Hillside cohort of first-episode schizophrenics (Chakos et al., 1996; Fig. 6.5). These show a

Table 6.8. *Estimated risk of persistent tardive dyskinesia (%) in the context of prior exposure. (After Glazer et al. 1993, with permission.)*

Years of prior exposure without tardive dyskinesia	Additional years of exposure				
	5	10	15	20	25
0	32.7	45.8	53.8	60.2	64.7
5	19.4	31.3	40.9	47.6	
10	14.2	26.7	35.0		
15	14.0	23.7			
20	11.3				

cumulative incidence for presumptive and persistent tardive dyskinesia respectively of 6.3 per cent and 4.8 per cent at one year and 17.5 per cent and 15.6 per cent at four years.

The Yale group has produced useful theoretical projections from its data on patients of mixed durations of illness (Glazer, Morgenstern and Doucette, 1993). On the basis of a sample of over 360 patients, the group calculated the likelihood of individuals developing tardive dyskinesia in the future, in relation to the number of years they had already been exposed to antipsychotics *without* developing disorder. This exercise reveals three things (Table 6.8). The first is that the theoretical risk in the first five years is, by this method, somewhat higher than would be expected from that observed in purely first-episode samples. The other two points are perhaps of greater interest. Over a 25-year period of exposure, the risk is *very* high, at more than 60 per cent. This is of interest in view of the fact that some of the earlier prevalence figures reported in long-stay populations were in this range (Owens, Johnstone and Frith, 1982) but at the time were criticised as being impossibly high. The third point to emerge from the Yale projections is that even after many years problem free, a not insubstantial risk remains.

Predisposing factors

The retrospective literature

Great effort has been expended in the retrospective literature in attempts to establish factors predisposing to the development of tardive dyskinesia, but while many have been called (Table 6.9), few have been chosen.

None of the variables relating to antipsychotic drugs has been conclusively shown to predispose. This is perhaps less surprising than at first

Table 6.9. *Factors proposed as predisposing to tardive dyskinesia (retrospective literature)*

Drug-related	Non-drug related
Type of antipsychotic (potency)	Age
Maximum daily exposure	Gender
Duration of exposure	Past physical treatments
Cumulative exposure	Leukotomy
Polypharmacy	Insulin coma
Antipsychotic blood levels	ECT
Antipsychotic-free intervals	'Organicity'
Previous EPS	Lateral ventricular enlargement
Anticholinergics	Cognitive impairment
Alcohol	Negative schizophrenic states
	Affective disorders
	Age at first exposure
	Metabolic disorders
	Diabetes
	Phenylketonuria

sight. A major consideration in interpreting this finding is the quality of the data. Anyone who has ever tried to work out precisely what a patient has been prescribed – let alone what he or she has taken – in the previous month will appreciate the problems of extending such an exercise back over 30 years. Furthermore, any relationships with drug variables may not be direct or linear, an assumption behind most of this work. Finally, associations that are weak may be lost in overzealous attempts to produce precise but ultimately arbitrary classifications of drug exposure.

Some recent attempts have pointed more consistently towards an association with drug variables, but to some extent such retrospective efforts are flawed from the start. Just because no clear relationships with antipsychotic variables can be inferred from this literature, however, does not mean that no such relationships exist. The meaning of this statement will become clear below.

An obvious candidate for predisposition would be unduly high antipsychotic blood levels. Wide interindividual differences in plasma antipsychotic levels, sometimes in the range of 100-fold, have been known for some years and are amongst the factors confounding investigation of dose–response relationships with these drugs. A current contender for explaining some of these differences is heterogeneity of genotypic expressions within the hepatic cytochrome system. However, no clear associations have been established between high plasma drug levels or variability in the P450 system and the likelihood of developing tardive dyskinesia (McCreadie et al., 1992b; Arthur et al., 1995).

The association with drug-free intervals emerged at a time when the idea of antipsychotic drug 'holidays' was widely advocated. The finding was that the best discriminator between patients with reversible tardive dyskinesia and those in whom it was persistent was the number of drug-free intervals of at least two months or longer, which was greater in the latter group (Jeste et al., 1979). The implication was that increasing numbers of drug-free intervals increased the risk over patterns of treatment that were continuous. The authors of this report provided an elegant theoretical explanation of their finding based on the electrophysiological principle of 'kindling'.

Despite subsequent replication with the 'off' period as low as one month (Branchey and Branchey, 1984), the issue did not penetrate clinical practice. Drug 'holidays' fell from fashion for purely practical reasons. Nonetheless, although this association came from retrospective methodology, it has long seemed to have resonance with the author's clinical experience, which has bred some worry about those whose therapeutic interventions are episodic. Whether this relates to 'kindling' or some other neurophysiological principle, or to characteristics of the illness itself in such non-compliant patients needs clarification, but it is still an observation that deserves to carry more weight with clinicians than it has hitherto. Recently, animal studies have found that rodents discontinuously exposed to antipsychotics show a significant, protracted increase in oral activity, a putative marker for tardive dyskinesia, compared to animals continuously exposed (Glenthoj et al., 1990), providing further presumptive evidence of a link. Most powerful of all, however, is the fact that the initial retrospectively derived observation appears to be gaining prospective support, as will be seen.

A previous history of extrapyramidal disturbance associated with the use of antipsychotic drugs has long been suspected and is certainly logical and in keeping with the common-sense view that vulnerability is vulnerability. Supportive evidence has been slow to accrue and has not come from retrospective investigation. However, the concern has been expressed that akathisia may represent a particular forerunner of later tardive dyskinesia (DeVeaugh-Geiss, 1982), though, while seeming increasingly likely, the issue remains to be resolved.

According to the predictions of the most widely held theory of pathophysiology (see below), anticholinergics should represent a clear predisposing factor. However, although anticholinergics may exacerbate the choreiform manifestations of the disorder, especially orofacially, there is no balance in the literature in favour of a primary role for these drugs in predisposition.

Alcohol abuse has recently been reported as predisposing in some

Table 6.10. *Gender ratios for tardive dyskinesia over time. (After Yassa & Jeste, 1992.)*

Decade	F:M
1960s	1.6:1
1970s	1.3:1
1980s	1.2:1

patients (Dixon et al., 1992) and although we have already seen that alcohol may in itself be associated with the development of involuntary movements, especially in withdrawal, it is not yet clear whether its role in tardive dyskinesia is a primary one or relates to some other common factor such as poor compliance and hence intermittent exposure.

Age is the one factor that stands out in this literature (Kane and Smith, 1982). Not only does the frequency of disorder increase with increasing age, it seems likely overall that so too does severity. In addition, there is considerable evidence that established disorder is less likely to reverse the older the patient is, especially if over the age of 40.

There has been much comment on the apparent consensus that tardive dyskinesia seems commoner in females, with a F:M gender ratio from early 'pooled data' of 1.6:1 (Kane and Smith, 1982). Some elegant theories, such as the sensitising effects on dopamine systems of circulating oestrogens, have been suggested to explain this observation.

It may not be necessary to go to such lengths, however, as this finding may not reflect a primary association. A female excess was certainly a frequent, though not universal, finding of the earlier studies, which were largely performed in long-stay, inpatient samples. Such samples tend to comprise a larger proportion of females who are on average older than the males (Owens and Johnstone, 1980). Furthermore, an interesting observation, little commented on generally but raised above, is that female schizophrenics, in the past at least, appear to have been more heavily treated with antipsychotics than males. The reasons for this would be fascinating to know but have not been explored, and whether the finding would stand today is unclear. However, the issues surrounding the use of milligram equivalents in males and females was mentioned in the context of acute dystonias. If treatment variables are important (see the prospective data below), this could be another factor in explaining the reported female excess. A further interposing effect in terms of age at first exposure is noted below. It is of interest that reviews of more recent literature show a clear narrowing of the overall F:M ratio (Yassa and Jeste, 1992: Table 6.10).

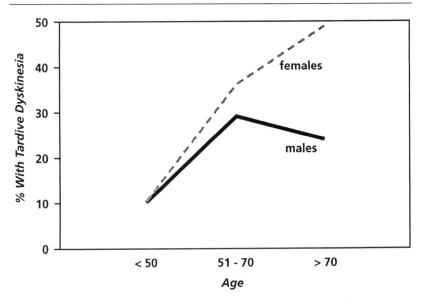

Fig. 6.6. Tardive dyskinesia: relationship between gender and age. (From Yassa and Jeste, 1992.)

What gender may do is interact with age and, in addition, severity. There is evidence that disorder may be more common in older females than in older males (Fig. 6.6). In one of our own studies, this relationship was most striking in relation to *severe* disorder (Fig. 6.7). In the youngest patients, severe disorder (AIMS single symptom criterion of 4) was confined to males, whereas in the older subjects, 85 per cent with severe disorder were female, a pattern also found by others. A continuing rise in the frequency of disorder in elderly females is compatible with prediction, but the fall-off in prevalence in elderly males, particularly of severe disorder, remains to be explained.

Past physical treatments had relevance in their own right at one time, but are mainly of importance now in relation to the question of whether organic brain change is a predisposing factor. Because of the varied treatment histories evident within the large sample that comprised the long-stay Shenley study, it was possible to address the role of such past physical treatments comprehensively. Many of those initially studied had been subjected to the three major modalities – insulin coma, ECT, and leukotomy – singly or in combinations, often over many years, while others had never received any. None of these treatments provided a basis for predisposition (Owens, Johnstone and Frith, 1982). This was surprising in that the degree of residual brain damage sometimes associated with, specifically, leukotomy could be substantial. One woman investigated with CT had a massive area of infarction on one side,

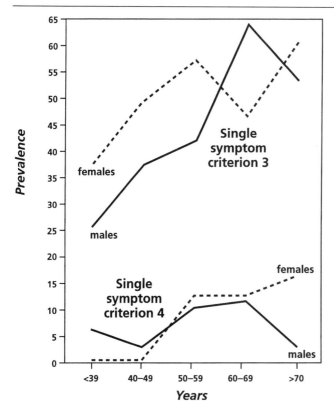

Fig. 6.7. AIMS: prevalence of involuntary movements by age at single symptom criterion of 4 and 3 in both genders.

compatible with postoperative spasm in the distribution of the internal carotid artery, yet had *no* objective neurological signs. Furthermore, she had the fourth highest score on cognitive testing in a sample of over 500!

Much of this literature is bedevilled by varying ideas of what constitutes the 'organic', but overall it has proved difficult to confirm what would seem intuitive: namely, that structural brain damage provides, as a general principle, predisposition to the development of drug-related involuntary movements.

A small literature does exist using imaging techniques, especially CT, to explore directly brain structure in patients with tardive dyskinesia. For obvious reasons, work of this sort is not easy to do in that, to some extent, if the patient can co-operate sufficiently to allow images of adequate quality to be taken, then his or her disorder is unlikely to be of degree that will show much. The author's group is one of the few to have found a significant relationship between ventricular–brain ratio (VBR) on CT and the presence of involuntary movements (Johnstone et al., 1989). While this remains one of the largest studies of the question to date, the balance of evidence does not as yet support structural change as a predisposing factor in patients with tardive dyskinesia. Better-quality (especially MRI) studies that apply volumetric and regional analyses are certainly required.

A different order of inference concerning the likelihood of brain disorder comes from cognitive testing, and here there is some evidence of an association pointing to heightened risk. A relationship with cognitive impairment does not stand as a unanimous finding, but has been reported sufficiently frequently to be of potential validity (Owens and Johnstone, 1980; Wegner et al., 1985; Waddington and Youssef, 1986; Waddington et al., 1990). A more recent suggestion is of an association with deficits on, specifically, tests of frontal lobe function (Waddington et al., 1995).

However, impaired cognitive performance may not be independent of another mental state variable for which a similar association has also been found, namely the 'negative' schizophrenic state. There is evidence that both cognitive impairment and involuntary movements may comprise integral parts of the 'negative' mental state complex (Owens and Johnstone, 1980; Crow, 1980), though once again a relationship between negative symptomatology and tardive motor disorder is not a universal finding (Iager et al., 1986).

This work addresses one aspect of an area of investigation that has been seriously overlooked in the literature on tardive dyskinesia, and that is the role of illness as opposed to treatment variables in predisposition. The above would point to aspects of the pathophysiology of the schizophrenic process as lending an element of risk in themselves (see Chapter 8). However, evidence from the USA would strongly suggest that rates of tardive dyskinesia may be higher in those with affective disorders than in patients in other diagnostic categories (Gardos and Casey, 1984).

There are several points to make in resolving these apparently contradictory observations. The first is that the association with affective disorders seems somewhat less robust than a decade ago, but even allowing for that, if the association with drug-free intervals noted above is valid, then this is likely to have a bearing, as affective disorders are par excellence disorders characterised by an episodic course and intermittent treatment patterns. Furthermore, involuntary movements are more likely to develop the older the patient is when first exposed to the offending medication (Yassa et al., 1986b; see Table 6.9), and, of course, affective disorders tend to have a later onset – and hence a greater likelihood of later first exposure to antipsychotics – than schizophrenia. This latter point could also account for some of the female excess reported in the literature, as the average age of onset of schizophrenia is significantly later in women than in men.

A further point to keep in mind is simply that the clinical Kraepelinian distinctions we adhere to today may bear little relation to the biology of the functional psychoses, with more similarities at the biological level shared by affective and schizophrenic psychoses than the dichotomous system of classification would suggest. This is a fairly radical suggestion, but one that has cropped up periodically over the last 20 years and one for which it is possible to make a convincing argument.

An addendum to the affective disorders story is that in these conditions tardive dyskinesia can sometimes express itself in a state-dependent fashion, being evident only during one phase of the bipolar cycle. The usual association reported is with depressed phases, the dyskinesias (with predominantly orofacial distribution) easing or disappearing during manic states or periods of euthymia (Cutler et al., 1981; dePotter, Linkowski and Mendlewicz, 1983). However, other relationships have also been described (Bhugra and Baker, 1990) and it is hard to know what such relationships tell us.

The author's single experience bears only indirectly on the issue in that the patient, a middle-aged man, had no apparent history of antipsychotic exposure so either had spontaneous disorder or involuntary movements related to tricyclics and/or lithium, which is unlikely. During phases of profound depression, he showed pronounced orofacial dyskinesia, which resolved completely when he was euthymic. To confuse things further, he suffered from a unipolar disorder!

Convincing evidence has been put forward in recent years indicating that patients with diabetes mellitus have an increased risk of developing tardive dyskinesia over the rest of the 'at-risk' population (Ganzini et al., 1991). One study has also suggested that children handicapped by phenylketonuria may present higher rates, but this was based on a very small sample (Richardson et al., 1986). Nonetheless, it does raise the possibility that generalised brain trauma consequent upon systemic metabolic disturbance may form a fertile substrate for the development of involuntary movements in a climate of dopaminergic antagonism.

If biological predisposition is taken seriously, it is surprising that the literature (prospective as well as retrospective) has so underplayed the role of genetic factors. There is reference to concordance for the presence or absence of tardive dyskinesia within families (Yassa and Ananth, 1981), though this is slim evidence indeed. The role of inherited predisposition is supported by associations with a positive family history of schizophrenia but not acquired damage in the form of obstetric complications (O'Callaghan et al., 1990; McCreadie et al., 1992a). This important issue clearly requires further exploration.

The author's experience of possible genetic 'programming' relates to a single pair of middle-aged identical twin sisters with schizophrenia,

Table 6.11. *Factors predisposing to tardive dyskinesia (prospective literature)*

Drug related	Non drug related
Antipsychotic dose	Age
prior to onset	Affective disorders (unipolar)
subsequent to onset	Alcohol abuse[†]
High potency[†]	Tremor[†]
Duration of exposure[*]	Race (Afro-Caribbean)
Drug-free intervals	
Prior EPS (especially akathisia[†])	

[†]In the elderly.
[*]Inverse relationship

long-term residents of the same ward, who both demonstrated an out-wardly similar pattern of tics, orofacial dyskinesias and bizarre backward 'kicks' in their walk. A systematic evaluation of these fascinating women was one of the many 'must dos' the author never quite did, indolence now much regretted.

The prospective literature

Clearly, the ideal way to establish factors predisposing to the development of tardive dyskinesia is by prospective methodology (Table 6.11). Few studies to date have adopted a sufficiently long time span and design complexity to tackle the questions, and what we currently have comes mainly from the work of the Yale and Hillside groups.

Both these groups confirm the strong relationship with advancing age. In addition, the Yale study clearly established a link with antipsychotic dose (Morgenstern and Glazer, 1993) This is an important finding and one that, although requiring confirmation, ought to be incorporated into all our management plans. Furthermore, this group also found an inverse relationship with duration of exposure, compatible with the non-linear risk noted above. It was, in addition, found that those of Afro-Caribbean origins had a greater risk than those of Caucasian origin. Indeed, in their sample, being black almost doubled the incidence rate for movement disorder (Glazer, Morgenstern and Doucette, 1994).

This touches on the area of racial difference, which is something the literature has largely ignored. In addition to the above, there is evidence of lower rates in Asian compared to Caucasian populations (Yassa and Jeste, 1992; Table 6.12). This mainly relates to Chinese patients, though in one Singapore sample, mixed Asian groups all had approximately

Table 6.12. *Geographical distribution of tardive dyskinesia. (After Yassa & Jeste, 1992.)*

	North America	Europe	Asia	Africa and Middle East
Prevalence (%)	27.6	21.5	16.6	25.5
F:M ratio	1.3:1	1.35:1	1.1:1	1.0:1

half the prevalence of Westerners, but numbers in the latter group were small (Tan and Tay, 1991).

Perusal of three studies adopting comparable methodology point to differences in treatment practices as the obvious explanation for reported racial differences, such as the use of clozapine and low doses of standard drugs in China, and high-potency and largely depot-based regimes in the predominantly Negroid population of Curacao (Table 6.13). The issue is nonetheless in need of systematic exploration.

The Hillside data confirm prospectively an association between the development of tardive dyskinesia and drug-free intervals. This is now an issue of sufficient concern to be discussed with patients and relatives when considering long-term treatment recommendations for both schizophrenia and recurrent affective disorders unresponsive to mono-therapy. This group's findings also support an association with an affec-tive (unipolar) diagnosis, though, by way of explanation, the same comments pertinent to this observation in the retrospective literature are also pertinent here.

A particular finding of note from the Hillside work is confirmation of the relationship between prior EPS and the development of tardive motor disorders. Over a five-year period, the incidence of tardive dys-kinesia was twice as great in those with acute/intermediate EPS as in those who had never shown these features. In a sample of elderly sub-jects, the presence of bradykinesia and, in particular, akathisia height-ened the incidence even further. In older patients without akathisia the incidence figure was about 26 per cent but this inflated to 71 per cent if akathisia had been present.

On the issue of race, this research has also suggested an increased risk in African Americans, but one apparently confined to those treated in the higher dose brackets.

Jeste and colleagues (1995) have recently shown the considerable risk run by older patients who have either never been exposed or whose exposure has been brief. In a prospective study of more than 200 patients over 45 years of age (mean 65.5 years) of mixed diagnoses who had a prior median cumulative duration of exposure of only three

Table 6.13. *Tardive dyskinesia and race: summary of three systematic studies*

Study	Sample	Recording method	Criteria	Prevalence (%)	Comment
Ko et al. (1989)	866 Shanghai Chinese Schizophrenia Mean age 42 years	AIMS	Jeste & Wyatt criteria +global severity >2	8.4	Low mean doses (311 mg/d CPZ equivalent) Extensive use of clozapine Correlates: age duration of exposure acute EPS +ve family history of schizophrenia antipsychotic dose
Chiu et al (1993)	572 Hong Kong Chinese Mixed diagnoses + non-pyschiatric and normals Age 55–103 years	AIMS	Schooler & Kane single assessment 'presumptive'	25.9 (n=274) (cf. 'spontaneous' 2.4%, n=249)	Brief exposures Psychogeriatric out-patients median 2.5 years Acute in-patient median 7 years Correlates: current dose (inverse)
Van Harten et al. (1996)	194 Dutch Antilles 94% negroid Mixed diagnoses In patients Mean age 53.1 years	AIMS	Schooler & Kane single assessment 'presumptive'	39.7	Tardive dystonia rated separately (13.4%) Low-potency drugs 6.2% Depots 64.7%

weeks, antipsychotic use was associated with a cumulative tardive dyskinesia incidence of 26 per cent at one year, which rose at two and three years to 52 per cent and 60 per cent respectively.

These figures are of interest when viewed in conjunction with the Yale projections as they might be taken to mean that the total pool of those liable to drug-related dyskinesia may not be higher in the elderly than in the population as a whole. It seems rather that the vulnerable within the population become symptomatic at a much faster rate if they are placed at risk by drug exposure when older.

In addition, this group found that, amongst other things, use of high-potency compounds, alcohol problems and, worthy of note, baseline tremor were predictors of heightened risk.

This work again emphasises the need for caution with the use of standard antipsychotics in the elderly, especially when exposure is for the first time or has been previously limited. It also suggests that the use of high-potency drugs in this situation should demand a deal of justification.

Onset, course and outcome

The projections from the Yale study confirm clinical experience: namely, that there often seems no rhyme nor reason to the onset of tardive movement disorders. In fact, no rigid time criterion can be applied to the concept as onset can follow from a few weeks to many years of continuous exposure (see Table 6.8). In view of the substantial implications of the diagnosis, however, one should be circumspect about symptomatology emerging within six months of first exposure, *except* when the features are exclusively or predominantly dystonic (see below). Onset tends to be gradual, though, again, this is frustratingly unpredictable, especially with chronic dystonia.

The basis of the professional concern about tardive dyskinesia that was so prominent in the early 1980s, especially in the USA, was largely due to worry about the course and outcome of the disorder. The perception was of a disorder of relentless evolution to maximal – and usually severe – expression. It is perhaps surprising that this 'worst case' scenario became so ensconced as the perceived norm, for it was never entirely compatible with clinical experience.

There is an important question to raise in considering the prognosis of any condition that is associated with the use of a necessary drug treatment, and that is whether the assessment of outcome should be in terms of what happens when the offending medication is stopped or whether it is more appropriate for this to take place in the context of continued exposure (Gardos et al., 1988a). The former tells us more about the question of reversibility, which is clearly one aspect of prognosis, but where no practical alternatives to the implicated medication are feasible, it is one of distinctly limited value. Furthermore, the question of reversibility may have little relevance to disorder that is mild, stable, non-intrusive and not in need of intervention.

Reversibility is, as was noted, dependent on age and is something that is to some extent still the stuff of myth. Some years ago, researchers in the USA asked 'experts' in the field of tardive dyskinesia in what percentage of patients they thought reversibility possible over different time scales. The opinions ranged from 100 per cent to 0 per cent (Gardos and Cole, 1980)! It may have been that, because of its generality, this question was pretty duff in the first place, but equally the 'duffness' may have resided with the opinions. Discontinuation studies of mixed age groups have suggested only a very gradual resolution of signs after stopping treatment. In one study, approximately half the sample showed a 50 per cent improvement in ratings over one year, but signs resolved completely in only 2 per cent of subjects (Glazer and Morgenstern, 1988). For many patients, however, discontinuation is not a practical option and, from what was said above, may not be a sound recommendation for reasons other than those relating to symptomatic relapse.

A very persuasive case can be made for the proposition that the prognosis of an iatrogenic disorder associated with use of a necessary drug treatment ought to be evaluated in the context of continued exposure. Seen in this light, the course and outcome of tardive dyskinesia are less unremittingly gloomy than was at one time thought (Fig. 6.8). Taking a mixed group of patients, some with and some without the disorder, the tendency is indeed for apparent progression within the group over time as new cases exert a greater impact on the symptomatic pool than established cases which undergo resolution. However, when groups comprising only tardive dyskinesia patients are followed – the more appropriate setting in which to study prognosis – the overall tendency is to improvement as the effects of those whose disorder progresses are offset by those whose disorder tends to amelioration (Gardos et al., 1988a).

Despite reporting the high incidence figure of around 5 per cent per year noted above, none of the Hillside patients had disorder rated as 'severe' during follow-up. Indeed, only 6 per cent were rated as 'moderately severe' and 37 per cent as 'moderate'. The bulk of the sample (57 per cent) continued to show disorder of only mild degree.

However, one factor that was associated with outcome was the modal dose of antipsychotic following establishment of the presence of tardive dyskinesia. Not only is it important to keep dose schedules low in order to minimise risk in the first place, it seems equally important to hold regimes to the lowest possible after emergence of the disorder – two intuitive practice principles now cemented by observation.

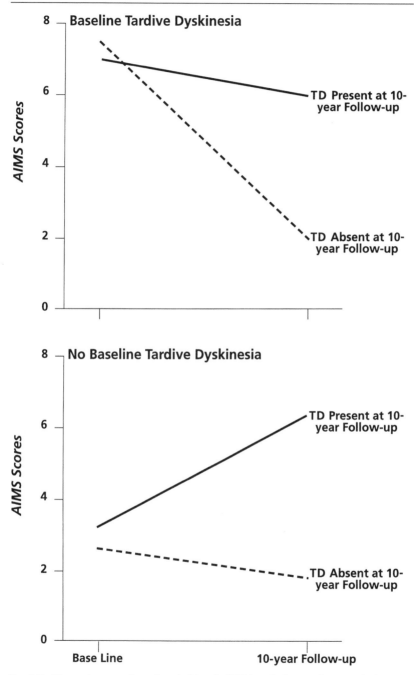

Fig. 6.8. The outcome of tardive dyskinesia (TD) in relation to the population status at baseline. (Reproduced with permission from Gardos et al., 1994.)

Notwithstanding the more favourable re-appraisal of the prognosis of tardive dyskinesia in recent years, the clinician is still left with the worrying fact that neither the course nor the long-term outcome can be predicted in the individual patient at point of onset. It is therefore necessary to bear in mind that tardive dyskinesia can add to the subjective experience of disability and to an objective appearance of 'oddness', either or both of which have the potential to exert a powerful negative influence on rehabilitation and re-socialisation.

Very occasionally, tardive dyskinesia can be associated with an outcome that can seriously threaten the patient's long-term health and indeed survival (Casey and Rabins, 1978). Profound motor overactivity can result in local trauma, including fractures (Szymanski et al., 1993), and breakdown in muscle tissue, which may cause myoglobinuria and consequent renal impairment and failure (Lazarus and Toglia, 1985). Patients can expend so much wasted energy that they may suffer profound weight loss and even descend into cachexia (Yassa and Nair, 1987). Oropharyngeal/laryngeal involvement may give rise to dysphagia with the risk of inhalation, and respiratory stridor (as noted) and, most importantly of all, the diagnosis may be associated overall with a slight but definite increase in mortality (Mehta, Roth and Lidz, 1978; McClelland et al., 1986; Youssef and Waddington, 1987)

There is certainly no room for complacency in relation to tardive dyskinesia, which can often be embarrassing, sometimes disabling and, very rarely, even life threatening. However, it is important that it is seen in context – and that includes the context of its overall course and outcome as well as the context of what an untreated psychotic illness means for its victims.

Treatment

The enthusiastic explorer of any medical topic can be sure of troubles ahead when textbooks begin their sections on 'Treatment' with long passages on primary prevention. This is not to belittle this domain of crucial importance to all doctors, but the proactive medical profession rarely *begins* with an emphasis on prevention when other treatment alternatives for an established disorder present themselves. There remains no satisfactory treatment for tardive dyskinesia and this section therefore begins with a tract on the crucial importance of primary prevention.

Primary prevention
The primary prevention of tardive dyskinesia incorporates three principles. The first is limiting the indications for offending

agents, the second is conservative utilisation in indicated conditions, and the third is avoidance of scenarios associated with heightened risk.

In the past, antipsychotic drugs were used for a range of clinical situations other than psychotic disorders, including anxiety states, neurotic depressions and personality disorders, as well as in patients with physical disorders, especially gastrointestinal. One North American group, seeking to assess the prevalence of spontaneous dyskinesias in the elderly, had difficulty in finding residential subjects who were not receiving a small dose of thioridazine to help them sleep! More worryingly, in a study of the disabling problem of tardive dystonia (discussed further below) Kang, Burke and Fahn, (1986) found that only one-third of the sample referred to their specialist centre was receiving antipsychotics for a clearly defined psychotic condition.

Nowadays, the indications for antipsychotics *must* be rigidly circumscribed. Their first-line use should be restricted to patients with psychotic disorders. 'Psychosis' was, of course, once a synonym for 'severe', although in recent years it has acquired a more restrictive usage, implying the presence of 'productive' psychotic symptomatology. In relation to the use of antipsychotic drugs, the latter meaning encapsulates the primary indications – the acute treatment and maintenance of schizophrenic disorders and all varieties thereof, including paranoid and delusional disorders, schizoaffective states, and affective disorders associated with 'productive' features, as well as the (usually short-term) management of some organic states.

However, in psychopharmacology, the older meaning may still apply, most obviously in bipolar disorders without hallucinations, delusions etc., for which antipsychotics continue to play an important role in both acute treatment and maintenance.

Other psychiatric disorders may, of course, be 'severe', and that includes conditions nowadays classified as 'neurotic'. This is particularly the case with some personality disorders, especially borderline states characterised by volatility of mood, misperception-like experiences and multiple self-harming behaviours. Although antipsychotics, especially in depot form, have been suggested as efficacious in such disorders, the evidence of benefit is weak, and any decisions to prescribe in this or other similar situations must be considered ones and come only after the failure of all other alternatives.

However, an emphasis on specific indications does not preclude the principle of a limited therapeutic trial in those patients in whom the balance of probability suggests a reasonable likelihood of benefit.

What antipsychotics are *not* is hypnotics or anxiolytics for the *non*-psychotic, something practitioners may be tempted to veer towards because of the negative pressures on prescribing benzodiazepines or their newer derivatives. Furthermore, antipsychotics ought to be used with care as non-specific agents of behavioural control, even if this can be an effect of their administration. This especially applies to those with learning disability and the elderly, for whom treatment plans incorporating antipsychotics require as much, or greater, thought as for those in other groups.

The principle of minimum dose utilisation is the second key element in primary prevention. This may seem obvious, yet there is a substantial body of evidence that, in schizophrenic disorders at least, psychiatrists still use antipsychotics in higher doses than are necessary to achieve the essential aim of resolution in psychotic symptomatology. In understanding this phenomenon, it is perhaps once again worthwhile stating some of the competing pressures psychiatrists must balance in formulating management plans. These are not the only reasons for excessive antipsychotic usage, but they may be important contributants.

The first pressure is the understandable desire to 'make things happen' – to achieve the predicted benefits as soon as possible. In countering this realistically, it must be remembered (as mentioned) that the therapeutic action of antipsychotics is associated with a built-in delay, probably to do with the development of changes in transmitter systems, and especially receptors, that lie behind the therapeutic effects – and these *take time* (see Fig. 4.8a). Non-specific benefits may be evident after a few hours or days, but it is the specific antipsychotic action that is inevitably delayed – a fact that cannot be side-lined by pushing doses rapidly in early phase management. All this is likely to achieve is the transformation of adverse actions that can be seen as beneficial, such as anti-anxiety effects and hypnosis, into symptomatic monsters that seriously compromise compliance (see Fig. 4.8b).

The second pressure is the need to contain disruptive or threatening behaviour and anticipate, and where possible avoid, psychiatric emergencies. These are justifiable reasons for tailoring regimes upwards but *not* for maintaining them high indefinitely. Furthermore, such steps should not be undertaken to satisfy the desire, from whatever source, for a 'peaceful' ward.

Third is the wish not to 'rock the boat'. When things have settled, why interfere? This exemplifies practice that is both timid and unrefined in that it fails to distinguish between the opposing principles of the different phases of management – especially the acute and the maintenance (see Fig. 4.7). Downward titration to the minimum effective and maximally tolerated dose is an essential component of maintenance management. Failure to undertake this will result in long-term exposure to unnecessarily high doses.

The decision to use a high-potency drug seems (as mentioned in Chapter 3) to carry with it an inherent risk of higher dosing. Baldessarini, Katz and Cotton (1984) showed that in clinical practice the mean chlorpromazine equivalent dose of haloperidol was almost four times greater than for chlorpromazine itself, and with fluphenazine it was six and a half times greater. This study once again emphasises the need for especial care in the selection of high-dose/high-potency regimes.

Finally, it must regrettably be said, there is ignorance. Some psychiatrists are simply determined to pursue their own autocratic course regardless of peer opinion. The author was once approached by a green but visibly alarmed junior enquiring about the 'normal' dose schedule for Depixol. Having explained the average in outline, she then asked 'What about 200 mg?' I explained that this would be in the high weekly range. 'Oh, not weekly,' she interjected. 'Three times daily!' An experienced patient admitted from another district had informed the trainee that when acutely unwell her regular doctor always prescribed Depixol – 200 mg *three times a day*! Such practitioners must expect what comes to them.

This does not mean that literature recommendations must be accepted slavishly. Advice based on clinical trial data is pertinent to the sorts of patients who enter clinical trials, who are as a rule unlikely to be entirely representative of psychotic patients in general. Nonetheless, the point is clear: doses of antipsychotics in all phases of treatment must be kept to the *minimum* necessary to achieve the primary aims of the management plan.

In a situation in which an element of risk is inevitable for even the most conservative prescriber, it is wise to minimise that component of risk that is amenable to treatment practice. Recommendations under this heading are unfortunately few and largely intuitive, as the literature reviewed above pointed to little of proven import. Nonetheless, avoidance of high-potency compounds, with their high liability to promote acute/intermediate EPS, would seem prudent, especially in older patients undergoing antipsychotic exposure for the first time. Although it is too early to be dogmatic, it might also be wise to eschew regimes which combine antipsychotics with SSRI antidepressants, a caution again most pertinent to the elderly. The safety of these newer antidepressants provides an understandable pull in such patients, but their known liability to promote neurological disorder at the acute end of the EPS spectrum might theoretically endow them with, in effect, a catalytic role in relation to the entire range of antipsychotic-related motor dysfunction, though this speculation requires confirmation. Advice on, and management of, alcohol abuse and the optimisation of diabetic control should also be offered when relevant.

Most importantly of all, every effort should be made to maintain compliance, especially in those whose relapsing pattern of illness has established the need for long-term medication. It has already been mentioned that compliance is not simply an issue that doctors can wash their hands of by dumping the entire responsibility on to patients. By keeping regimes and modes of administration simple, by educating patients on the reasons behind treatment plans, both acute and long-term, by close monitoring, by acknowledgement of adverse effects, and by vigorous efforts to eradicate them where possible – by these means and more – doctors can bring to bear a powerful impact on compliance. Improvement in this may in itself be rewarded by reducing the risk of tardive movement disorders.

Specific interventions

Having ensured, by good practice, that the above steps are (and always have been) in place, the next decision when confronted by the patient with tardive dyskinesia is not what specific intervention you might recommend, but whether any intervention is necessary at all. As seen in other contexts, the diagnosis should not automatically impel one to intervention. The overall well-being of patients with mild, non-intrusive and especially non-progressive disorder may be best served by industrious non-intervention. This means, of course, that when suspicions are first raised or the diagnosis is first confirmed, it is necessary to observe the situation over time to establish the pattern and course of the condition, after which the decision specifically to intervene should, wherever possible, be consensual. None of the following recommendations offers great prospects and so the decision to apply them should take account of the patient's perception and that of others involved in executing the management plan.

In view of the importance of affective tone in modifying tardive symptomatology, it is worth considering – before proceeding to specifics – whether the situation might not be helped by attention to co-existing anxiety/depression/dysphoria along conventional lines.

When it comes to specifics, it seems that virtually every centrally acting drug in the pharmacopoeia has been tried as a treatment for tardive dyskinesia (Table 6.14), yet it remains one of medicine's paradoxes that, in controlled trials, the drugs most effective in diminishing signs of the disorder are the ones that promote it in the first place – antipsychotics! This undoubtedly relates to the 'suppression' phenomenon described above, and whether it can truly be considered as 'therapy' is debatable. Escalating antipsychotic doses should certainly not be considered a routine treatment strategy as there is the risk – largely, it must be said, theoretical – of breakthrough at a later stage and possibly at greater levels of severity. Also, of course, it runs the risk of exacerbating other extrapyramidal symptomatology in the form of akathisia and parkinsonism. This tactic should be reserved for those with expertise in cases of potentially life-threatening disorder

Table 6.14. *Treatment of tardive dyskinesia: average rates of improvement from controlled trails of different drug types. (After Jeste et al. 1988.)*

Strategy	Average rate of improvement (%)
Antipsychotics	66
Noradrenergic antagonists	63
Anticholinergic withdrawal	60
GABA-ergics	48
Non-NA-ergic catecholamine antagonists	42
Cholinergic drugs	38
Antipsychotic withdrawal	37
Miscellaneous	37
Catecholaminergics	25
Anticholinergics	7
Average (*n*=3614)	43

characterised by cachexia, dysphagia/inhalation, myoglobinuria etc., when all else has failed.

As far as psychiatry's other efforts are concerned, these have been diverse and, it must be said, to some extent hypothesis driven, based largely on the dopamine supersensitivity theory discussed below. These efforts have been reviewed by Jeste and Wyatt (1979) and Jeste et al. (1988) covering the 1970s and 1980s respectively.

Although the quality of work in the field has improved, there are still major difficulties in undertaking therapeutic studies in tardive dys-kinesia that have not yet been adequately addressed. The varied and complex symptomatology of the condition, its inherently fluctuating nature, the effect of alterations in antipsychotic and incidental drug treatments, the intimate relationship it bears to the mental state, and its amenability to alteration by non-specific actions of both the test agent and the trial circumstances all conspire against a simple study design. The ideal investigation would need to consider:

the type of recording instrument (multi-item versus global impression) in the light of what the information is required for;

sample homogeneity (orofacial versus peripheral disorder and coincidental motor pathology, particularly parkinsonism);

the stability of routine treatment regimes (antipsychotic regimes unchanged for at least three months before and continuously throughout the study period, with avoidance of other drugs, especially benzodiazepines and anticholinergics);

a fixed assessment time (morning *or* afternoon);

coincidental psychiatric symptomatology (especially variations in potentially distressing productive and non-specific symptomatology);

the question of using an active placebo (for test compounds with sedative or other confounding actions);

an adequate 'run-in' (to allow subjects to adapt to the trial circumstances);

an adequate sample size (to detect an effect);

an adequate trial period (to ensure that any changes are substantive and not merely transient and non-specific);

the method of analysis (total scores versus means or other measures of change).

It can be seen that the comprehensive trial of a potential therapeutic agent in tardive dyskinesia is no mean undertaking.

Early interest focused on attempts to augment cholinergic transmission in the striatum by use of choline, which had the unfortunate effect of making the patients smell a bit like fishwives – and it didn't work to boot! The choline precursor, lecithin, was equally unhelpful. The alternative approach of reducing breakdown of acetylcholine by intravenous administration of the anticholinesterase physostigmine, was reported as beneficial and was one of the 'tests' proposed as forming a basis for the pharmacological classification of tardive dyskinesia. However, these drugs do have other central effects that may indirectly modify the motor signs.

A particularly elegant theory of this time related to modification of the proposed pathophysiological mechanisms. If, the argument went, involuntary movements result from dopamine supersensitivity (see below), then a successful treatment strategy would be to desensitise the supersensitised receptors by, for example, long-term, low doses of L-dopa (Friedhoff, 1977). There was evidence that this could happen in the laboratory but as the eminent Victorian biologist, Sir Thomas Huxley, pointed out, 'The tragedy of science is the staying of a beautiful hypothesis by an ugly fact' – in this case, the fact that in patients it did not work (Casey, Gerlach and Bjorndal, 1982)!

The use of a presynaptic depleting agent such as tetrabenazine could achieve the same effect and has been recommended and reported as successful. However, these compounds need delicate handling in view of their own profile of side-effects, and the author's patients have not been able to share in their reported benefits to any great extent. In addition, their tendency to promote parkinsonism makes it hard to know if symptom reduction really represents symptom substitution through a masking of the hyperkinesia by its clinical opposite.

The other main theory to gain vogue in the late 1970s involved facilitation of GABA transmission following from evidence of a decrease in dopamine neuronal activity with augmentation of GABA-mediated transmission. Hence, it was argued, boosting GABA inhibition might bring unruly supersensitised dopamine mechanisms to heel.

A full exploration of this hypothesis has been hampered by the limited availability of agonists suitable for clinical application, because existing drugs tend either to undergo tolerance or to have unacceptable side-effects. Studies have been undertaken of muscamol, the prototypic GABA-A agonist, baclofen, which has preferential effects at GABA-B sites, and gamma vinyl GABA, a GABA transaminase inhibitor that acts as an indirect agonist. While benefits have been reported with, especially, the latter of these compounds (Tamminga, Thaker and Nguyen, 1989), results overall were, and have remained, somewhat equivocal and certainly nothing of clinical utility has yet emerged from this field. However, the hypothesis remains underexplored rather than disproven.

As has been mentioned, benzodiazepines facilitate GABA inhibition and can reduce the severity of tardive movements, but it remains unclear whether this is merely a non-specific consequence of anxiolysis. However, benefits claimed for clonazepam might suggest that the action is indeed rather more specific.

A further strategy involves modification of noradrenergic transmission, with some favourable reports concerning the use of both the beta-adrenergic blocker propranolol and the alpha-2 agonist clonidine (Jeste et al., 1988). However, the doses suggested for the former (up to 800 mg daily) are beyond what most clinicians would be comfortable with, and even then benefits seem slow to accrue, while those for the latter (usually up to 0.45 mg per day) may be associated with their own profile of adverse effects. In addition, both these drugs are significantly active against affective symptomatology and have been reported to reduce productive psychotic features, though this is somewhat more problematic. Nonetheless, the specificity of any improvements in movement disorders must again be open to question.

In recent years, an alternative approach has attracted attention. This is the use of so-called free-radical scavengers. Free radicals are ultra-short-acting, highly reactive chemical species that are powerfully pathogenic to biological systems, especially membranes (Lohr, 1991). Their role in disease is an increasing focus of medical interest, in line with which it has been proposed that their excess production may underlie the pathophysiology of tardive movement disorders. This might occur as an integral part of antipsychotic action associated, for example, with increased dopamine turnover, which may stimulate formation of an excess of dopamine quinones and hydrogen peroxide, through the activity of monoamine oxidase (MAO).

A number of compounds are known to 'mop up' or neutralise the effects of free radicals, including vitamins C and E. Alpha tocopherol, or vitamin E, appears to be a major lipid-soluble scavenger, operating within membranes, and has been the subject of a number of investigations as a treatment for tardive dyskinesia. It has been reported to reduce formal ratings, though results are not unanimous (Elkashef et al., 1990; Adler et al., 1993b; Lohr and Caligiuri, 1996; Shriqui et al., 1992; Egan et al., 1992a). Even where positive effects have been found, the benefits overall do not appear to be striking, with reductions on AIMS totals in the range of 20 per cent. It may be that benefits are restricted especially to those with disorder of relatively brief duration (Egan et al., 1992a), which may go some way to explaining why such a strategy should work at all.

It does still seem somewhat strange that a pathophysiological process resulting from neurotoxicity can be reversed 'after the fact'. In addition to this intuitive concern, no difference has been found in vitamin E or lipid peroxide levels, or vitamin E/cholesterol ratios in patients with, compared to those without, tardive dyskinesia (McCreadie et al., 1995).

This approach is nonetheless of some interest, and does have additional support in the observation that alpha tocopherol may reduce antipsychotic-induced dopamine supersensitivity in chronically treated laboratory animals (Gattaz, Emrich and Behrens, 1993). It would be particularly interesting to see whether its long-term adjunctive use, starting early in antipsychotic exposure, could minimise the eventual development of tardive dyskinesia. No such studies have yet been reported, although the coincidental administration of multivitamins (containing alpha tocopherol) has been reported to have such an effect (Hawkings, 1989). In doses up to 1200–1600 mg (i.u.) per day, vitamin A is safe, but more clinical investigation is required to establish its place.

One of the licensed indications for the prescription of clozapine is EPS intolerance, and tardive dyskinesia can be considered under this rubric. Two cases of tardive dyskinesia have been reported in association with clozapine use, although one of these could be seen as withdrawal-emergent disorder, the origins of which lay in previous standard medication (Dave, 1994).

However, it may as yet be premature to conclude that this drug has no action at all in promoting tardive movements. Kane et al. (1993) found that two patients in a sample of 28 converted from 'questionable' to mild 'definite' tardive dyskinesia over a 12-month follow-up. Both had taken clozapine for nine years. In one animal model, vacuous chewing, clozapine appears to produce a lower rate of disorder than haloperidol, but is not devoid of liability (Tamminga et al., 1994). Despite this, the evidence remains that, as with shorter term administration, clozapine's long-term neurological tolerability is very favourable. Gerlach and Peacock (1994) reported a 14 per cent prevalence of tardive dyskinesia during clozapine treatment, but in this retrospective/ prospective study, absence of disorder at the start of clozapine was based on chart review, which might have meant that mild abnormality was under-recognised. Furthermore, a component of withdrawal-emergent disorder might also have been attributed to clozapine.

In support of its value in patients with established tardive dyskinesia, Lieberman and colleagues (1991) found that 43 per cent of their sample showed a 50 per cent reduction in AIMS ratings during follow-up. This study also showed, however that such benefits may take some time to filter through, as these reductions were evident after an average of 27.8 months of follow-up. This group also suggested that the greatest benefits may pertain in those with tardive dystonia, an observation of interest in view of clozapine's potent anticholinergic action and the reported efficacy of anticholinergics in idiopathic chronic dystonia (see Chapter 7).

These data raise the important question of whether clozapine's undoubted advantages in this regard are the result of a specific antidyskinetic action. The time sequence of resolution would seem to make this unlikely, and what seems more probable is that clozapine, with its diminished potential for promoting or sustaining disorder, holds mental state stable for a sufficient time to allow a degree of spontaneous resolution to take place. Having said this, recent evidence has suggested that clozapine may suppress dyskinesias in patients receiving treatment for Parkinson's disease (Bennet et al., 1994). So the issue remains open.

Clozapine must, therefore, be seen as a legitimate and potentially valuable tool in the management of tardive dyskinesia.

The place of the other 'new-generation' drugs remains to be clarified. Although there is evidence from one arm of the Phase III risperidone studies that this may possess an antidyskinetic function (Chouinard, 1995), the study was not ideal for addressing the question, the answer to which must also remain open. However, if early EPS predicts late EPS, then a lowered liability to tardive dyskinesia is a reasonable proposition with the new drugs.

An outline plan for the management of tardive dyskinesia is shown in Figure 6.9. This is not presented as the definitive strategy, but merely as one which emphasises the crucial element in the approach to treatment – that it be systematic.

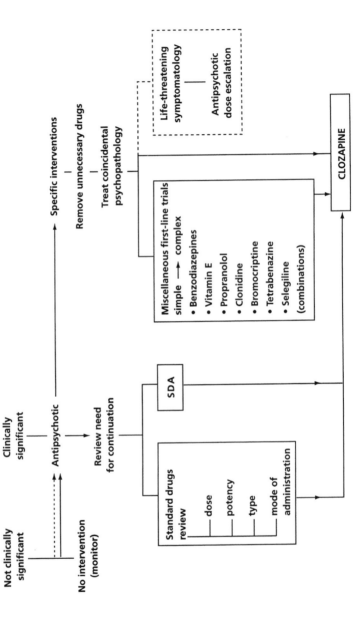

Fig. 6.9. Outline management of tardive dyskinesia. (SDA, serotonin–dopamine antagonist.)

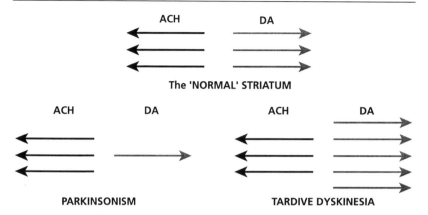

Fig. 6.10. The pathophysiology of tardive dyskinesia: the post-synaptic dopamine receptor supersensitivity hypothesis. (ACH, acetylcholine; DA, dopamine.)

Pathophysiology

The most widely propounded theory of the pathophysiology of tardive dyskinesia invokes striatal post-synaptic dopamine receptor supersensitivity as the underlying mechanism (see Fig. 3.8). This was formulated in 1970 out of speculations on the possible pathophysiological basis of the hyperkinetic disorders that had by then been clearly established in patients receiving long-term L-dopa for Parkinson's disease. To explain the outwardly similar tardive motor disorders, Klawans and colleagues and Carlsson separately suggested that protracted blockade of dopamine receptors by antipsychotics resulted in denervation supersensitivity of post-synaptic receptors which manifest clinically as hyperkinesias.

In naive form, the control of voluntary movement in the striatum might be viewed as representing a balance between the opposing actions of dopaminergic and cholinergic mechanisms (Fig. 6.10). A loss of dopaminergic input, as in parkinsonism, results in an imbalance in favour of the cholinergic side of the equation, modifiable by either anticholinergics or dopamine agonists – or both. The situation in tardive dyskinesia would, to some extent, represent the functional 'opposite'. Here, post-synaptic supersensitivity induced by chronic exposure to antipsychotics tips the balance in the other direction, resulting in dopaminergic excess.

This theory has proved remarkably durable, but must be seen for what it is: namely a hypothesis that can accommodate some, but by no means all, of the observations on tardive dyskinesia. In fact, its persistence for a quarter of a century does not speak of its robustness in the face of challenge, but rather of the absence of a more explanatory alternative. It can clearly account for the suppression and withdrawal phenomena described above, and therefore perhaps also for that awkward fact that antipsychotics remain the most effective drugs in reducing symptomatology. However, it leaves even more of the facts unaddressed.

Supersensitivity appears to be a universal response to antipsychotic exposure and, furthermore, can, in animals at least, be shown to develop early. In rodents, its behavioural effects can be demonstrated after a single parenteral dose (Christensen et al., 1976). This is clearly not compatible with late – sometimes very late – onset of hyperkinetic signs that afflict only some of those exposed. Neither does the hypothesis explain the unpredictable relationship between tardive dyskinesia and parkinsonism. The initial chemical denervation might reasonably be seen as the basis for parkinsonism, but the distributions of this are widely variant and bear no relationship to those of subsequent dyskinesias. Furthermore, the theory does not provide an adequate explanation for the striking relationship with age and the greater risk of disorder in the elderly, and it does not explain the heterogeneous response to pharmacological probes (dopaminergic/cholinergic agonists/antagonists), nor, of course, why anticholinergics cannot be shown quite unequivocally to be a causative as opposed to a modifying factor.

For these and other reasons, the post-synaptic dopamine receptor supersensitivity hypothesis is, in its straightforward form at least, certainly an oversimplification, which ignores both the complexities of neurotransmitter pharmacology and the chemical jungle that is the striatum. It may be that disruption of *presynaptic* mechanisms involving dopamine and possibly also noradrenaline is more important than the theory credits (Jeste and Wyatt, 1981a), as may be disturbed relationships with other modifying systems such as those utilising GABA and even acetylcholine.

It is unlikely, however, that any single theory of pathophysiology can account for a syndrome that is clinically and probably pharmacologically heterogeneous, and it is likely that our understanding of the mechanisms underlying tardive dyskinesia will have to await a more comprehensive appreciation of those individual factors imparting vulnerability, and a clearer elucidation of the neurochemistry of the striatum.

Clinical subtypes

Some authors, especially in the USA, have been eager to promote 'micro-classification' – that is, defining subsyndromes of tardive movement disorders on the basis of the predominant or lead type of movement comprising the disorder.

In general there is – with one exception – little evidence that this is a fruitful endeavour. Tardive akathisia, which is not strictly in this category as it is not defined in terms of a specific movement type, has already been discussed. The exception – tardive dystonia – is of sufficient import to be given separate and more detailed consideration in the next chapter.

Cases in which motor and vocal tics dominate the clinical picture have been described in association with long-term antipsychotic exposure and referred to as tardive Gilles de la Tourette's syndrome. Such cases may exhibit echolalia and coprolalia in addition to more rudimentary grunting and barking, but the more complex obsessional behaviours of the idiopathic state do not appear to have been noted. Less than a dozen such reports have been published and, in some, multiple tics have occurred in association with other involuntary activity (Lieberman and Saltz, 1992). A number of these cases have emerged following discontinuation or reduction of antipsychotic medication. Reports have invariably been deficient on background details such as whether these abnormalities were ever evidenced prior to starting antipsychotics, the family history, and the extent of other associated pathology. Such cases are clearly extremely uncommon and while they may demonstrate some symptomatic overlap with the idiopathic disorder, this is hardly justification for allocating them to a separate nosological category. The same is true of tardive Meige's syndrome (blepharospasm – oromandibular dystonia).

A tardive myoclonus has also been reported in association with the use of standard antipsychotics. In one study, 24 per cent of subjects exposed for more than three months developed postural myoclonus, with 34 per cent of the males but only 13 per cent of the females affected (Tominaga et al., 1987). This high prevalence flies in the face of clinical experience (at least the author's), which would suggest that disorder of this type is extremely rare. This is supported by the fact that, apart from this single publication, only one other case report has been published.

The issue of myoclonus is important, however, especially in relation to its undoubted, if infrequent, occurrence in the course of established treatment with clozapine. It may be that this association is a consequence of close monitoring rather than a particular adverse effect of this drug. It would certainly seem prudent for psychiatrists to be more familiar with myoclonus as a neurological sign rather than simply attributing its rapid, jerky appearance and its precipitation in some circumstances by noise and other sensory stimuli to the mental state of a twitchy, anxious patient.

Other 'syndromes' described include tardive tremor and tardive parkinsonism, but these are concepts that go beyond the present author's experience (and indeed comprehension), and extend greatly beyond what is likely to be useful to the present reader.

7

Tardive and chronic dystonia

Introduction

The term 'dystonia tarda' was first used by Keegan and Rajput (1973) to draw attention to persistent dystonic postures, which, although mentioned in previous reports on tardive dyskinesia, had been largely ignored. Even this effort was less than successful, and it was only after a decade that the problem began to attract serious attention. However, interest has come largely from neurologists, and psychiatrists still seem to deal with the issue with either neglect or bewilderment.

The reasons for considering tardive dystonia separately from 'classical' tardive dyskinesia are threefold. This particular presentation has somewhat different associations, is much more functionally incapacitating, and may have somewhat different treatment characteristics. Indeed, the strong implication is that the pathophysiology may also differ, but as the details of this are unknown, no specific comments can be made on the underlying mechanisms. It must be emphasised though, that in terms of our present knowledge, tardive dystonia remains essentially just one rather specific subtype of the general disorder we call tardive dyskinesia.

However, one must in all frankness admit that the literature is not always clear about when the term tardive dystonia is appropriate, especially as mixed types of abnormal movements may be found together, as has already been suggested. The term (or diagnosis) is best reserved for situations in which chronic dystonia is either the sole or dominating manifestation of disorder in patients treated with antidopaminergic drugs. An important part of the judgement in this latter situation is the level of functional disability that the patient experiences.

It could be argued that in many of its characteristics, tardive dystonia has more in common with the idiopathic dystonias than with 'classical' tardive dyskinesia, and for this reason a lucid exposition of the issue is perhaps best approached from the perspective of chronic dystonias in general.

Definition and classification of chronic dystonia

The confusing origins of the concept of dystonia have already been explored, origins that led to diverse applications of the term in neurology, as elsewhere. In 1984, an ad hoc committee of members of the Scientific Board of the Dystonia Medical Research Foundation defined dystonia as 'a syndrome dominated by sustained muscle contractions frequently causing twisting and repetitive movements, or abnormal postures' (Fahn et al., 1987b). While this might be adequate for a neurological perspective, and that would include tardive dystonia, it does omit the possibility of dystonia occurring as a sign, as, for example, in tardive dyskinesia in general where it may, as has been seen, form but one of a range of movement types. Hence, the 'expert' definition is, for our purposes, somewhat restrictive.

In the earlier account, the origins of the concept were traced back to Hammond's idea of 'athetosis' and this was not without justification, because phenomenologically, dystonia and athetosis do not differ. Indeed, the two terms have traditionally been used almost interchangeably, with the only distinction being on the basis of distribution. Thus, Marsden has referred to athetosis as 'distal dystonia', while Wilson called dystonia 'proximal athetosis' (Owens, 1990). In the context of chronic drug use, dystonia is the universally applied term.

With regard to clinical typologies, Wechsler and Brock's (1922) distinction of 'kinetic' disorders, in which the movement aspect predominates, and 'myostatic' disorders, in which the postural distortion is the predominant manifestation, has already been commended to the reader. However, although of clinical utility in bringing together two outwardly different presentations, this does not amount to a classification as such.

Chronic dystonias may be classified on the basis of the age of the patient at onset, by the presence or absence of definable cause, or by the distribution of disorder (Fig. 7.1). Age of onset is an important classificatory tool as it relates to prognosis. The earlier the onset, the more likely dystonia is to generalise and hence to be associated with greater disability and poorer outcome (Marsden, 1976). The same relationship is seen with acute, drug-related dystonias, and it is equally true of chronic disorder. Generalisation is, by contrast, rare after the age of 40. However, psychiatrists are unlikely to encounter chronic dystonia with a very young age of onset, even in the context of long-term antipsychotic drug use, as these conditions usually have clear neurological antecedents.

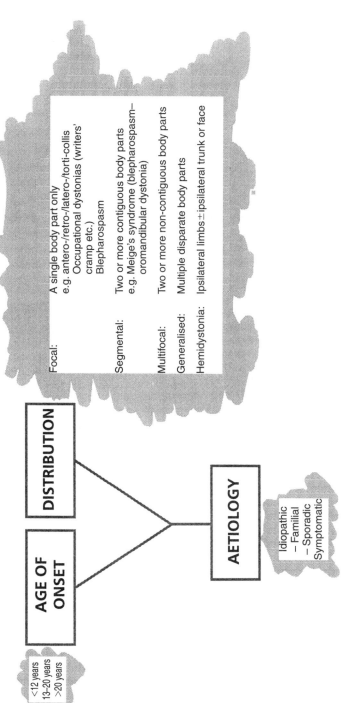

AGE OF ONSET

<12 years
13–20 years
>20 years

DISTRIBUTION

Focal: A single body part only
e.g. antero-/retro-/latero-/torti-collis
Occupational dystonias (writers'
cramp etc.)
Blepharospasm

Segmental: Two or more contiguous body parts
e.g. Meige's syndrome (blepharospasm–
oromandibular dystonia)

Multifocal: Two or more non-contiguous body parts

Generalised: Multiple disparate body parts

Hemidystonia: Ipsilateral limbs±ipsilateral trunk or face

AETIOLOGY

Idiopathic
– Familial
– Sporadic
Symptomatic

Fig. 7.1. The classification of chronic dystonia.

A wide range of neurological afflictions can result in dystonia, though thankfully only a few of these are likely to confront the psychiatrist (see Table 7.2). But a broad, aetiologically based classification is of clear relevance to psychiatry, and especially to the present context. Thus, dystonia may be considered simply as idiopathic or symptomatic (i.e. secondary to some identifiable cause). Clearly, tardive dystonia is one type of symptomatic, chronic dystonia.

What is perhaps most useful to psychiatrists, however, is a descriptive classification based on distribution. This is clinically both straightforward and practical as it helps to bring together a number of differently named entities under a recognisably similar banner. Focal dystonias are restricted to one body part, while segmental disorder involves two or more contiguous body areas. Multifocal refers to disorder affecting two or more non-contiguous body parts, whereas in generalised abnormality, multiple, disparate body parts are affected. Hemidystonia is used for disorder of ipsilateral limbs ± ipsilateral trunk and/or face, and is a manifestation that strongly implies a contralateral focal brain lesion, especially of caudate/lenticular nucleus or thalamus. As has been emphasised, any drug-related movement disorder, including dystonias, can present unilaterally, though this usually involves abnormality of a restricted distribution only (e.g. focal or segmental).

Using these easy principles, it should be possible for those dealing with drug-related, symptomatic dystonia to provide a more specific classification of disorder based on distribution, which will not only aid clarity but, in particular, will be of value in charting progression.

Clinical features

Any of the dystonic abnormalities described as a part of either acute, drug-related dystonia or of tardive dyskinesia in general, can form the clinical presentation of tardive dystonia, but it is again worth emphasising that in this situation these features will either form the exclusive or dominating abnormality. Furthermore, while the disorder with acute dystonias is overwhelmingly myostatic in type, that seen in chronic dystonia of whatever cause may also be kinetic.

Although it is likely that in some patients chronic, drug-related dystonia may be associated with the same early affective symptomatology as described under acute dystonias, there has been no systematic appraisal of this. In idiopathic disorders, symptoms of pain or aching discomfort antedating signs, appear to figure in only a minority of cases (Owens, 1990). It is, therefore, possible that early subjective symptomatology is a function of the speed of onset of the disorder, and hence may be more likely in cases of tardive dystonia that develop over a short time scale of, say, a few weeks or so rather than in those exhibiting a more gradual course to completion.

While the prominence of premonitory discomfort may be a matter of debate, the distressing nature of established disorder is not. Patients frequently experience considerable pain and aching discomfort in areas affected by established disorder, symptomatology that may emanate from the muscles themselves or from their origins/insertions or, with long-standing disorders, from secondary degenerative joint changes.

Most of the obvious objective manifestations have already been described and will probably remain more familiar to clinicians under their long-established clinical names (Fig. 7.1). However, by the above method of classification, blepharospasm and torticollis might now be considered as focal dystonias, while more widespread facial involvement may be segmental if, for example, blepharospasm is combined with oromandibular dystonia. This latter presentation is sometimes referred to as tardive Meige's syndrome, in that it resembles idiopathic blepharospasm–oromandibular dystonia, which, although given a number of eponyms, is now most commonly known as Meige's syndrome. Truncal leans may be the consequence of either focal or segmental involvement.

A precise pattern of abnormality in tardive dystonia – if such a thing there be – is difficult to elicit from the literature, because almost all the systematic work on the subject has been undertaken by neurologists working in tertiary referral settings. Referral to such centres is more likely in those with marked disorder and, in particular, those with abnormality which is either socially or functionally incapacitating. Hence, such reports may only be informative in relation to specific types or severity of disorder. Nonetheless, from these data, disorder seems to start most often in the face and neck (Burke and Kang, 1988). This would, therefore, appear to mimic idiopathic disease where, of the non-generalised forms, craniocervical dystonia is the most common (Duane, 1988). Retrocollis has been reported in one study as being particularly common, affecting up to 40 per cent of cases (Kang et al., 1986), but any sort of neck displacement can be found, including anterocollis and laterocollis as well as the better known forms, retrocollis and torticollis.

The complexity of the disorder underlying torticollis ought to be appreciated, for this is one bastion against misattribution. It is quite simply extremely difficult to simulate. Although sternocleidomastoid is the most commonly affected muscle, there is in fact no characteristic presentation. The pattern of muscular involvement is usually highly complex, as a result of which the disorder invariably comprises more than just the simple rotational tilt implied by the name. In addition to the obvious head displacement, it can also be helpful to look for a compensatory kyphoscoliosis, which may be the best clue to the presence of subtle disorder. In even mild cases, this is usually betrayed by an elevation in the shoulder on the side of the rotation or by the fact that the hand on that side does not extend as low as the one on the other side. Unequal prominence of the sternomastoid insertions is another clue.

Despite the craniocervical origins, the majority of cases reported from neurological clinics spread to other areas to some extent, with the most common end pattern being a segmental one (Kang et al., 1986). A possible exception to this would seem to be oculogyric dystonias, which may sometimes occur as a tardive phenomenon (Fitzgerald and Jankovic, 1989). In the author's experience, such tardive oculogyric spasms tend to remain as an isolated manifestation of chronic dystonia without spread to other areas. Even in tardive form, these episodes are in most cases far removed phenomenologically from the 'crises' of old (see Chapter 4).

In addition to these generally quite well-known manifestations of dystonia, it is worth emphasising again the typical inward rotations of the arms resulting from hyperpronation of the forearms and distal flexion/extension movements of the fingers. Flexion/extension can affect all lower limb joints, with the addition of adduction/abduction of the thigh and rotation/version movements around the ankles.

It is particularly important to evaluate dystonia with the patient walking, when movements may emerge or accentuate (see below). The limbs are an especially fruitful focus of attention. Finger filliping, 'piano playing' and other finger movements may only be evident on walking, and the arms may show a grotesque, accentuated swing that looks almost like a parody of the norm. The excursion of the swing is increased, largely due to an exaggerated extension of the pronated arm round the back combined with a compensatory increase in forward movement. Gait may assume the stiff, mechanical quality of an automaton.

The potential for distress and functional incapacity associated with chronic dystonia cannot be overestimated, and this is the first reason for considering tardive dystonia separately from tardive dyskinesia in general. The distress sometimes associated with tardive dyskinesia has already been noted, but this pales in relation to that found in patients with established chronic dystonia. These disorders have much less the characteristics of 'release' phenomena but much more those of actively imposed abnormality. This applies as much to patients with focal or segmental abnormality in the face as to those with other distributions, but the high prevalence of truncal and limb disorder is a major factor contributing to incapacity. The intrusive and distorting effects of dystonia in these peripheral sites can represent severe assaults on independent functioning.

Table 7.1. *Factors modifying the expression of chronic dystonia*

Mental state	Level of arousal
	Concentration
Periodicity	Diurnal
	Day to day
Severity	Action only
	Overflow
Selectivity	Movements not muscles

Characteristics of dystonia

Chronic dystonias are vulnerable to modification by the same psychological influences as all the extrapyramidal disorders discussed in the present volume. In addition, however, they have certain characteristics that are frankly peculiar, and may be reasons why they are still sometimes considered 'hysterical'. These are as relevant to drug-related as to idiopathic disorders (Table 7.1).

The influence of 'arousal', as described previously, may be one factor behind a certain periodicity in expression of dystonia over time, so that abnormal postures or movement activity may be evident one day but not the next. Furthermore, patients with chronic dystonia often exhibit a striking diurnal variation with disorder worse in the latter part of the day, in line with what has been noted in other contexts above. Indeed, especially early in its course, sufferers may be free of disorder on waking, only for the abnormality to impose itself as the day progresses. However, other associations are more unique to dystonia.

In the early stages of the disorder, dystonia may not be evident in the resting or passive state and may only emerge when the affected part is specifically brought into movement. This represents so-called 'action' dystonia, which may or may not progress eventually to abnormality evident in the resting state also. It, nonetheless, emphasises the importance of incorporating a component of evaluation during activity into routine examinations (see Chapter 10). With progression, the phenomenon of 'overflow' may be noted – that is, when activity in *distant* muscle groups can precipitate dystonia in a specifically affected area, something we have also seen the value of (with qualification) in examination.

What can sometimes be striking about dystonia is the way in which disorder can affect particular movements rather than specific muscles (Owens, 1990). Furthermore, the motor action precipitating the disorder can be highly specific. Thus, a patient unable to walk forwards normally may have a perfectly fluid backwards gait. This is not a justification for considering the disorder to be 'hysterical' – quite the opposite.

One of the most noteworthy characteristics of dystonia, at least in its early stages, is the fact that patients may 'learn' that certain behaviours on their part can, to some extent, alleviate their disorder. The folded arms of the patient with axial hyperkinesis have already been referred to. Another, perhaps more common, example is seen in patients with torticollis who touch their chin or, in particular, hold the back of their neck with the hand on the opposite side to the direction of the rotation. One man with Meige's syndrome found that the functional blindness resulting from an almost total blepharospasm on walking could be sufficiently improved to allow a degree of independence by rubbing or exerting pressure on his upper dental margin.

Actions of this sort may actually attenuate the disorder or, if it is of more advanced degree, at least relieve some of the subjective distress, and are so characteristic across patients that they have been considered virtually diagnostic of dystonia (Fahn et al., 1987b). These behaviours, which seem to be effective by recruiting tactile or proprioceptive stimuli, are referred to as 'sensory tricks' or, more technically, 'antagonistic gestures'.

Diagnosis

The diagnosis of tardive dystonia should emerge from the balancing of two sets of probabilities. The first is that the dystonia is symptomatic and the other that it is secondary to specific drug treatment.

The first issue can never be addressed with confidence because chronic dystonia is a not uncommon disorder in the general population. Indeed, when mild postural distortions are taken as a sufficient diagnostic criterion, it is a much commoner disorder than is generally appreciated, as estimates of the gene frequency would indicate. With the development of an interest in the field, the author was able to diagnose a relative's mild torticollis, long held to be 'just a habit'.

The history of one 30-year-old schizophrenic patient illustrates the problem of certainty in a clinical context. This young man developed a very severe torticollis to the left, with a profound compensatory kyphoscoliosis and other disorders, after many years on standard antipsychotics – a seemingly straightforward scenario to interpret. However, on reviewing his medical records, it emerged that his first contact with professional services was when still a schoolboy, at the age of 16, some four years before the onset of his psychosis and the start of specific treatment. At that time, he had been referred to an educational psychologist because when he went to bed at night, his head would 'jerk' to the left! The problem appeared to respond to whatever it was

Table 7.2. *Causes of chronic dystonia that*
may be encountered in psychiatric practice

Huntington's disease
Parkinson's disease
Multiple sclerosis
Post-infarction/haemorrhage
Post-trauma
Post-encephalitis
Neoplasm/A–V malformation
Wilson's disease
Idiopathic dystonia
Carbon monoxide poisoning

the psychologist had implemented, at least insofar as the patient could recall, because he defaulted after a few sessions and the whole thing was forgotten – even by him. It may seem reasonable, 'on the balance of probabilities', to attribute a subsequent precipitating role to anti-psychotics in a case such as this – but who knows?

Having decided that the disorder is symptomatic and not idiopathic, the second set of probabilities is somewhat easier to juggle. An extensive list of primarily neurological disorders can give rise to a presentation dominated by chronic dystonia, but most of these are mercifully rare and, more mercifully, only a few impinge on psychiatric practice (Table 7.2). As some do, however, it is important to remember that there is always, as we have always noted, a differential diagnosis.

The author is willing to admit to having been caught out here, too. On regular sojourns around the grounds of the hospital housing my long-stay beds, I had been particularly struck by the gross generalised dystonia of one middle-aged man, and indeed had videoed him as part of a salutary lesson on the risks and 'nasties' of long-term antipsychotic medication. The sequence never failed to impress. When putting together clientele suitable for a research ward, I was delighted to see that the nurses who were consulted put his name high on the list, and he was duly transferred. Unfortunately, the author only undertook a review of his case-notes *after* the patient was happily ensconced in the shiny new facility, and discovered to my chagrin that the man in question suffered from multiple sclerosis! The reasons why he was on long-term antipsychotics – let alone in long-term psychiatric care – were mysteries lost to time. There is *always* a differential diagnosis.

Burke et al. (1982) have proposed guidelines for diagnosing tardive dystonia encompassing four areas for consideration: (1) that the dystonia is chronic; (2) that it occurs in the context of a history of antipsychotic exposure preceding or concurrent with onset; (3) that no other cause of secondary disorder can be established; and (4) that there is no family history of dystonia.

Epidemiology

There are few hard data on the frequency of tardive dystonia. The 'accepted wisdom' is that situations in which this type of disorder is the sole or predominating abnormality are rare, affecting no more than 1–2 per cent of patients (Yassa et al., 1986a; Friedman, Kucharski and Wagner, 1987).

This would seem to address the question only partially, however. Psychiatry has become concerned with this issue relatively recently and, if the history of tardive dyskinesia in general is to be repeated – which is likely – increasing awareness will probably be associated with increasing recognition. It is certainly the author's impression that, while it may be correct that in only a small number of patients chronic dystonia forms the sole or dominating picture, this is nonetheless a much more common disorder than the above figures would suggest. In saying this, one is referring to disorder that is either mild and easily overlooked or misattributed, as well as to that which is insufficiently prominent to be seen as diagnostically other than part of a varied clinical mix.

In line with this suggestion, van Harten and colleagues (1996) found a prevalence of 13.4 per cent. What is important about this study, conducted in the Dutch Antilles, was the use of a specific instrument to rate dystonia (the Fahn–Marsden Scale) and operationalisation of the diagnosis. While disorder in a proportion of these patients would clearly be part of mixed symptomatology and hence would not conform to the concept of tardive dystonia used here, this work clearly illustrates that chronic, drug-related dystonia is not an uncommon phenomenon. There are no data available on the incidence of tardive dystonia.

It is, therefore, worth searching out the bizarre postures, the truncal leans, the 'silly' walks. Look for the ominous stares, the twitching eyes, the arms that are held in slight hyperpronation. Listen for the strained or whispered speech and observe the conversation that comes from a mouth that is tense and appears full when it is not. You may well be surprised at what is there to be seen!

Predisposing factors

Age is an important factor in the clinical expression of tardive dystonia, as it is in other varieties of dystonia and chronic, drug-related dyskinesias in general. The prevalence appears to increase with increasing age. However, it also seems that patients who develop exclusive or predominant dystonia tend to be younger than those with 'classical' tardive dyskinesia. Thus, the cumulative distribution curve for tardive dystonia is shifted to the left (Kang et al., 1986). This earlier age of onset is the second powerful reason for considering chronic, drug-related dystonia separately from other tardive motor disorders.

The literature has fairly consistently reported tardive dystonia to be about twice as common in males as in females. This may reflect interposing influences and the special populations that have, to date, formed the bulk of the study material, though it is perhaps less easy to convince with such 'special pleading' than it is in relation to the gender differences reported for tardive dyskinesia in general (see Chapter 6). The possibility of predisposition imparted by African descent (van Harten et al., 1996) is also unresolved.

Some idiopathic dystonias have been associated with local trauma, hyperthyroidism, a history of essential tremor, and repetitive use of the affected part, and dystonia musculorum deformans may be familial, so there can also be a genetic component (Owens, 1990). Indeed, a dystonia gene appears to be quite widely distributed in the population at large.

Apart from an isolated report of an association with prior essential tremor (Sachdev, 1993a), none of these factors has been established as predisposing to chronic, drug-related dystonia, though none has been adequately investigated. A genetically determined predisposition would be of particular interest to explore, which should be possible with developments in molecular biology. It is likely that drugs with a generally high EPS liability and regimes that incorporate higher doses predispose to tardive dystonia, as they do to the more 'classical' presentations of tardive dyskinesia, but these remain to be established. A further possibility is susceptibility, evidenced by prior extrapyramidal symptomatology, and in particular a previous history of acute dystonias that has been suggested in the literature (Sachdev, 1993b).

Onset, course and outcome

The onset of chronic dystonia, of whatever sort, is highly variable. Symptomatology may evolve slowly over months or years or progress to completion in a matter of weeks.

In line with the relationship to activity noted above, disorder may be first noted only in executing specific tasks. One young man, retrained in computer skills after a severe, early-onset schizophrenia, noted a slight hyperpronation of the right forearm after operating the keyboard for a quarter of an hour or so, which presumably represented disorder being 'released' by relative fatigue. His hand signs did not progress, but after a few months he noted that an inversion of the right foot accompanied the arm signs. Fortunately, his dystonia stabilised at a level that was non-intrusive and did not impair his competency, and was helped by the 'trick' of resting his wrist on a support. Interestingly, he was a keen cyclist, but this did not precipitate either his hand or foot dystonia, again reflecting the very specific nature of the task affected. This is probably the tardive dystonic equivalent of the occupational dystonias such as writers' cramp, and the focal dystonias that can affect musicians, dancers and sportsmen. It is, of course, always possible that this young man would have developed such an 'occupational' disorder anyway, had his illness permitted an occupation.

This case also illustrates a further point about onset in that the patient had been treated for six years without incident. Chronic dystonia, like other forms of tardive dyskinesia, can start after a brief exposure interval of weeks or only after many years of uneventful treatment. However, this type of disorder does appear to be disproportionately represented amongst cases with an onset early in the exposure period. In one study, 50 per cent of cases had an onset within five years of starting antidopaminergic medication (Kang et al., 1986; Fig. 7.2). Although these data come from a tertiary referral setting and hence are most pertinent to the more severe or disabling disorders, they nonetheless would seem to reflect clinical experience.

The point at which tardive dystonic abnormalities will stabilise and the degree of generalisability cannot be predicted, nor can the level of functional disability. The severity of the disorder, once plateaued, tends to remain stable, apart from the inherent fluctuations described above. In fact, a further distinguishing characteristic may be that, in comparison to tardive dyskinesia in general, tardive dystonia may show little or no tendency to resolution (Burke et al., 1982; Gimenez-Roldan, Mateo and Bartolome, 1985).

The outcome for seriously psychotic patients (especially those with schizophrenia) who develop tardive dystonia has not, until recently, been good. One group found that the only patients in its series in whom dystonia resolved completely were those who could come off, and stay off, antidopaminergic medication (Burke and Kang, 1988) – clearly something that is not an option for most schizophrenics. However, clozapine has changed this gloomy outlook for the better (see below).

Treatment

The final, and perhaps most important, reason for giving special consideration to tardive dystonia is that it may differ to some extent in its

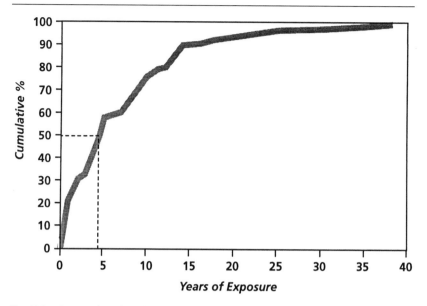

Fig. 7.2. Onset of tardive dystonia in relation to duration of drug exposure.
(After Kang et al., 1986, with permission.)

treatment characteristics. The words 'may differ' are important, however.

The questions surrounding the importance of primary prevention and the decision to treat noted in connection with tardive dyskinesia in general are relevant to tardive dystonias also, as are any of the specific regimes proposed, with the exception of antipsychotic dose increment, which should *not* be undertaken in this situation. However, the expectation of success cannot be great. Simple interventions designed to stabilise mood disorder, such as benzodiazepines for anxiety/agitation and antidepressants for coexistent depression, should not be overlooked.

As was noted, until recently, persistence of antipsychotic medication seemed to be almost inevitably associated with continuation of dystonic symptomatology. The exception to this rule now is clozapine. There is, in fact, some evidence that this compound's remarkable profile of extrapyramidal tolerability may be particularly effective in allowing resolution of chronic dystonic abnormality as opposed to other types of tardive motor disorders (Lieberman et al., 1991). Currently, therefore, clozapine should be immediately considered as soon as the diagnosis of tardive dystonia has been made in those for whom on-going antipsychotic medication is necessary. However, one must not expect – nor lead the patient to expect – dramatic results. Lieberman et al.'s study would suggest that a 50 per cent reduction in the severity of tardive disorders (which, of course, include dystonias) can be expected over approximately 30 months on clozapine, with no evidence that the dystonia resolves quicker. The position of the newer compounds remains to be seen, though in situations in which clozapine is impractical or cannot be maintained, these would be the obvious next choice.

The mechanism whereby clozapine may bring about such a therapeutic benefit, possibly targeted on dystonic abnormality, is unknown, but its potent anticholinergic actions may be relevant, especially when we note one of the additional interventions that 'may' justify us viewing the treatment characteristics of the disorder as being slightly different.

This additional intervention is high-dose anticholinergic. The possible merits of this spring from extrapolation of results from controlled trials in the treatment of idiopathic dystonia. In this situation, there is evidence that very high doses of the anticholinergic benzhexol (trihexyphenidyl) are associated with significant symptomatic improvements (Burke, Fahn and Marsden, 1986). Starting with low doses of 2 mg per day and increasing no more than twice weekly, very high regimes of up to 130 mg per day or more have been tolerated in nonpsychotic sufferers of idiopathic chronic dystonia and have been found to be beneficial. Open studies in patients with tardive dystonia suggest an improvement rate of up to 50 per cent (Kang et al., 1986). The risk noted above, of exacerbation of choreiform disorder, may be less than theoretically predicted, at around 10 per cent (Kang et al., 1986).

Nonetheless, for the reasons expounded previously, high-dose anticholinergic medication regimes should only be implemented with care in those suffering from psychotic illness.

At several points in the present volume, considerable pains have been exerted in trying to urge the reader to caution in the use of anticholinergics, and even mentioning the above finding may seem to smack of contrariness. However, chronic dystonia – tardive or otherwise – can be such a distressing development that it is incumbent on practitioners to be aware of every possibility.

Presynaptic depleting agents such as tetrabenazine have also been reported as helpful – indeed, in the group reported by Kang et al. (1986), the most helpful drugs of all. Two-thirds of this sample did not have a clear psychotic diagnosis, and these agents require careful use, especially in those with unstable mood. The author's experience has not been favourable.

In recent years, local injection of botulinum A toxin has become the least ineffective treatment for idiopathic dystonias of especially focal distribution. As one's last-ditch therapeutic endeavour in otherwise treatment-resistant and severely disabling cases of limited distribution, it might be worth trying to persuade a friendly and enthusiastic neurological colleague to attempt this, though such a request is likely to be met with some – perhaps justified – scepticism!

An outline of treatment strategies in tardive dystonia is shown in Fig. 7.3.

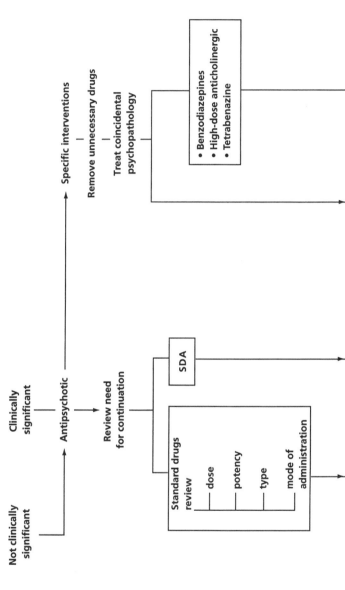

Fig. 7.3. Outline management of tardive dystonia. (SDA, serotonin–dopamine antagonist.)

8

Involuntary movements and schizophrenia: a limitation to the concept of tardive dyskinesia?

Introduction

When the concept of tardive dyskinesia was first mooted, appraisals of the supportive evidence ranged from 'thoroughly convincing' (Marsden, Tarsy and Baldessarini, 1975), through 'compelling' (Kane and Smith, 1982), to die-hard scepticism (Crow et al., 1983). How could such diversity of opinion have been sustained?

It has already been seen that antipsychotic drugs are neither necessary nor sufficient to 'cause' involuntary movement disorders. Individuals never exposed to these drugs can develop identical disorder, but not everyone comparably exposed does so. The divergence in appraising the initial evidence arose from a conflict between the wish to understand the disorder as opposed to merely establishing its validity. Those who wished to understand were strongly influenced by the lingering recollection of a literature suggesting that schizophrenia may be a condition that can itself be associated with the development of involuntary movements.

The descriptive evidence

The early descriptive writers on schizophrenia clearly recognised that all was not well in their patients' motor domains. Kraepelin and Bleuler both acknowledged the importance of motor signs and both went along with the inclusion of Kahlbaum's 'Katatonie' as one subtype. Beyond this however – in the realm of movement disorders of hyperkinetic type – they parted company fiercely.

Bleuler (1911; pp. 185 and 191) described patients: 'performing all kinds of manipulations with their teeth ... (with) grimaces of all kinds, (and) extraordinary movements of the tongue and lips.' He classified these as manneristic/stereotyped disorders – as largely something in need of interpretation – and chastised those who called them, 'quite mistakenly', choreiform. However, Bleuler was at best neurologically inconsistent and at worst confused, as at different points he himself used words such as 'involuntary' (p. 191) and 'unco-ordinated' (p. 215) to describe some of these movements. In addition, in describing other motor activity, he wrote 'I cannot immediately differentiate many (such) acts from organic apraxia.', yet concluded, 'I am convinced that all these various elements represent concomitant influences' (p. 196).

Thus, Bleuler was hooked on unconscious mechanisms (i.e. 'concomitant influences') and there was no doubt against whom his chastisement was directed.

Kraepelin (1919) was very much in the descriptive tradition. Not for him the analytical speculations of Bleuler. What Kraepelin saw from his medical perspective was what his medical readership got. He also noted movement disorders and, although his inferential neutrality precluded him adopting Bleuler's firm explanatory posture, there is no doubt what side of the fence he was on (p. 83):

> The spasmodic phenomena of the musculature of the face and of speech, which often appear, are extremely peculiar disorders. Some of them resemble movements of expression which we bring together under the name of making faces or grimacing; they remind one of the corresponding disorders of choreic patients. Nystagmus may also belong to this group. Connected with these are further, smacking and clicking with the tongue ... (and) we observe especially in the lip muscles, fine lightening-like or rhythmical twitchings, which in no way bear the stamp of voluntary movements ... The outspread fingers show fine tremor. Several patients continually carried out peculiar sprawling, irregular, choreiform outspreading movements, which I think I can best characterise by the expression 'athetoid ataxia'.

Over the years, a number of authors have reported involuntary movements in psychotic patients never exposed to antipsychotics, most *after* the delineation of dementia praecox (Table 8.1). These studies were either done in the pre-antipsychotic era or referred to patients who remained unexposed for administrative or other reasons.

This literature is clearly small, especially when placed in comparison to the reams of paper filled with reports on disorder of 'tardive' sort. However, this need not concern us too much. The climate of psychiatry for most of this century was quite definitely not in the direction of a neurology

Table 8.1. *Historical accounts of involuntary movements in (psychosis and) schizophrenia*

Griesinger	1857
Diller	1890
Bleuler	1911
Kraepelin	1919
Farran-Ridge	1926
Reiter	1926
Jelliffe	1926
Kleist	1936
Jones	1941
Leonhard	1957
Jones and Hunter	1969
Yarden and Discipio	1971
Brandon et al.	1971

for schizophrenia – in that sense, Bleuler won the early part of the day. Furthermore, it is highly likely that any motor disorder that might have been present in populations of a previous generation either would have remained buried amid the behavioural chaos that was the pre-antipsychotic long-stay ward or would have been interpreted out of existence as a neurological sign. As seen earlier from the study of Weiden and colleagues (1987), even at a time when involuntary movement disorders were a priority area given maximum exposure in the professional literature, recognition was still appalling. The roots of 'tramlining' run deep. Thus, the absence of a dominating theme of involuntary movements in association with schizophrenia prior to the introduction of antipsychotics cannot be taken as evidence that such disorders did not exist.

A further criticism that came from neurology was that such patients as were brought to attention were more likely to have originally suffered from encephalitis lethargica. This is certainly possible with some of the earlier reports, but can hardly be proffered as a serious explanation for cases comprising more recent publications. The fact is that by the application of operational criteria, such cases can be shown to conform to what we now call schizophrenia.

Although free from exposure to antipsychotics, cases showing involuntary movements were invariably not free from exposure to all physical treatments, but again there is no evidence that those physical interventions that they might have received were contributory (Owens et al., 1982).

Reference is made at several points in the present volume to an early study of the author's that comprised the first comprehensive review of the long-stay schizophrenic population of a large psychiatric hospital to apply systematic and standardised methodology. As findings within this population were instrumental in reviving the question of the relationship between involuntary movements and the disease process itself, it may be of interest briefly to review this study.

The Shenley Study

Shenley Hospital in Radlett, Herts, was one of the last of the large, purpose-built psychiatric hospitals constructed in Britain. It was opened by King George V in 1934 to serve north-west London – latterly, the boroughs of Brent and Harrow.

It was, in its day, a place of innovation. Dr Russell Barton published his still-quoted monograph on 'Institutional Neurosis' while acting as its superintendent, and it was there that Dr David Cooper, one of the doyens of the so-called 'antipsychiatry' movement of the late 1960s, ran the famous (or infamous) Villa 21, a much publicised and controversial therapeutic community devoted to the management of schizophrenia. From the mid-1970s, it provided the patients for the first CT scan study in schizophrenia, the material on which the Type I/Type II hypothesis was proposed, the first of the modern studies of chronic schizophrenia, and more. It is one aspect of the last of these that will be concentrated on here (Owens and Johnstone, 1980).

This study concerned all inpatients resident for at least one year who conformed to the St Louis Criteria for Schizophrenia – a total of 510 subjects. A detailed array of personal and historical information, including past treatments, was extracted from the case notes and the patients were examined in terms of their mental state, cognitive ability, behavioural competence and neurological status, including involuntary movements. What was novel about this study was that, for the first time, standardised methodology was applied to a severe and comprehensive long-stay population.

The core finding of relevance to the present considerations was that involuntary movements (recorded on a simple present/absent basis) did *not* correlate with positive mental state features but *did* correlate strongly with negative features, cognitive impairment and behavioural disorganisation, the latter three of which were also strongly inter-correlated (Fig. 8.1).

In the course of this investigation, it became clear that in one section of the hospital, physical treatments, including antipsychotics, had been eschewed and that a number of patients remained who had been

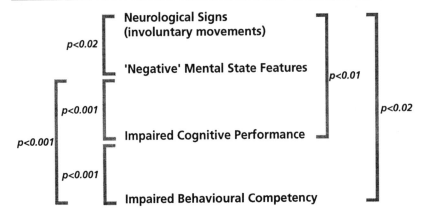

Fig. 8.1. The Shenley Study: relationships between domains of disability. (From Owens and Johnstone, 1980, with permission.)

kept drug free throughout the entire duration of their illnesses. Initially, this group comprised 65 subjects. By this time, standardised schedules had become available for recording involuntary movements and it was felt important to repeat these examinations using two such scales, the AIMS and the Rockland, or Simpson, Dyskinesia Scale (see Chapter 11).

A total of 411 patients was available for re-examination, but junior doctors being as they are, 15 of the original drug-naive sample had in the interim been started on antipsychotics. Using data from this second examination (Owens et al., 1982), movement disorders – recorded on either scale and however analysed – were indistinguishable in those with a history of antipsychotic exposure compared to those with no such history (Fig. 8.2). The prevalences, severities and patterns did not significantly differ.

Thus, at a straightforward clinical level, the mere presence of a history of antipsychotic exposure would not in itself have been sufficient to confirm a diagnosis of tardive dyskinesia.

On further analysis, however, the antipsychotic 'virgins' were, at 66.7 years of age, on average about 10 years older than the antipsychotically 'ravaged' (mean age 56.9 years) and in this sample, as in others, movement disorder was related positively to age. Taking age into account, a significant effect of drugs was evident. However, this emerged from a baseline of disorder inherent to the untreated illness that, at around 45 per cent was very high (Fig. 8.3).

To say that these data did not set the psychiatric world alight would be an understatement. Collective somnolence is more the impression that springs to mind! Nonetheless, they do imply that, in older schizophrenic patients at least, involuntary movements may emerge as part of

■ Antipsychotic treated patients
■ Non-antipsychotic treated patients

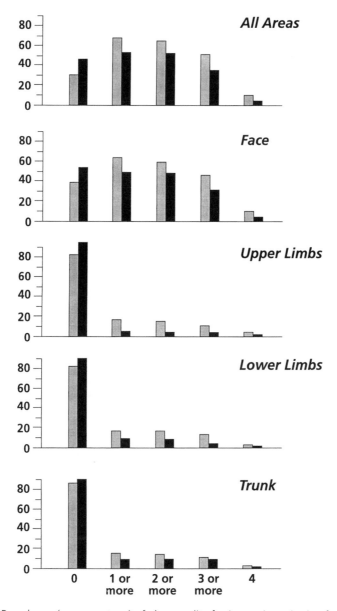

Fig. 8.2. Prevalence (as percentage) of abnormality for increasing criteria of severity on AIMS. (From Owens et al., 1982, with permission.)

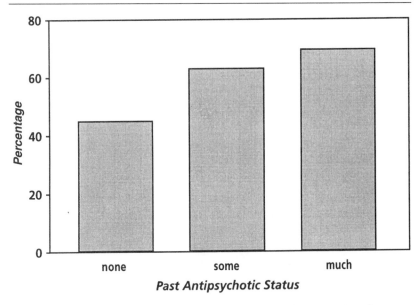

Fig. 8.3. AIMS: prevalence of abnormality (two or more) by categories of past antipsychotic exposure.

the evolution of the unmodified disease process. This may be the result of chronic illness-related pathophysiological changes in the striatum interacting with or potentiating normal changes associated with ageing.

The population from which these data were obtained was to some extent unique in being an anachronistic hangover from a bygone therapeutic age. Around the world, schizophrenic patients who remain antipsychotic free over many years of illness are increasingly rare even in non-industrial societies. Shortly after our finding emerged, one of the author's junior colleagues announced his intention of devoting two years to voluntary service in a part of the Western Pacific where, so it seemed from London, there would be an excellent opportunity to recruit long-standing, drug-free schizophrenic patients. The junior was duly trained up in the assessment of extrapyramidal function and sent packing with a wad of schedules and a lot of expectation. Unfortunately, it transpired that the only things the islands in question possessed in abundance were coconuts and chlorpromazine!

Two attempts to replicate the Shenley findings, one in Morocco the other in Nigeria, were unsuccessful (Chiorfi and Moussaoui, 1985; McCreadie and Ohaeri, 1994). However, these studies comprised relatively small numbers of drug-naive patients – but, most importantly, concerned younger schizophrenics.

Recently, other studies have supported the original Shenley findings. In a retrospective review of the uniquely detailed records of Chestnut

Lodge, Fenton, Wyatt and McGlashan. (1994) found motor abnormalities documented in 23 per cent of 100 operationally defined schizophrenic patients never exposed to antipsychotics, and in 15 per cent orofacial dyskinesia was described with sufficient clarity to be considered 'nearly certain'. Furthermore, the presence of orofacial disorder correlated with lower IQ level, more in the way of negative symptomatology, and greater symptomatic disturbance at follow-up, which was on average 23 years later.

McCreadie and colleagues (1996) have taken on board the fact that the Shenley sample was relatively old. They have reported on a population of chronic, drug-naive schizophrenics from Madras, in South-East India, who, with a mean age of 65 years, were comparable to our own sample and certainly elderly by the standards of their society. These authors similarly found, using the AIMS, a prevalence of movement disorder in the drug-naive schizophrenics that was not only indistinguishable from that in patients treated with antipsychotics (38 per cent versus 41 per cent respectively), but was also remarkably similar to our own. Provisional findings from a further on-going study in Morocco are pointing in the same direction.

The limitations of the concept of tardive dyskinesia

Data of this sort cannot, and ought not to, be used in futile attempts to deny the epidemiological validity of the concept of tardive dyskinesia. They do indicate, however, that the role of drugs in some schizophrenics at least may be more one of promotion rather than 'cause' de novo. It has already been mentioned that a model of 'neuro-medical' disposition has been proposed to explain the higher prevalence of spontaneous involuntary movements in the physically ill elderly – that the movements may emerge as a consequence of illness-related effects on critical brain areas. It would not seem too radical to suppose that certain pathophysiological changes integral to some forms of schizophrenia may operate similarly. If it can be accepted without controversy that antipsychotic medication can act on a pathophysiological substrate to reveal an individual patient's tendency to parkinsonism, a similar hypothesis in relation to hyperkinesias would not seem to represent a giant leap in the dark.

In support of such an 'integrated' hypothesis, reference has already been made to recent findings showing that between one-fifth and one-sixth of first-episode, drug-naive schizophrenics have extrapyramidal signs at presentation (Caligiuri et al., 1993; Chatterjee et al., 1995). The Hillside group has further shown the prognostic significance of these in that such patients took a longer time to reach remission, had a generally

poorer outcome, showed more negative features and – most significantly, from the point of view of the present discussion – were more
likely to develop drug-related extrapyramidal symptomatology
(Chatterjee et al., 1995).

It certainly seems the case that the 'causes' of involuntary movements
in association with antipsychotic drug use are multifactorial and that, if
we wish to *understand* this complex problem, as opposed to merely
establishing the validity of the epidemiological concept, we must look
beyond the obvious drug factors to others inherent to the conditions for
which the drugs are being given in the first place.

To this extent, the heated debates of the early 1980s were an essential
element in sustaining the breadth of perception necessary to address a
question more complex than was originally thought.

9

Special populations

Children and adolescents

In adults, the major indications for the use of antipsychotic medication are, for the most part, agreed. They may not in practice be universally applied, but at least on the written page it is possible to obtain some element of consensus on those categories of illness in which their use ought to be recommended.

The position in children and adolescents has been much more open and controversial. Concern has especially focused on the use of antipsychotics as agents of non-specific behavioural control rather than as drugs active against specific disorders of the mental state. In recent years, however, a number of specific indications have been identified on the basis of clinical research and it is therefore the case that these compounds will continue to be used in the very young.

The literature on extrapyramidal side-effects of antipsychotics in children and adolescents is poor. Studies are few and often methodologically flawed, limiting the conclusions that can be drawn. There is an uncomfortable component of surmise in what is to follow.

However, it is important to acknowledge the problems that recognition of disorders of this type present for those involved in paediatric practice. Patients are less able to articulate, far less understand, symptomatology, which is more likely than in adults to show solely in behavioural terms. As a result, formal examination in children requires much greater levels of expertise and ingenuity than in adults, a particular issue for those whose background and inclination may be towards predominantly psychological mechanisms. It is, therefore, all the more important for those in paediatric practice to maintain an even higher index of suspicion than colleagues whose work is with adult patients.

Table 9.1. *EPS in children and adolescents: the prevalence of acute dystonias*

Study	Sample	Age (years)	Prevalance (%)
Polizos & Engelhardt (1978)	Schizophrenia with autistic features	Mean 8.8	5.75
Chiles (1978)	Acutely psychotic	13–18	63.6
Campbell et al. (1984)	Aggressive/conduct disorder	5–13	16.4
Spencer et al. (1992)	Schizophrenia	Mean 8.8	17.5 (35 including symptoms)

Acute dystonias

The very young are not immune to acute dystonias, which can be caused by the same range of drugs as in adults. In addition, those in paediatric practice must be alert to the extensive range of widely advertised proprietary 'cold cures' containing antihistamines and non-antipsychotic phenothiazines that may promote disorders of this type.

Pre-emptive intervention is extremely difficult in children owing to their inability to articulate the subjective component that represents early or mild disorder. This can only be seen in behavioural terms, with increasing restlessness, querrulousness or clinging dependency, which is even more likely than in adults to be confused with symptoms of the condition for which medication is being given.

Thus, in the young, one is more likely to be confronted by the sudden onset of signs in the form of gross postural distortion, which, it is again worth emphasising, is likely to adopt a generalised (i.e. whole-body) distribution. The sudden onset of such gross disorder, perhaps interspersed with periods of relief from a naturally fluctuating course, in a child terrorised into muteness can easily be misdiagnosed as seizures, a particular trap to be wary of. One wonders how many children with flu-like illnesses medicated by their parents have gone down the diagnostic road to febrile convulsion when a drug history might have alerted to another, less sinister, explanation.

Only half a dozen studies have reported on acute dystonias in the very young. Only four were systematic and in none was this the primary focus of investigation (Owens, 1995), so only a vague stab can be aimed at prevalence (Table 9.1). From what was said previously about the strong inverse relationship between acute dystonias and age in adults, one could be forgiven for assuming that the risk curve might extend backwards to reveal an even greater, if not universal, prevalence in the very young. Fortunately, this does not appear to be so. Reported prevalences range from 6 per cent to 63 per cent, suggesting a wide, but at least not a universal, constituency. These studies certainly allow us to conclude that at least some of the same risk factors operate in children as in adults, in that the very high figure came from a high-dose/high-potency study (Chiles, 1978).

The best figures come from the New York group of Campbell and colleagues (1984; Spencer et al., 1992), who found a figure of 16.4 per cent in children aged 5–13 diagnosed with conduct disorder and treated with relatively modest doses of haloperidol. In a later prospective study of children with early-onset schizophrenia, they reported an incidence of 17.5 per cent though this figure doubled to 35 per cent with the inclusion of equivocal cases.

Acute dystonic episodes, therefore, can and do occur in children and adolescents with probably the same frequency as in young adults exposed to similar medications, though their recognition requires the exercise of particular awareness.

The principles of treatment for drug-related acute dystonias in the young are the same as for adults.

Parkinsonism

The literature on drug-related parkinsonism in the young is truly meagre (Owens, 1995), as a result of which it is not possible to comment accurately on any of the issues discussed above in connection with adult patients.

Again, the condition presents particular challenges for diagnosis. Affected children may be no more than somewhat withdrawn or disinterested and may be thought to be 'depressed'. Motor behaviour may be crude and unrefined, with the child considered 'clumsy'. Two studies have reported drooling to be the most frequent feature (Engelhardt and Polizos, 1978; Spencer et al., 1992), but whether this means sialorrhoea is a genuinely more prominent sign in the young or merely that the relatively less sophisticated social behaviour of children makes it more evident is unclear. Alternatively, if observations from adults can be transposed, it may mean that disorder has to be more pronounced before it can be recognised.

The positive association of drug-related parkinsonism and age in adults may once again allow one to ask whether children might not be immune – or even relatively immune – from the disorder. This is clearly *not* the case, although just how commonly the problem occurs cannot be stated with any confidence. It seems likely that it is to be found with the same frequency as in young adults, but even this is an assumption. Similarly, nothing can be added regarding predisposing factors, course and outcome etc., though it is safe to conclude that management principles are the same.

The lack of data on the characteristics of drug-related parkinsonism in the young is a glaring omission from the psychiatric literature and, with specific indications for the use of antipsychotics in childhood psychiatric disorders now being established, is one that needs urgent addressing.

Akathisia

The difficulties of diagnosing extrapyramidal dysfunction in children are encapsulated in the problems associated with akathisia. As has been seen, akathisia in its 'classical' or acute form is more of a dysphoric mood state than a motor disorder, and in populations who lack the verbal facility to describe the symptomatology, the diagnosis becomes problematic. Furthermore, some of the conditions for which antipsychotics are prescribed may themselves be associated with non-goal-directed overactivity.

There is little advice the author can give those in paediatric practice to promote a heightened recognition of akathisia, except to remind them yet again of the need for the highest index of suspicion in 'at-risk' patients. Indeed, a useful principle in approaching the problem might be to assume its presence unless and until one can be convinced of its absence.

Again, one is confronted with a desert – or perhaps, in fairness, a semi-arid zone – in attempting to derive even a prevalence figure from the literature. Only some six studies have broached the question (Owens, 1995), and although these include the largest sample sizes of any of the studies looking at EPS in the young, the work is not of the greatest quality. The figures vary from 0 per cent to 13 per cent, with an average at around 5 per cent.

Clearly, this is an extremely low figure in comparison to that from the adult literature. Even if this figure is genuine and not a spurious consequence of the poor-quality data from which it is derived, it is likely to reflect more modest exposure patterns in children rather than any protective influence of young age itself, though this assumption must be clarified.

There is nothing to suggest that approaches to the management of akathisia in children should be any different from those set out for adults.

Tardive dyskinesia

It is in the field of tardive movement disorders that the paediatric literature is strongest with over a dozen published studies (Owens, 1995). A number of these studies suffer the same problems of retrospective design, sample heterogeneity and unstandardised evaluation as the early adult literature, though several are of good quality.

Table 9.2. *Tardive dyskinesia in children treated with antipsychotics: the New York prospective studies*

Study	n	Age (years)	Prevalence/ incidence	Treatment or withdrawal emergent
Campbell et al. (1982)	33	2.3–7.9	12	T/E+W/E
Campbell et al. (1983)	36	2.8–7.8	22	T/E+W/E (3+5)
Perry et al. (1985)	58	3.6–7.8	22	T/E+W/E (4+9)
Campbell et al. (1988)	82	2.7–11	29	T/E+W/E (5+19)
Malone et al. (1991)	104	2.32–8.22	28	T/E+W/E (6+23)
Locascio et al. (1991)	125(73)*	2.3–8.2	29	?

* Long-term treatment group.

The particular problem for the evaluation of childhood tardive movements is ensuring the distinction from repetitive stereotyped movements that form an integral part of the symptomatology of a number of the childhood disorders for which antipsychotics are given (Campbell et al., 1982; Meiselas et al., 1989). This can only be satisfactorily addressed in prospective studies in which baseline levels of such disorders can be accounted for. Only the New York group has taken this issue on board to date (Table 9.2).

Tardive movement disorders *do* occur in children exposed to antipsychotics, and with a prevalence that is probably comparable to that in adults. The reported prevalences range from 8 per cent to 45 per cent, with an average of 28.3 per cent. At one level, this is worrying for those who work with and treat children suffering from major psychiatric disorders. However, this literature does provide some contrasts with that referring to adults, which may form a basis for militating the pessimism.

Firstly, it is clear that tardive disorders in children are overwhelmingly withdrawal emergent. Table 9.2 summarises the prospective data from the New York group, which are to be interpreted in the context of haloperidol use. These data show that approximately 30 per cent of patients developed involuntary movements during the course of haloperidol treatment (these are not strictly incidence figures because subjects left and joined the cohort over time). This is clearly comparable to the prevalence for adults discussed above. In the early years of follow-up, when numbers were relatively small, between 30 per cent and 40 per cent of disorder was treatment emergent. However, in more recent follow-ups with larger numbers, the figure has settled at 20 per cent. That is, overall, only about 5–6 per cent of these children developed involuntary movement disorder recognisable in terms of its adult counterpart. In the largest single study to date, 5.8 per cent of patients demonstrated disorder that was definitely treatment emergent (Malone et al., 1991). Indeed, some of the motor abnormality in these children seemed to represent an exacerbation of pre-existing stereotyped disorder, so the de-novo contribution of antipsychotics was therefore even less than the 'raw' figures would imply.

It has also been reported that treatment-emergent disorder is usually of mild severity, with only around half of cases conforming to operational (Schooler and Kane) criteria (Richardson, Haugland and Craig, 1991).

The second point of consensus is probably not unrelated, and that is that these movement disorders appear largely reversible. The vast majority resolve within 3 to 12 months of discontinuing antipsychotics (Owens, 1995). Where the clinical condition is such that the cessation of antipsychotics is associated not only with the emergence of movement disorders but with psychotic relapse, the neurological signs seem readily suppressed on restarting treatment. What is not clear, however, is the long-term outcome in such cases – whether they remain suppressed or whether they eventually become treatment emergent.

The evidence to date is that orofacial disorder is a less prominent part of the total disorder in children, being the sole focus of abnormality in only 16–40 per cent of cases (Owens, 1995). This is in keeping with speculations from multivariate analyses of adult ratings that orofacial disorder is more directly related to the changes associated with ageing that were mentioned above.

No specific predisposing factors have been established, and it is worth noting that, in the paediatric literature, this applies to intellectual level.

While there is no room for complacency, and more work is certainly required, it might be concluded thus far that tardive dyskinesia is indeed generally less severe in children than in adults. The immature brain may, therefore, possess sufficient reserve to at least partially absorb the adverse effects of antipsychotic medication and/or sufficient plasticity to compensate for any changes that may result. It will be of particular interest to see, from long-term follow-up of childhood tardive cases, what happens to this differential in severity through the synaptic pruning of early adult life.

Learning disability

It is in the field of learning disability that the ethical and legal challenges to the use of antipsychotics have perhaps been most contentiously brought. Indeed, in the early 1970s the US Federal Drug Administration was petitioned with a request that, on the basis of lack of evidence of efficacy, their use should be suspended in institutions for the mentally handicapped. Objections then and since have revolved around the use of these drugs to control disruptive behaviours, which, it has been argued, are infrequently a constituent of illness and therefore ought more properly to be tackled by environmental, social and other interpersonal means that reflect more accurately their origins.

It is beyond the scope of our present deliberations to explore these arguments further, but on largely empirical grounds, antipsychotics continue to be a major plank of management in those with learning disability who exhibit impulsive, aggressive or injurious behaviours. In addition, however, it is clear that psychotic disorders can develop in the learning disabled and, indeed, there is evidence that the risk may be greater than in the population at large. It has been found, for example, that schizophrenia has a prevalence approximately three times that of the general population (Turner, 1989). Indications for the use of antipsychotics in these populations are being increasingly defined.

Thus, notwithstanding concerns about their inappropriate prescription, antipsychotics will continue to have a place in the management of patients with learning disability, and hence a risk of extrapyramidal disturbance is something to which we must be alert.

Motor disorders are an integral part of many states that give rise to learning difficulties, and the systematic evaluation of those superadded abnormalities associated with the use of antipsychotic drugs, especially the tardive disorders, requires particular skill. As with children, assessment is heavily predicated on observation without the dimension of patient subjectivity, and as such the clinician is once again heavily reliant on a high index of suspicion.

Despite the importance of the issue, research-derived information is alarmingly rudimentary, with published work focusing largely on tardive dyskinesia. In fact, it is not possible to provide a systematic review of the literature on disorders of the acute/intermediate type in such populations because there is no substantive body of literature to compare and review. This is not because such individuals are immune. In one study of almost 1300 patients, 13 per cent were rated as having akathisia (Stone, Alvarez and May, 1988), though, in view of the communication problems that so blight the diagnosis, reported figures as low as 3.7–7 per cent come as no surprise. Stone and colleagues also reported a prevalence of parkinsonism of only 3 per cent, a figure that should in itself have stimulated interest. These figures are certainly lower than those reported for general adult populations, but derive from too flimsy and narrow a base to allow of any definite conclusion.

With regard to tardive dyskinesia, the data are stronger. In a detailed review of early studies, Kalachnik (1984) calculated a mean prevalence of 29 per cent for persistent dyskinesias and of 36 per cent for with-drawal-emergent disorder. The study of Richardson et al. (1986) is of interest in that it applied comparable methodology to that utilised in general psychiatric populations. In a group of over 200 develop-mentally disabled, long-stay residents (mean age 35 years), the authors found a point prevalence of 24 per cent applying operational criteria to data from the Abbreviated Simpson Scale (see below) which is compar-able to that reported by Woerner et al. (1991) with the same instrument in general adult samples, as discussed previously. However, the preva-lence did rise to 49 per cent attaching the same criteria to AIMS data.

Overall, it can reasonably be concluded that figures from adult populations with learning disability are within the range reported for patients without learning disabilities – that is, between 20 per cent and 30 per cent. Furthermore, the suggestion is of disorder that is again pre-dominantly orofacial.

While acknowledging the potential confound of motor disorders inherent to the varied states comprising learning disability, Bodfish et al. (1996) have claimed that it is possible to distinguish these from tardive disorders on the basis of topography. Stereotyped movements involved predominantly whole-body rocking, whereas movements designated 'tardive' were largely orofacial. The presence of stereotyped abnormality was associated with an increased prevalence of tardive dyskinesia, with higher levels of dyskinesias in those also exhibiting stereotypies who had been drug free for three years. This would support the promotional rather than de-novo causative role for antipsychotic medication.

Despite this, it is hard to escape the criticism that *all* studies of move-ment disorder inevitably make some a priori assumptions about aetiol-ogy, which in populations afflicted by multiple symptomatologies, may oversimplify a complex situation.

The dominance of motor disorder in those with learning disability was demonstrated by Rogers et al. (1991) using the so-called 'non-prejudicial' recording method – in other words, an approach which does not involve prior assumptions about the aetiology of *any* abnormalities. Rogers et al. found that although some degree of motor disorder was virtually universal, ratings for these correlated with the severity of mental handicap. Effects of antipsychotic exposure *were* evident, but all those types of disorder found in the treated patients were also to be seen in those who had remained drug free, which again the authors interpreted as indicating a promotional action of the medication.

In a similar vein, Dinan and Golden (1990) reported orofacial dyskinesias, defined on the basis of at least one '3' (moderate) rating on the pertinent items of the AIMS, in 70 per cent of a population with Down's syndrome who were aged between 30 and 60 years. In line with other findings in adult females (Farren and Dinan, 1994), the authors found an association with intellectual impairment but not with age. The intriguing possibility from these data is once more that of biological predisposition inherent to the underlying disorder.

Drug-related extrapyramidal dysfunction in the learning disabled exposed to antipsychotic drugs is a field ripe for meticulous exploration. Basic demographic information is urgently required for disorders at the acute/intermediate end of the spectrum, while clarification of associations with tardive motor disorders could open further the window on mechanisms of pathophysiological predisposition. As in other populations to which reference has been made, however, clear relationships with levels of intellectual impairment are not universally found, and the explanation of this discrepancy will be of interest beyond the boundaries of learning disability.

Undoubtedly, the would-be researcher in this field must confront major problems, but if it is not beyond the ingenuity of our species to place a man on the moon, these must surely be surmountable. In particular, the use of video to record the sign-based symptomatology that lies at the heart of most of the relevant syndromes would seem particularly suited to work in this patient group. The complexities of motor function in the naturalistic state, however, also emphasise the need for studies incorporating drug-naive control groups.

The elderly

Several issues raised at other points in this volume in themselves justify this heading, as do one or two other important considerations, in order to emphasise the vulnerability of the elderly to extrapyramidal adverse effects.

As has been noted, all the extrapyramidal syndromes associated with antidopaminergic use, with the exception of acute dystonias, increase in frequency with increasing age, and while the effect of age on severity has only been formally investigated and established for tardive dyskinesia, it is possible that a similar relationship pertains with parkinsonism and akathisia. These facts in themselves urge conservatism in exposing older patients to antipsychotics.

There is, however, a particular concern in relation to tardive dyskinesia, and that is the observation referred to previously that vulnerability may increase with increasing age of first exposure, especially if this occurs after the middle of the sixth decade. This, combined with the fact that the likelihood of reversibility decreases with advancing years, underlines the need for caution in starting treatment with antipsychotics for the first time in older patients. In particular, it argues powerfully for avoiding, wherever possible, their use to achieve non-specific treatment goals such as improved sleep pattern and control of agitation in those suffering from dementia (see below).

This enhanced vulnerability to tardive dyskinesia with late first-time exposure in effect amounts to a decrease in the duration of exposure to antipsychotics necessary for the development of the disorder, as already noted. A similar phenomenon operative in parkinsonism and akathisia would certainly seem logical. The impact of both of these disorders in the elderly can be profound, but may affect domains of functioning not readily apparent to the unwary. A major source of morbidity and a contributing factor to mortality in the elderly is locomotor instability, which, regardless of its primary causes, may be more likely to result in falls if parkinsonism and/or akathisia supervene. It is all too easy to confuse the features of parkinsonism with 'just old age' or to assume their origins in the therapeutically bleak terrain of idiopathic disease.

This latter point was illustrated in one recent study in which the prior use of antipsychotics was evaluated in matched groups of elderly patients who had or had not been newly prescribed an antiparkinson drug (Avorn et al., 1995). Those receiving antipsychotics were 5.4 times more likely to start antiparkinson treatment, which is hardly surprising. What was surprising, however, was the fact that they also had a twofold increase in likelihood of starting a dopaminergic drug. Indeed, in those receiving dopaminergic medication, 37 per cent of such therapy could be attributed to previous antipsychotics, continuation of which occurred in 71 per cent!

It might be expected that such a therapeutic muddle could be avoided when the definitive diagnosis of Parkinson's disease and the decision to treat are collaborative and involve specialist services. Nonetheless, with a steady increase in the classes of drug implicated in the promotion of extrapyramidal disturbance, a number of which are likely to be used specifically to treat age-related illnesses, the importance of *always* obtaining a drug history in such patients cannot be overemphasised.

In recent years, interest has developed in the prevalence of extrapyramidal signs in patients suffering from Alzheimer's disease. Although differing methodologies probably underlie the differing figures reported, it is suggested that about one-third of patients with dementia of Alzheimer type show such, predominantly parkinsonian, features (Ellis et al., 1996). While these patients may to some extent be 'extrapyramidally' predisposed to the adverse effects of anti-dopaminergic medication, particular attention has focused on patients in whom this may be part of a defining clinical characteristic.

Lewy bodies have been known for some time to be the characteristic neuropathological finding in Parkinson's disease, in which they are classically described in a subcortical distribution. However, Lewy bodies are difficult to visualise in traditional preparations. The development in the late 1980s of an immunocytochemical technique using anti-bodies against a neuronal protein, ubiquitin, which is identified with the intracytoplasmic inclusions, allowed them to be readily visualised for the first time. This has sparked considerable interest in the role of Lewy body pathology in dementia, in which the inclusions can be seen to have more of a cortical distribution, and the relation between this and extrapyramidal symptomatology.

It is clear that Lewy body dementia comprises a considerable proportion of the dementing population, though just how much remains unclear. Post-mortem figures range from approximately 5 per cent to 25 per cent, with an average of around 18 per cent (Kalra, Bergeron and Lang, 1996). It does appear that a definable clinical pattern can be identified, and indeed operational diagnostic criteria have been proposed which have satisfactory reliability and specificity, although they remain modest with regard to sensitivity (McKeith et al., 1994)). Lewy body dementia is characterised by fluctuating, though usually not pronounced, cognitive impairment without sustained plateaux, prominent hallucinations (especially formed visual misperceptions of creatures or people), and established features of parkinsonism (especially rigidity), which are usually symmetrical, may be associated with a striking tendency to fall and that may develop in advance of the cognitive disability.

One of the clinical points of relevance in trying to make the distinction with Alzheimer's disease is the focus of our present concern. Such patients seem to be sensitive to a range of medications and, in particular, to antipsychotics (McKeith et al., 1992). It has been suggested that up to 80 per cent of patients with Lewy body disease will experience significant adverse effects to antipsychotic medication and that in at least half of these the effects will be severe, with a twofold to threefold increase in the mortality risk (McKeith et al., 1992). In addition to exacerbation of extrapyramidal symptomatology, such potentially terminal declines may also be contributed to by sudden, profound sedation, increasing confusion and, in some instances, a clinical complex resembling neuroleptic malignant syndrome.

There is, therefore, a need for great caution in the use of anti-psychotics in those suspected clinically of having Lewy body disease – so the differential is one that is worth attempting. However, caution is not the same as proscription and, in patients suffering the consequences of florid and fearful psychotic phenomena, antipsychotics may need to be considered.

Depots, because of their prolonged duration of action, have obviously no place, a ban that should similarly extend to high-potency oral compounds. Thioridazine, often favoured in the elderly and in doses not that much lower than those used for a younger clientele, has the added problems of potent anticholinergic actions, which may compromise cognition, and calcium channel antagonist properties, which may promote cardiac dysrhythmias in those predisposed by virtue of age-related cardiac disease. Despite its entrenched role in geriatric psychiatry practice, thioridazine has often struck the author as an unusual drug to occupy such a position.

Recently, clozapine has been reported as useful in treating the psychotic features associated with Lewy body disease (Chacko, Hurley and Jankovic, 1993), but more firm data are required before this can be generally endorsed. Once again, the potent anticholinergic actions of this drug may be responsible for as many problems as its other actions solve. The value of other, new-generation, drugs remains to be seen, though if early expectations are borne out, this may be a particular area in which their enhanced neurological tolerability has benefits to offer.

Antiparkinson medication has been found to be helpful, though its effects are usually fairly short lived, and the potential risks of both L-dopa and anticholinergics in this population should not need to be expounded. Chlormethiazole has been raised from prolonged psychiatric entombment and suggested as a treatment on the basis of a 'neuroprotective' effect demonstrated in animals (McKeith et al., 1995). This amounts to little in itself, and the only valid reason for the re-introduction of this drug in this context is empiricism. Until its benefits can be demonstrated in clinical trials, the reasons why it was largely eschewed by psychiatry in the first place should be borne in mind.

While the literature may be short of therapeutic options for this patient group, there is no doubt about the principle – ultra-low starting doses and slow, careful increments under close observation. Those dealing with such patients should be familiar with the 10 mg strength tablets of chlorpromazine, or its equivalent.

Acquired immune deficiency syndrome

Neurological complications associated with human immunodeficiency virus (HIV) infection are well known, with up to one-third of patients showing signs of neurological deficit at the time when acquired immune deficiency syndrome (AIDS) is first diagnosed. This may encompass signs of extrapyramidal disturbance, including abnormal involuntary movements that have been described as a presenting feature in those converting to full-blown AIDS (Nath, Jankovic and Pettigrew, 1987). Of particular concern to us, however, is the fact that patients with AIDS appear to comprise another group that is particularly vulnerable to the extrapyramidal side-effects of antidopaminergic medications.

Antidopaminergic medication is frequently indicated in AIDS patients. Metoclopramide and prochlorperazine are widely used in the management of the nausea that can be a common accompaniment of treating *Pneumocystis carinii* pneumonia with cotrimoxazole or pentamidine, while antipsychotics are clearly indicated for the control of psychotic symptomatology of whatever cause and specifically have been shown to be the most effective approach to treating patients with delirium (Breitbart et al., 1996). However, there is a growing literature pointing to a heightened vulnerability to EPS.

Much of the evidence continues to reside in the form of case reports, but in one controlled retrospective evaluation, patients with AIDS who had taken antidopaminergic drugs were found to be 2.4 times *more likely* to develop extrapyramidal symptomatology overall than age-matched psychotic patients without AIDS who had received antipsychotic medication. The increased risk applied across the 'acute' end of the spectrum, with the AIDS patients 2.4 times more likely to develop akathisia, 1.7 times more likely to develop dystonia, and 1.5 times more likely to develop 'rigidity'. Those most vulnerable were the patients treated with haloperidol, whose overall risk was 3.4 times that of those who did not receive it (Hriso et al., 1991).

This study does have the limitations of all retrospective designs, though the authors did address the obvious criticism that the psychotic patients would be more likely to have had prior exposure by excluding those treated for more than one month in the past. It does, nonetheless, produce data worthy of note. The study concerned younger patients (under 50 years) and was limited to the month after starting relevant medication, which restricted it to the early risk period only. It is possible that some of the differences in, for example, akathisia and parkinsonism might have been even more striking with an older population followed for longer. Furthermore, the results must be seen in light of the fact that the AIDS patients had received significantly lower mean chlorpromazine-equivalent doses than the psychotic patients (a calculation valid only for antipsychotics, which comprised the bulk of agents), and that this finding held even when their lower average body weight was accounted for.

Most of the literature on the heightened susceptibility of AIDS patients to EPS concerns dystonias, parkinsonism and akathisia, perhaps a reflection of antidopaminergic exposure that is relatively time limited. However, 'classical' tardive dyskinesia of very rapid onset over a two-week period has also been described in a patient treated with oral then depot fluphenazine in unexceptional doses for only six months (Shedlack, Soldato-Couture and Swanson, 1994). Dyskinesias in this patient were initially withdrawal emergent, but swiftly progressed and subsequently proved irreversible. Thus, it cannot be assumed that the liability to EPS in those suffering from AIDS is restricted to the 'acute/intermittent' end of the spectrum, and the prudent assumption would be that the risk of tardive disorders is also increased.

The mechanism whereby increased susceptibility is imparted in such patients is unclear. In some instances, opportunistic infections, such as cerebral toxoplasmosis, are likely to play a role. Another factor may be altered pharmacokinetics resulting from a lower body fat, with consequently less distribution of active drug to tissue stores. However, also of relevance are likely to be encephalopathic changes consequent upon the direct neurotropic actions of the virus itself (Factor, Podskalny and Barron, 1994). In the tardive dyskinesia case noted above, the clinical signs developed in consort with an advancing diffuse multifocal leukoencephalopathy consistent with AIDS (Shedlack et al., 1994). Although in this case the basal ganglia were not grossly involved, there is evidence from functional (PET) studies that AIDS encephalopathy is associated with early metabolic changes in these structures, changes that precede clinical signs and that are dynamic in line with progression over time (van Gorp et al., 1992; Hinkin et al., 1995).

This is a literature that is in need of – and that is likely to receive – expansion, but there is sufficient information available at present to alert all those who treat patients with HIV/AIDS to a potentially major therapeutic issue. The alert is incidentally also one that may apply to neuroleptic malignant syndrome (Breitbart, Marcotta and Call, 1988).

There is evidence, however, that, with parsimonious use, antipsychotics can remain a valuable part of the therapeutic armamentarium in this patient group (Breitbart et al., 1996) – a conclusion that could probably, with justification, also be extended to other antidopaminergic compounds. But, as with Lewy body dementia, this is another situation in which awareness of the heightened liability is an essential quality-of-care issue.

10

The clinical examination

Introduction

There is little point in having a sound theoretical knowledge of the constituent features comprising drug-related extrapyramidal disorders and the issues surrounding them, if one is a novice in their clinical evaluation. Hands-on expertise is an essential clinical skill.

Of all the components of medical evaluation, the neurological examination is the one about which general clinicians are invariably least confident. Even those junior doctors who can wield a stethoscope with at least a semblance of confidence turn into quivering wrecks when presented with a tendon hammer. If asked to evaluate extrapyramidal status, most would barely get past a tentative tweaking of the wrists as a token evaluation of rigidity. While some might view neurological skills as some sort of medical astrophysics, the routine neurological examination is, in fact, less taxing intellectually than it is physically.

The key to gaining useful information is to approach the examination *systematically*. Too often, non-neurologists 'do' a cranial nerve or two, test for a bit of weakness, tap a couple of tendons, check a few more cranial nerves and so on – ending with the plantars, the international neurological 'full-stop'! Such a confused approach to examination produces understandably confused results. This is the major reason why neurologicals performed by non-neurologists are often sorry affairs – this and, of course, ignorance.

Ignorance must not be underestimated. At an MRCP exam, the author recalls a cocky candidate being asked by a neurologist of international repute to exam infraspinatus. 'Certainly, sir,' replied the candidate, quite unfazed. 'Could you tell me precisely where it is, please?'

By this point in the present volume, the reader should be acquainted with 'where' the neurological symptomatology associated with antipsychotic drug use 'is'! It remains for the present section to provide some structure for eliciting it.

The following is not presented as 'the' definitive examination of extrapyramidal status. No such creature exists. Different practitioners will have different methods for eliciting different features. This section is offered merely to provide an organised approach to assessment within which the major abnormalities can be found. It may be that not all its components will be necessary for all circumstances, but if followed through systematically, it should provide comprehensive information of clinical value and certainly sufficient for completion of most, if not all, of the standardised recording instruments. However, the following is based on a methodology suitable for subjects able to participate to at least a limited degree, and would require modification for a direct transfer to young children or those with significant learning disability. Finally, and purely for reasons of simplicity of presentation, the description of the formal examination assumes the majority of clinicians to be right handed.

Preliminaries

Although the bulk of the time and effort will go into the formal examination, in a thorough assessment this will be sandwiched between two periods of unobtrusive evaluation, when the patient is observed without knowledge of the examiner's presence or purpose. This is necessary to remove from the symptomatology the modifying influences of the examination environment and procedure. Despite the greater commitment of the formal part of the examination, it is sometimes the case that as much, or more, information will come out of these informal 'peeks' at what is a more naturalistic situation, so the unobtrusive periods should be seen as an essential part of the whole exercise.

The first period of unobtrusive observation is prior to contact. One should try to watch patients as they sit in the waiting area or in other circumstances where they may be at a loose end, *before* your introduction. Observe, indeed, whether they can sit at all, and if so whether any postural, positional or other static disorders can be seen, or whether there is any hyperkinetic activity. If they cannot sit, try to gain some impression of reasons why this might be so.

Initial unobtrusive observation should be extended to include a period of general conversation after first introduction but before the start of the formal procedures. This chat is at the level of enquiries about overall well-being, social bits and pieces and, of course, in Britain at least, the weather. It is not a symptomatic enquiry, but merely a 'setting at ease' exercise that allows for a further dimension of assessment.

Observation will also be carried through the symptomatic enquiry, but this is obviously not strictly unobtrusive.

Thus, the first preliminary is to manipulate the circumstances such that an adequate period of unobtrusive observation is possible.

The environment in which the examination is conducted is important. Try to avoid poky, cluttered rooms with oppressive atmospheres in favour of bright and spacious surroundings with a more relaxing feel.

Offer patients a firm, high chair, with no arms. This denies them the temptation of leaning on the arms, which they may use as a ploy to support their posture or control involuntary activity. The arms may further act as an aid to standing. Even the most agile of individuals may require more than one attempt to extricate themselves from the soft, low chairs so popular in psychiatric clinics, which, furthermore, produce a stilted posture with use of the arms unavoidable, so these should be given a miss.

If there is a desk in the room, the patient should be seated to one side of this, with the examiner 'side on' so that there is an unobstructed view of all body parts. In fact, a better arrangement is to dispense with the desk altogether and have no physical obstructions between examiner and patient.

Whether this is done throughout the interview, or just during the motor examination itself, consideration should be given to the placing of the chairs. Do not sit directly facing the patient, which is too confrontational – as is sitting too close. Place your chair at approximately 45 degrees to the patient's and about a metre apart.

The second preliminary, therefore, is to ensure that the environment in which the examination is to be conducted is conducive.

Obviously, you are going to tell patients what you are up to, especially prior to the motor examination. But you would be well advised not to tell them too much. This is nothing to do with devious doctors withholding information, but more mundanely relates to the fact that if patients know what you are about, they will invariably try to 'help' you. With extrapyramidal symptomatology so amenable to extraneous influences, that is just what you do not want. Most of all, never ask a patient to relax, which in the author's experience seems to be inevitably interpreted as an instruction to tense up! Experienced patients will, of course, become familiar with your techniques, but even here – and especially initially – keep your comments general, such as that you would like to see how well the patient is tolerating the medication etc.

There are three final questions prior to launching the formal proceedings: the first involves asking patients about their dental status; the second is about whether they have anything in their mouth; and the third is if they would mind removing their shoes.

The reasons for the first have already been noted, while the second avoids a snare for even the most experienced. The author recalls his delight that one patient's 'bon-bon' sign was so clearly evident during the making of an educational video. Unfortunately, I had omitted to ask the second question. The 'bon-bon' sign in this case was the consequence of a rather large 'bon-bon'! Removal of shoes is often overlooked but is important, firstly to provide the means for whole-body assessment, and secondly because it can allow appraisal of dexterity.

The final preliminaries therefore concern the instructions you provide to the patient.

The standardised examination

Phase I

Unobtrusive assessment (1)
As above.

Phase II

Introduction
The standardised examination will incorporate the following principles:

- a combination of formal and unobtrusive examination;
- a comprehensive approach covering the major syndromes and all body parts;
- a symptomatic enquiry which should extend to subjective symptomatology and activities of daily living, i.e. interference in domestic and social skills;
- a frame of reference that views the body by component areas – orofacial, facial expression, upper/lower limbs, trunk, internal;
- formal evaluation in both active and passive states;
- specific 'activation' or 'reinforcing' procedures;
- assessment of 'core' parkinsonian features in all body parts;
- the principle of 'scanning' – a specific focus at any point complemented by continuous whole-body appraisal.

Having completed the preliminaries, you are then in a position to begin formal examination. It is not conducive to the 'flow' of the examination to record positive features as you go along. Furthermore, a representative impression of a number of features may be best fostered by continuous appraisal throughout the examination. In order to avoid forgetting potentially important signs or confusing their sites, it is useful to see the patient as a 'combination' of different body areas rather than a single whole. In view of the frequency distribution of disorder, a useful breakdown is: (1) orofacial; (2) facial expression; (3) upper and lower limbs; (4) trunk, including neck; (5) 'other', including oropharynx, larynx, diaphragm etc.; with a special 'mental' category (6) reserved for walking, as this can be so revealing.

Despite what some scales recommend, there is no fixed time that can or should be allocated to each component of the examination. Each part should be as long or as short as is necessary for the examiner to be confident that he or she has gained a firm enough knowledge to comment on what is representative for that body part.

The symptomatic enquiry

It is necessary with the symptomatic enquiry to be sure that positive responses do, indeed, refer to extrapyramidal symptomatology because a number of the symptoms, such as stiffness, for example, may have other origins (e.g. orthopaedic). It is also important, if possible, to explore the impact of any features on practical domestic and social skills such as personal hygiene, dressing, using implements, ability to get about, including dealing with stairs etc. However, it is equally important that you do not jeopardise your assessment at this early stage by either protracting the enquiry unduly or turning it into an interrogation. While the importance of a symptomatic enquiry has been emphasised throughout the present volume, if that is all you get, it stands for little! In the face of the 'mother' of rambling interviewees or a querulous individual whose resistance is palpable, cut down on the verbiage.

Enquiry should cover subjective restlessness, weakness and slowness, and clumsiness with routine tasks, as well as stiffness and lack of suppleness, especially proximally in the mornings. Awareness of any 'cramps' or muscle spasms should be sought, along with twitches and any activity clearly recognised as involuntary, including 'shakes' and tremors. Patients should be asked about difficulties they may have noticed with posture or balance and any problems with walking and turning, and also about whether they have noticed a change in their voice, or in salivation and swallowing. The impact on activities of daily living is highly variable, and the clinician must use his or her ingenuity. The important point to be emphasised is that not all disability in your target population will be psychogenic.

The symptomatic enquiry allows one a further opportunity for observation. This is obviously not strictly unobtrusive, but it does allow for an overview of disorder that is evident without the patient being aware of a specific focus of examination. It also provides a basis for evaluating skin texture, resting tremor, should such be present, speech in terms of pitch, power and intonation and articulation, and for gauging the ebb and flow of interactive expression and gesture in both the face and more generally. In appraising hypomimia, one is looking for a loss of mobility, a flattening of facial contours and the reduction in blink rate that lies behind the rather glazed and distant eyes. During breaks in the conversation, the partially open, 'gormless' mouth may be seen. Speech and facial expression, like many of the features of interest, will undergo continual assessment throughout the examination.

Phase III

The orofacial area

The third phase begins with silent observation of patients in the passive state. Ask them to make themselves comfortable and to rest their hands gently on their lap and sit quietly, looking ahead (i.e. beyond the examiner) for a few moments. Remember to avoid the 'relax' word! Scan the body slowly several times, looking for any signs referable to any of the drug-related syndromes. From now on, *any* features that emerged during unobtrusive assessment should provide a valuable focus for particular attention. You are not only looking for involuntary movements, including tremor, but for any features worthy of note, from restless, fidgety behaviour to static disorders of posture.

Proceed by focusing on the orofacial area, to be assessed both passively and actively. Ask the patient to drop his or her mouth partially open while continuing to sit comfortably. One is particularly concerned with whether or not the tongue displays any of the types of movement described above and whether involuntary activity can be seen in the perioral musculature. This also provides an opportunity to evaluate the moistness of the oral cavity. Again, the whole body should be scanned several times for abnormal activity.

Then ask for the mouth to be actively opened and the tongue forcibly extruded. Assess for involuntary activity and undue moistness or drooling. Be wary of what appears a simple instruction being executed in a far from simple way. For example, some patients may be overcompliant and open their mouth and protrude their tongue to its limits, which makes for rapid fatigue and a quick breakdown of voluntary control. Also, be alert to manoeuvres to stabilise the tongue such as 'pinching' the protruded tongue between the lips or supporting it by curling it down over the chin. What is sought is forward, unsupported but *not* maximal protrusion. One must not be diffident about demonstrating to the patient exactly what is required – in fact, the author would commend such histrionics where appropriate throughout the examination, as they create an air of joint participation that helps keep the patient involved.

It has been suggested that an inability to sustain active tongue protrusion for 30 seconds is characteristic of pronounced tardive dyskinesia, but this is *not* a finding unique to this condition. In the course of orofacial evaluation, scan the whole body.

The above steps are then to be repeated during performance of an 'activating' procedure. There are a number of these that can be utilised at this point. The author's preferred one is bilateral opening and closing of fists raised to the side of the head, as this seems 'do-able' by even the most impaired patient. A task employed in my earlier days – opposing thumb and alternating fingers in regular sequence – seemed, for many, a painfully ponderous exercise that consumed remaining reserves of concentration. Never assume that what you as the examiner consider easy will be such to the patient. One is once again focusing on the orofacial area while scanning the whole body.

Phase IV

Motor tasks

The next step is to assess fluidity and dexterity of movement. Impairment here is one of the major manifestations of bradykinesia and is best evaluated comprehensively on a series of tests, with disorder rated 'globally' as a composite of your findings. There is no fixed number of these tests that must be done; again, the requirement is to ensure that one gains an impression of disorder that is representative. The first line of evaluation is from speed and ease of performance on a series of *natural* actions, such as rapid alternating supination/pronation, or rapidity of finger/thumb opposition, or, alternatively, touching dorsum and palmar surfaces of each hand in turn with the palmar surface of the other. At an even more rudimentary level, the patient can be asked to perform a simple tapping task such as finger tapping or tapping the heel on the floor, or lifting the foot off the floor and tapping with the toe.

Then ask the patient to move to the desk (if not already there). Watch how he or/she gets up from the chair and manipulates it to the desk. Do not intervene, but let the patient do this unaided. Then add to your evaluation of dexterity by asking the patient to perform a couple of *specific* tasks, like rotating a small object such as a match-box or pen in each hand in turn, or removing and lining up some matches, or, in these smoke-free days, placing multicoloured plastic counters in piles by colour. What you are looking for is slow or impaired initiation of movement, clumsy or hesitant execution and, in more severe cases, perhaps even interruption in the form of 'freezing'. As always, scan.

Next, ask the patient to write a short passage – his or her name and address are often recommended. A well-known nursery rhyme copied from a boldly typed sheet is another alternative the author used to use. There are concerns, however, that holding to the structure of name and address or a verse may allow the patient to 'tap into' an overlearned behaviour in militating against alterations in handwriting. The author has tended to abandon these in favour of a short prose passage dictated to the patient, such as 'I came to the hospital by car today because the buses are always full'. Remember that the public's abilities in tasks of this sort might not be up to those of the average medical practitioner and, for reasons that should by now be clear, one wants to avoid causing undue embarrassment – so keep it simple. Then, on the same page, ask the patient to draw a spiral (having first demonstrated what it is you want), with the dominant then the non-dominant hand.

As has been noted, alterations in handwriting have long been considered a subtle sign of drug-related extrapyramidal dysfunction, and this should be given weight. One is looking for a reduction in the size of writing and the space covered on the page. In addition, look for the rhythmic intrusions of tremor (see Fig. 4.4). Individual handwriting is, of course, hugely varied and one may not have previous examples of an individual's writing available for comparison. If there is no obvious point of comment, however, it is well worth asking patients if *they* have noticed any change. An alteration in writing is something most people are very aware of.

In examining the spiral, one is looking for loss of symmetry in the circular form from clumsiness in execution and a sinuous rather than a smooth line. This sinuosity will usually reveal the strikingly regular pattern of the tremor that underlies it (see Fig. 4.4).

It is important to note that, even in the absence of specific abnormalities of writing or drawing a spiral, one may still gain valuable information on dexterity by observing the way the patient executes the tasks – how fast, how flexibly, how smoothly – in short, how much the task is indeed a task as opposed to an elementary, almost automatic function.

Throughout this section, the importance of constant whole-body scanning is emphasised, and it is *crucial* that this is undertaken during a writing exercise. Writing is a skill that calls on not just motor but also cognitive assets and is particularly likely to be associated with some modification of involuntary activity in different body parts. The conventional teaching that this is activation must be borne in mind, but so, too, must the caveat to this discussed previously. The safest approach to evaluating the effects of writing on involuntary movements elsewhere is open-mindedness.

Phase V
For the next stage, one is going to ask the patient to take up his or her chair once again and move away from the desk. Some

examiners may prefer to have only one move, with everything at the desk being done either at the beginning or the end, but the author has found it useful in assessing mobility to have patients make, as it were, a double move. This is clearly a flexible component of the procedure.

Glabellar tap

The merits or otherwise of the glabellar tap have already been discussed. This can be a striking sign in idiopathic disease, but in psychiatric patients a positive response, if there at all, usually only allows non-specific inferences. Nonetheless, it may be required for some standardised ratings and it is as well not to compound the lack of specificity with bad examination technique.

Stand to the right of and slightly behind the patient and hold any floppy hair away from the forehead with your right hand. Even if the patient is bald as a coot, the right hand on the upper forehead is a useful 'trick' to help stabilise the head and standardise the procedure. Tell the patient that you are going to tap his or her forehead gently. Then, using the index or, preferably, the middle finger of the left hand, tap firmly and regularly about twice per second over the glabellar prominence in the midline, making sure that the other digits of the left hand do not intrude into the field of vision. This tapping movement should be a wrist action, producing a regular force with each tap. This should be done for 10 to 15 seconds and, in psychiatric patients, especially those who are clearly anxious, should be repeated after a short pause. The test is deemed positive if the initial blink response fails to habituate after six to eight taps. Strictly speaking, however, one does not require full eyelid closure to qualify as a blink; any on-going reflex contraction of orbicularis oculi, even without full eye closure, would be sufficient. Such minor movement is usually best seen inferomedially. It would seem, however, that in view of the risk of contamination of this feature with change that is non-specifically mediated (e.g. anxiety), it is best to veer on the side of conservatism in judging when a response is indeed positive. Again, scan.

Limb rigidity

The next task recommended for assessment is rigidity. The word 'task' is well chosen, for in the author's experience it is this feature above all others that clinicians make a four-course meal of! Tell the patient that you would like to examine the muscles and that all you require of him or her is to sit comfortably and let you do all the work. It is most of all here that the 'R' word – relax – is absolutely forbidden. At this point you are going to focus on the limbs (axial musculature will follow), and although proximal sites are the most sensitive sources of signs the technique is easiest for more distal muscles, so start there – with the wrist.

Stand to the right of the patient and take the lower third of the forearm, palm down, in your left hand. Then, grasp the patient's hand with your four fingers to its palm and your thumb over the dorsum to anchor the hand. Resistance to passive movement is assessed in the course of both a simple passive flexion/extension and a similar movement into which is incorporated an element of elliptical rotation. These should be alternated at random.

Do not assess rigidity immediately, but start with general movements that are merely designed to put patients at ease and to familiarise them with what you are about. Make conversation to distract them from the formality of the examination and, when you are convinced that the patient's responses are indeed passive, then make a mental note of your findings.

Tone at the elbow can be assessed by simply moving your left hand from the forearm to the lower third of the upper arm while still holding the hand as before. Alternatively, your right hand can also be moved to grasp the lower third of the patient's forearm. This latter position gives better overall control. The evaluation procedure is passive elbow flexion/extension, with the forearm in the neutral position, i.e. thenar eminence 'up'.

For supinators and pronators, rest the elbow in your left hand and hold fast with your thumb in the antecubital fossa over the flexor tendons and grasp the patient in a 'handshake' with your right hand and rotate clockwise and anticlockwise. This is also a useful position from which to evaluate rigidity in the shoulder muscles. For this assessment, the movement is again not just a backwards/forwards one, but should incorporate rotation and abduction, all in random order. As with the wrist, rigidity should be assessed only when you are convinced that movement is indeed passive.

Having completed this sequence of assessment in the resting state, it should then be repeated with patients performing a reinforcing exercise. Two possible choices are asking them to make a tight fist on the left while the examination is conducted on the right, or getting them to draw an imaginary circle in the air with their left index finger. If choosing the latter, however, be sure the circle is a large one and described from the shoulder, not the wrist. For the left side, the positions are simply reversed.

Rigidity of the legs requires the generation of a bit more sweat, often, it has to be said, for little proportionate return in terms of information. Drug-related rigidity is usually relatively mild and can be hard to elicit in the legs. Nonetheless, thoroughness requires it be attempted. This can be done by lying patients on a couch, though the author prefers to keep them seated in the chair. The best technique involves the examiner getting down on one knee. For the lower limbs start with the proximal, girdle muscles – that is, around the hip – as, unlike in the upper limb, it is probably easier to detect change there. Starting from the right, support the patient's knee from behind with your left hand and take the lower leg above the ankle in your right hand. Then, in a co-ordinated action, flex and straighten the whole leg, incorporating at the hip an element of abduction/adduction and gentle rotation. This position can clearly also be used for the knee, but for this it is perhaps better, rather than actively supporting the knee with your hand, to allow it to rest passively on the back of your wrist. The movement here is a simple flexion/extension. For the ankle, grasp the lower leg above the ankle with your left hand and lift the limb off the floor. Place your right hand as for the assessment of wrist rigidity – that is, the fingers of your hand on the patient's sole, with the foot supported on the dorsum by your thumb. Flexion/extension is again combined with random elliptical rotation.

The same reinforcement techniques may be utilised as were described for the upper limbs or, additionally, you might ask the patient to pull maximally against interlocked, cupped fingers.

If the examiner does not feel up to all this effort, there are two technically much simpler methods that can be used to assess tone in the limbs. For the upper limbs, the patient is simply asked to raise the arms horizontally to the side. The examiner then holds them at the upper arms/elbows and tells the patient to let him or her support the weight. When the examiner is sure that the patient is indeed resting the arms completely (a process helped by the examiner gently and irregularly 'rocking' the arms up and down), support is suddenly withdrawn. Rigidity is gauged by the rate at which the limbs fall and the noise they make on slapping against the patient's side.

For the legs, the patient is asked to sit on a couch with the legs dangling freely over the edge. It is important to be certain that the knees are not supported in any way by the edge of the couch, which is best ensured by having the lower third of the thighs overhanging. The legs are then grasped at the ankles and lifted forward (either singly or together) and, when resting fully in the examiner's hands, allowed to fall under gravity. The degree of rigidity is assessed on the basis of the degree to which gravity is thwarted and the duration and excursion of residual swinging.

The author has never felt comfortable with these regionally insensitive and essentially crude methods, which most importantly deny the examiner the expertise that comes uniquely from the 'feel' of the disorder. This expertise is especially important in categorising severity, a basic requirement of most standardised rating scales and one which cannot be adequately addressed other than by 'hands on' contact.

However, particular opprobrium is reserved for a related method of assessing upper axial and neck rigidity, which requires patients to lie comfortably on a couch, with the examiner then lifting their head and letting go! The degree of rigidity is assessed by the loudness of the whack with which the unsuspecting napper touches base. Such a technique may yield valid information at the first try, but is hardly conducive to repeated use.

Restlessness, axial rigidity, postural tremor, postural stability

A far more acceptable method of evaluating truncal rigidity comes in the next part of the formal examination. At this point, ask the patient to stand away from the chair in the 'at ease' position – that is, feet slightly apart, hands limp at the sides. Facing the patient, ask him or her to perform some simple cognitive task such as reciting the days of the week or months of the year backwards, or serial threes. Note any shifting of weight or dancing restlessness – and scan the whole body.

Then grasp the patient's shoulders firmly with your hands and tell him or her you are going to give them a shake. Rotate the shoulders back and forward resolutely, starting slowly and increasing in speed and force. This, in the Glasgow parlance, 'shoogle' method is as likely to raise co-operation – and a laugh – in the patient as the head bombing method is to precipitate them – parkinsonism notwithstanding – towards the door!

Next, ask the patient to extend the arms out in front, with the fingers apart, and to close his or her eyes. Observe the patient for a short period (at least 30 seconds and preferably longer), looking for postural tremor of the outstretched arms/hands/fingers. Note also the patient's ability to maintain the neutral position without signs of incipient hyperpronation. Tremor should also be sought in the eyelids, as, of course, should any other involuntary activity in any body part.

Now ask the patient to stand 'to attention' – that is, erect with feet together. You are going to test for postural instability, something that may be localised by direction, so all four must be looked at. First, stand in front of the patient and reach out to him or her with your hands at the level of the patient's upper arms and some 7–10 cm away. Explain that you are going to give the patient a tap. With your right hand, tap firmly on the upper arm. Instability can be seen in displacement excessive to the force applied and, in marked disorder, complete loss of balance. Hence, the function of your left hand is to provide a psychological and, if necessary, a physical support. However, instability may also be seen in delayed recovery of the erect position from the point of maximum displacement. After allowing the patient to re-adopt the neutral position, repeat two or three times, increasing the applied force slightly each time. The tap should be brisk, firm and a combined wrist and shoulder action. Repeat on the other side.

Then stand to the patient's right side and place your hands in front and behind, opposite the midsternum and the interscapular area, again a few centimetres away. Tap the sternum as above, noting the displacement and, if necessary, supporting the patient. After repeating this, then switch to tapping from behind on the upper back between the shoulder blades. In severe cases, patients may only be able to maintain the upright position against their displaced centre of gravity by forward (tapping on the back) or backward (tapping on the sternum) motion giving rise to anteropulsion or retropulsion respectively.

Phase VI

Walking

The final part of the examination is the most important – so it should be done properly. This is your appraisal of walking. Asking the patient to 'walk' a few steps in a cluttered, poky office is hopeless. An unbiased appraisal of all the features you wish to assess in this phase can only be undertaken with the patient walking free from all psychological as well as physical obstructions. What you are trying to achieve is to get the patient to move in as natural and uninhibited a way as possible, so unless you have the benefit of an exceptionally large room, get him or her out into the corridor.

Ask the patient to walk up and down in his or her normal walk, just as if out in the street. Allow the patient to walk *at least* 10–15 metres away from you before asking him or her to return. On the first occasion, patients are likely to be understandably rather self-conscious, so get them to repeat this two or three times, initially without, but latterly with, encouragement. Be sure they are not holding something in their hand and be most careful that they do not walk with their hands in their pockets, or hold them in any other way except by their sides. If they do, specifically ask them to walk 'hands by your side'.

First look at their speed of movement and seek out any distortions of posture not evident when they were stationary. Observe gait itself in terms of both the length and height of step and for evidence of loss of the normal heel-to-toe sequence. Look closely for any hyperkinetic movements, including tremor, in any body part that you have not seen before, especially periorally and in the hands and fingers. Watch how fast and with how much confidence they can turn on command. As they approach, look for signs of expressive masking, which may be more evident in this emotionally more distant situation. Most of all, look at the arms – for evidence of flexion, abduction, pronation and especially reduction in pendular swing.

Phase VII

Unobtrusive assessment
Once this is completed to your satisfaction and the patient takes his or her leave, do not think that your work is finished. Again, observe patients unobtrusively after you take your farewells. This is likely to be a slightly different emotional situation for patients than that which pertained before the interview because the element of being 'examined' – that element of enforced submission that, for even the most experienced patient, is psychologically intrusive – is now over. Something may emerge in this climate that did not before. Thus, this second period of unobtrusive observation is providing information about a *new* context and is not merely duplicating the earlier circumstances.

Phase VIII

Recording
It now rests with you to record your findings in your chosen format, a process that should be aided by the systematic recall to memory of the separate body areas – though, regretfully, this will not help you to classify one funny twitch from another. Some issues relevant to the major recording instruments are the subject of the next chapter.

Summary of the standardised examination of extrapyramidal status

Phase 1

Unobtrusive assessment prior to introduction, looking at posture, involuntary and other purposeless, non-goal-directed movements.

Phase II

Procedure: general greeting/conversation.

Purpose: essential to set patient at ease.

Seat patient in a firm, upright chair with no arms, away from desk.

General explanation: avoid specifics – patient's perception of the purpose of the examination may influence responses.

Ask patient: to remove shoes; if anything in mouth; about teeth (dentures/fit etc.); to place hands on lap.

General conversation leading to:

Symptomatic review:

weakness	walking/turning/balance
fatiguability	talking
stiffness/lack of suppleness	swallowing/drooling
clumsiness	shakes/tremors
slowness with routine tasks	restlessness
cramps	twitches/jerks/involuntary
postural disturbance	movements.

Subjective impact:

    domestic
    social.

Note:

    voice:
      pitch
      tone
      volume
      articulation
    facial expression
    resting tremor.

Phase III

Silent, passive observation with examiner seated approx 3 feet away and slightly angled (45 degrees) to avoid direct face to face contact.

Observe all body areas.

Note:

    posture
    involuntary activity
    restlessness
    resting tremor
    skin texture.

Ask: patient to open mouth partially.

Observe: tongue and all body areas.

Note:

    lingual/perioral/periorbital movements
    salivation
    any body movements.

Ask: patient to protrude tongue.

Observe: tongue and all body parts.

Note:

      lingual/perioral/periorbital movements
      salivation
      any body movements.

Additional observation: *note:* whether patient can maintain tongue in forced protrusion for 30 seconds or more.

Repeat the above with **'Activation' procedure.** For example:

Ask: patient to perform rapid thumb/alternating finger opposition.

Note:

      lingual/perioral movements
      any body movements

or

Ask: patient to open and close raised fists rapidly.

Phase IV

Ask: patient to perform rapidly alternating movements. For example:
      rapid supination/pronation *and/or*
      rapid finger/thumb opposition *and/or*
      rapid tapping dorsum/palm *and/or*
      rapid finger tapping *and/or*
      rapid tapping of heel on floor

Note:

      slow initiation
      clumsy/slow execution
      any body movements

Ask: patient to perform a simple motor task. For example:
      rotating matchbox rapidly in each hand *and/or*
      rotating pen/pencil rapidly in each hand *and/or*
      lining up matches removed from a box *and/or*
      placing coloured plastic counters in piles

Note:

      manual dexterity
      any body movements

Ask: patient to write a short passage, e.g. name/address/date etc. *or* nursery rhyme copied from bold-type sheet.

Note:

        writing

        any body movements

Ask: patient to draw a spiral (first demonstrate)

        with dominant hand

        with non-dominant hand

Note:

        irregularity, especially from tremor

        any body movements

Phase V

Stand to one side of patient

Additional examination: Glabellar tap.

Note: positive if periorbital muscle 'blink' fails to habituate after 6–8 taps.

Assess tone:

        at wrist

        forearm

        at elbow

        around shoulder

        around hips

        at knee

        at ankle

Note:

        hypertonicity

Continue full body scan.

Repeat with reinforcement.

Phase VI

Ask patient to stand – 'at ease'. **Face** the patient. **Apply** a simple cognitive test:

        months backwards

        serial threes.

Note:

        restlessness

        walking 'on the spot'

Continue scan.

Ask patient to outstretch arms in front, spread fingers and close eyes.

Note: postural tremor upper limbs, eyelids.

Continue scan.

Ask patient to **stand** – 'neutral position'. **Face** the patient. **Grasp** shoulders firmly and shake.

Note:
> axial rigidity
> resistance to movement
> 'floppiness' of arms

Ask patient to **stand** – 'at attention' (feet together). **Face** the patient.

Assess postural stability:
> to the right (left force)
> to the left (right force)
> backwards (force to sternum)
> forwards(force to interscapular area)

Note:
> excess displacement
> delayed recovery
> loss of position
> retropulsion
> anteropulsion

Continue scan.

Phase VII

Ensure adequate space for unrestricted walk (minimum 15 yards)

Ask patient to walk up and down
> in their normal walk,
> hands by side
> and not holding any objects

Note:
> truncal posture
> arm posture
> arm swing
> speed of walking
> length of step
> height of step

stability: turning on command
facial expression
any involuntary movements

Repeat several times.

Phase VIII

Patient departure.

Unobtrusive observation.

Note: any abnormal feature.

Record findings.

11

An overview of some standardised recording instruments

Introduction

Having systematically examined the patient, one is then left with the decision as to how to record the information for posterity – although, in fact, this decision is one that will have, or *ought* to have, been taken well in advance.

It may be that in routine practice one opts for simply describing what one has observed. If so, the author wishes you well! As far as the *signs* are concerned, not only does this result in pages of script that few are ever likely to read, it presents data that are unstandardised and of limited meaning to others, and that do not allow reliable comparisons of findings from serial evaluations. It is also an extremely inefficient method, with the very real risk that important information will be omitted or inadequately presented. Furthermore, there are quite simply no words – in the English language at least – to describe much of what you will encounter in patients with drug-related movement disorder.

One is on surer ground using descriptive methods to note *subjective* symptomatology and the impact of features on, for example, the activities of daily living, not least because, in a psychiatric context, standardised recording schedules afford little opportunity for noting information of this sort at present.

There are few things more hazardous in this world than an 'expert' with little expertise, and the use of standardised recording instruments does require *some* expertise. These instruments were, of course, all devised to serve the needs of clinical research, but the merits of them – or, perhaps, the demerits of the long-hand method – are such as to justify a recommendation that their use should be extended to routine clinical situations also.

The following is an overview of some of the major techniques for recording extrapyramidal dysfunction in standardised fashion. Not every author who hoped for professional immortality by devising his or her own scale will find a mention. A degree of selectivity is essential. Furthermore, although an 'overview', it is one containing a bias, for the emphasis is on scales and techniques that have been developed, or may be of use, within a psychiatric context, even if in practice there is little legitimacy in maintaining a 'neurological' versus a 'psychiatric' split in this field. The schism has arisen because scales tend to have been developed in response to issues surrounding particular disorders – that is, they have been largely diagnosis generated rather than problem generated. As in so many instances, psychiatry and neurology have, like the galleons of old, sailed on the same winds by different courses to the same destinations, each largely oblivious to the other's aims – which were, in fact, always the same anyway!

The origins of rating scales for movement disorders

The development of rating scales for movement disorder is in reality the standardisation of rating clinical disorder in Parkinson's disease and tardive dyskinesia. Everything else came later. However, the emphasis on each came about in response to two different imperatives.

Until the 1950s, the treatment of Parkinson's disease was largely empirical and of limited efficacy, and protracted and progressive disability not infrequently resulted in long-term institutional care. In this situation, there was little need for refinement of clinical assessment.

This changed following the first stereotactic basal ganglia surgery by Dr Russell Meyer in 1946. From 1952, this was enthusiastically adopted as a treatment of Parkinson' disease, especially by Dr Irving Cooper in New York. Despite the views of neurosurgeons that these were not invasive procedures and that the outcome was excellent, a pall of scepticism settled over the techniques. Those who harboured doubts pointed to the fact that cross-sectional evaluation of outcome provided limited and sometimes misleading information in a condition with an inherent tendency to fluctuate and progress. The need for some sort of standardisation of the assessment of disability was clear.

Hence, the imperative behind the development of standardised methodology for recording symptomatology in Parkinson's disease was the need to evaluate treatment efficacy. Initially, this was in relation to surgical procedures, but the great flowering in the field came with the introduction of L-dopa a decade later.

The imperative for developing standardised recording techniques for tardive dyskinesia was different – and emanated from the needs of psychiatry and not neurology. The first accounts of this apparently new syndrome were anecdotal and did not in themselves stimulate great interest. Much of the credit for raising awareness lies, as was mentioned, with Dr George Crane and colleagues at the Psychopharmacology Research Branch of the National Institute of Mental Health in Washington, who, in a series of studies, described the clinical features and attempted to link their development to antipsychotic exposure and other correlates.

Even these efforts were indifferently received. Most neurologists had other concerns, and psychiatrists (at least those who were aware of the issue) could not agree on whether this was indeed a new phenomenon. Written or verbal accounts reminded many of an older generation of the motor disorders that had been so evident in the pre-antipsychotic era. In order to support the view that this did, indeed, represent a new development in the face of a sceptical or indifferent profession, it was necessary to strengthen the quality of the data by providing some standard framework. Crane introduced the first rating scales for separate recording of hyperkinetic movement disorders on an arbitrarily defined nominal scale.

Thus, the imperative behind the introduction of rating scales for tardive dyskinesia was epidemiological. The scales were a necessary prerequisite to defining boundaries and establishing reliable prevalences in a complex syndrome characterised by marked interindividual variability.

Principles involved in rating scales

Rating scales for extrapyramidal disorder tend to adopt one of two main principles.

1. *Multi-item (symptom/sign) scales.* Such scales focus on the presence of specifically defined clinical features recorded on a severity continuum that is usually arbitrary. They are conventionally ordinal, providing data in numerical form that is readily amenable to statistical analysis.

2. *Global impression scales.* These assess the presence and severity of any abnormalities, not specifically defined, and focus either on the whole body or on different anatomical areas. Such scales may be nominal (or categorical), placing disorders in particular groupings on the basis of their being, for example, mild, moderate or severe, or they may adopt an ordinal structure.

Although ordinal formats have become the norm, it is important to bear in mind that these scales make no claims to being proportionate. Higher points on the scale represent greater 'degrees' of disorder but do not bear a mathematical relationship to one another. A score of 4 can be taken as representing a greater level of abnormality than a score of 2 – but *not* necessarily 'twice' as much.

A further distinction to be borne in mind is the basis of scale construction, be it largely theoretical or practical from observation of clinical material, as this impacts on item composition. Instruments that are theoretically derived tend to be more restricted, whereas observationally derived ones are frequently syndromally contaminated.

The defined symptomatology of Parkinson's disease lends itself to a multi-item recording format and to an assessment technique based on routine, if standardised, clinical examination and, despite some confusion, these principles lie behind many of these scales.

The confusion, often encountered in these instruments and that has transferred to most of those utilised in drug-related disorder, is whether the focus of rating should be the 'core' features themselves or regional manifestations of core abnormality. A number of the scales discussed below have adopted a hybrid of the two that is conceptually unsound and results in a mix that is, in practice, uncomfortable.

The position for tardive dyskinesia is somewhat different from that of parkinsonism. This is a relatively recently described disorder and, at the time when scales were being developed, had no clearly agreed symptom profile or method of evaluation. This is reflected in the heterogeneity of recording techniques and their accompanying recommendations. The scales themselves cover both global and multi-item formats, and although evaluation based on a standard clinical examination has become the most widely accepted assessment method, it is not the only one recommended, as will be mentioned.

Multi-item scales for hyperkinetic abnormalities, especially if regionally ordered, have strong scientific appeal. They allow a detailed profile of disorder that is symptom-specific or sign-specific and offer the prospect of organising detailed symptomatic typologies that can then be tested by, for example, pharmacological probes. By breaking down complex aspects of motor activity into component parts, they are, however, fundamentally unphysiological. This can place uncomfortable burdens of choice on raters. This issue has already been touched on in relation to the component parts of orofacial dyskinesia (see Chapter 6), but the point is worth emphasising. A patient with forced tongue protrusion must clearly open his or her mouth to execute the movement, so is mouth opening to be rated as a specific part of a complex dyskinesia or ignored as a normal reflex response to a primarily lingual disorder? It is certainly phenomenologically different from someone exhibiting forced mouth opening as part of an oro-mandibular dystonia. The more detailed the scale, the more such dilemmas arise. More than other types of formalised recording, multi-item scales demand a careful selection of constituent items, with clear and detailed definitions of their material and of the anchor points adopted for severity.

Scales based on global impressions minimise some of these problems but do not abolish them altogether. Those which, in order to enhance sensitivity, are broken down into separate body areas may cause similar debate about rating movements that overflow into adjacent areas. Furthermore, they preclude analysis of detailed movement types and relationships and hence cannot be used to construct and test typologies. However, they do provide an overview, which in many clinical situations may have greater relevance than data produced by the more molecular approach of their multi-item counterparts.

In addition to the standard clinical examination for eliciting hyperkinetic disorder (see Chapter 10), an alternative proposal involved a numerical count of abnormal movements in specific areas. This frequency count method has a number of attractions. It is simple and, with the focus of the count clearly defined, has an excellent inherent reliability. It is sensitive to change and needs no particular expertise or equipment. It can also be easily done unobtrusively.

As it is simple, however, so too is it crude. It does not allow the detailed components of movement to be analysed and, indeed, of greatest concern, it may actually produce misleadingly unrepresentative data, particularly in a condition such as tardive dyskinesia that is so susceptible to short-term and long-term variation. Good inter-rater reliability may therefore be attained at the expense of test–retest reliability.

Little attention has been paid to the methodology of frequency counts, but there is evidence that this is crucial. It has been shown, for example, that counts made for one minute every hour for ten hours produced a mean variation from baseline of only 5 per cent, while ten counts of one minute each equally spread over one hour produced 25 per cent variability (Delwaide and Hurlet, 1980). On the other hand, five counts of one minute every two hours were associated with an intermediate degree of variation of 15 per cent. The investigators, having established these important data, opted for the first method on the basis of scientific rigor. On the basis of pragmatism, however, they took weekends off!

The choice of a recording instrument for rating drug-related extrapyramidal disorders needs, therefore, to be determined by the nature of the information required and the purpose for which it is intended to use that information – and is a choice that needs thought.

Standardised rating scales for Parkinson's disease

It is beyond the scope of this volume to present a comprehensive critique of all the proposals in this field. The major examples are listed in Table 11.1. There is clearly no shortage of choice, which in itself suggests inadequacies with all. In fact, it is fair to say that neurologists did not approach the challenges of standardising this aspect of practice in a systematic or particularly collaborative spirit. At one point, it seemed as if the development of a new scale was a prerequisite for undertaking a treatment response study. These scales presented no clear rationale for their choice of items nor for their sign versus disability emphasis and, most damning of all, after years of often widespread use, most had never been subjected to any statistical analysis. An evaluation of the statistical properties of four of them showed an understandable lack of consistency and consensus (Diamond and Markham, 1983). It was clearly impossible for data from different centres based on different recording scales to be adequately compared.

With the dawning of a new era of combination and early intervention packages, a radical overhaul of the standardised methods of recording was deemed necessary, and between 1984 and 1987 a group of experts devised what has become known as the Unified Parkinson's Disease Rating Scale (UPDRS; Fahn et al., 1987a). This is an extremely comprehensive instrument with 44 ratings comprising a balance of signs versus symptoms divided into five sections. It can also account for adverse effects. It includes evaluation of features of the mental state, although the lack of psychiatric input is evident (in the original draft, hallucinations were referred to as a thought disorder!).

There is legitimate concern that the discriminative power of tests based on what are essentially *examiner-subjective* ratings is probably inherently limited, which is a problem not necessarily obviated by extending the number of items comprising a recording instrument. This is a conceptual problem pertinent to all the scales mentioned here, but the UPDRS has become widely accepted as some sort of 'gold standard' in treatment-response studies. It has not been widely applied in drug-related disorder as yet, but could be with only minimal modification.

The important point is that neurology was ready to acknowledge a problem and eager to attempt to rectify it. Psychiatry, on the other hand, does not yet seem ready to acknowledge a similar and major problem within its own realm, far less attempt rectification.

Table 11.1. *Rating scales for Parkinson's disease*

Scale	Reference	Sign	Symptom
		Orientation	
Northwestern University Disability Scale	Canter et al. (1961)		+
Webster Scale	Webster (1968)	+	
New York University Scale (MK I)	Alba et al. (1968)	+	
Activities of Daily Living Scale	Schwab & England (1969)		+
Modified Columbia Scale	Calne et al. (1969)	+	
Columbia University Scale	Duvoisin (1970)	+	
Cotzias Scale	Cotzias et al. (1970)		
King's College Hospital Scale	Parkes et al. (1970)	+	+
McDowell (Cornell) Scale	McDowell et al. (1970)	+	+
Anden Scale	Anden et al. (1970)	+	+
UCLA Scale	Treciokas et al. (1971)	+	+
New York University Scale (MK II)	Lieberman (1974), Lieberman et al. (1980)	+	+
Larsen Scale	Larsen et al. (1984)		+
Unified Parkinson's Disease Rating Scale (UPDRS)	Fahn et al. (1987a)	+	+
Self Care Scale	UK Bromocriptine Research Group (1989)		+

Table 11.2. *Rating scales for drug-related parkinsonism*

Scale	Reference
Neurological rating scale	Simpson & Angus (1970)
Modified by, for example	Lehmann et al. (1970)
	Rifkin et al. (1978)
	Perenyi et al. (1984)
	Caligiuri et al. (1989)
Mindham Scale	Mindham et al. (1972)
Scale for Targeting Abnormal Kinetic Effects (TAKE)	Wojcik et al. (1980)

Standardised rating scales for drug-related parkinsonism

The first attempts to quantify and correlate a feature of drug-related parkinsonism were H.J. Haase's efforts to establish a 'neuroleptic threshold' using changes in handwriting. This research did not set the world on fire, though it is of interest that the concept of a 'threshold' has been revived by some authors in recent years.

The most widely used scale for recording drug-related parkinsonism (Table 11.2) was also the first (Simpson and Angus, 1970), two facts that are probably not unconnected. The reader will come across a substantial body of literature whose results are based on data from this scale, and so a critical look is justified.

The Simpson–Angus Scale is the result of an extension to an earlier attempt by the same group to standardise the recording of certain parkinsonian features (eight extended to ten) for use in drug studies. The scale is entirely sign led. It is based on a clearly described examination procedure and the anchor points on its 0–4 severity scale are also clearly defined.

The Simpson–Angus Scale is, however, an exception to the rule that longevity of rating scales in psychiatric practice speaks of some face validity. As a system for rating drug-related parkinsonism, it is deeply flawed.

First, is the choice of items (Table 11.3). In a condition dominated by bradykinesia, this scale devotes six of its ten items to – rigidity! By contrast, bradykinesia can only be rated under the first item, which is, in fact, a compound one incorporating gait and posture as well as loss of pendular arm swing. In addition, glabellar tap is viewed as of comparable importance to 'core' items.

Table 11.3. *Neurological Rating Scale (Simpson & Angus, 1970)*

Item	Description	Comment
1	Gait	Compound item
2	Arm dropping	Anchor point 'a stout slap'
3	Shoulder shaking	?Different from (2)
4	Elbow rigidity	
5	Wrist rigidity	
6	Leg pendulousness	
7	Head dropping	Anchor point 'a good thump'
8	Glabella(r) tap	?Non-specific. (in ψ population)
9	Tremor	?Resting ?Postural
10	Salivation	

Then there is the examination method, which hardly seems designed to cement an on-going professional relationship. Upper trunk/neck rigidity is to be assessed by the 'bombing' head method described in Chapter 10, with the item rated on the basis of the force of the 'thump' with which the head hits the couch – although, mercifully, it is recommended that this should be 'well padded'! With arm dropping, the severity of rating is based on the recognition of a 'stout slap', an anchor that even by the standards of psychiatry is somewhat vague.

Surprisingly, the Simpson–Angus Scale is not possessed of the psychometric properties that might redeem this widely used scale from its manifest inadequacies. For four of its items, the mean inter-rater correlations in the original publication are below 0.66, with ranges from as low as 0.16, and only glabellar tap, the least valuable and probably valid sign in drug-related disorder, has a mean coefficient above 0.80.

The persistence of this scale must not be interpreted as an endorsement of the excellence with which it performs the task required of it. It is, in fact, a reflection of sterility in the field of scale development over the past quarter century. The Simpson–Angus Scale was a noble pioneer, but now deserves a decent burial. Few clinicians – and no researchers – should shed any tears at its passing.

The Simpson–Angus Scale has also become psychiatry's 'Lego' scale, to be built on and demolished by individual workers on the basis of their individual studies of the moment (see Table 11.2). Indeed, no scale in the history of medicine has been so ruthlessly beaten up and mutilated, yet still refused to die. Such 'modifications' are too numerous to mention but, despite their frequent appearance in the literature, the principle cannot be condoned. Unless such manipulations result in a new instrument of proven clinical and statistical merit, the value of the data provided by the hybrid is of dubious scientific merit, based as it is on little more than a shared name. Merely adding the prefix 'modified' does not alter this fact.

The dearth of standardised recording scales dedicated to drug-related parkinsonism is illustrated by the fact that the only other one to receive any substantial airing (and that comes a long way behind the Simpson–Angus) is the Scale for Targeting Abnormal Kinetic Effects (TAKE; Wojcik et al., 1980). The idea behind this was to produce an instrument for parkinsonism that paralleled in format and style the AIMS, of which, more later. The examination technique recommended for the AIMS needed only to be slightly amplified to elicit the necessary additional information, and the two could be seen as providing a simple yet comprehensive assessment package.

The TAKE rates the three 'core' parkinsonian features of bradykinesia, rigidity and tremor wherever they occur and hence is conceptually uncontaminated. In addition, one item pertains to autonomic disturbance and one to akathisia. In line with the AIMS, three global impression items for 'awareness', 'severity' and 'incapacitation' are included. Ratings are on a five-point (0–4) severity continuum, which also parallels that of the AIMS. Akathisia is assessed on the basis of subjective symptomatology and hence the concept adopted is that of 'classical' or acute disorder.

This scale has excellent statistical properties and the authors largely succeeded in producing a practical instrument complimentary to the AIMS. In criticism, it might be said that although rating all the many manifestations of bradykinesia but the relatively few manifestations of rigidity, each on a single item, is conceptually sound, this compromises the scale's sensitivity and masks the relationship between 'core' symptomatology.

The author's affection for this scale has been fostered over a number of years of usage, though it has to be admitted that he seems to be one of only a small band of acolytes.

Standardised rating scales for tardive dyskinesia

The benchmark scale in this category is undoubtedly the AIMS (Table 11.4). This was introduced by the National Institute of Mental Health in response to the need for a simple and widely acceptable method for recording drug-related hyperkinesias (Guy, 1976).

The AIMS is a global instrument, divided by seven body regions, with each item rated on a five-point ordinal scale. Four of its seven items refer to the face, and hence it has a clear regional bias. In addition, global ratings of 'overall severity', 'incapacitation' and 'patient awareness' can

Table 11.4. *Rating scales for tardive dyskinesia*

Scale	Comment	Reference
Abnormal Involuntary Movement Scale (AIMS)	Global impression	Guy (1976)
Barnes–Kidger Scale	Global impression (counts)	Barnes & Kidger (1979)
Rockland (Simpson) Dyskinesia Rating Scale	Multi-item	Simpson et al. (1979)

be made and, as noted, dental status can be recorded. In line with its theoretical origins, tremor is specifically excluded.

The AIMS comes with a detailed examination protocol and scoring system that includes the so-called 'one less rule'. This is the requirement to rate movements only evident on activation at one point *less* on the severity continuum than movements evident without activation. To the author, this has always seemed conceptually unsound. Unequivocally abnormal types of movement such as dystonia may frequently show only on activation when mild, which would require their rating at point '1' on the severity continuum. But this category is by definition reserved for movements *not* considered pathological in either type or degree. Furthermore, although the scale was introduced in advance of its statistical properties being established, these were subsequently shown to be satisfactory in a series of studies by Smith and colleagues in which the 'one less rule' was suspended (Smith et al., 1979a; 1979b).

Several workers (including the author) have also suspended the rule, but most authors do not state how they operated and it cannot be assumed that all have done so similarly. However, it is up to those who advocate retention of this illogical condition to show that, with it intact, the AIMS produces as good or better reliability data than with it suspended. Because maintaining the rule could materially alter results, especially those based on mean scores, it would seem important that authors should state in published work what their position in relation to the 'one less rule' was, something referees and editors should insist upon.

In itself, however, the AIMS justifies its place as the 'market leader' scale for recording drug-related dyskinetic disorders.

It is probably correct to say that the benchmark multi-item scale is that devised by Simpson and colleagues (1979) and variously referred to as the Simpson (after the principal author) or Rockland (after the institute)

Dyskinesia Rating Scale (see Table 11.4). This scale was devised on practical as opposed to theoretical foundations, bringing together the commonest movements observed in patients exposed to antipsychotic drugs and assuming these to represent 'tardive dyskinesia'. However, the authors do acknowledge the risk of contamination with this methodology.

The full scale is an extremely comprehensive instrument, with 34 separate defined movements to be assessed on a six-point (0–5) continuum. In addition, nine unspecified items are reserved for rating any other (essentially uncommon) disorders not covered by the specific items. With 14 specified and two unspecified ratings referring to the face, it has less of a regional bias than the AIMS.

This scale adopts a somewhat ambivalent approach to tremor, excluding 'obvious parkinsonian tremors of the extremities' but including tremors of the upper lip ('rabbit syndrome'), tongue and eyelids and, somewhat paradoxically in view of its initial prohibition, 'pill-rolling movements'. In addition, item 17 ('head nodding'), despite the authors' assertion that this is slower than tremor, sounds suspiciously like 'affirmation', found particularly in essential tremor.

The confusion that highly comprehensive multi-item scales can engender is illustrated by this scale's approach to lower limb movements. Akathisia is defined as an inability to sit or stand still, but without the necessity of subjective distress, which, in terms of the definitions, may or may not be present. In addition, however, specified items to be rated also include 'restless legs', 'crossing/uncrossing legs – sitting' and 'stamping movements' both standing and sitting. Furthermore, item 29 refers to 'caressing or rubbing face and hair', while item 30 is devoted to 'rubbing thighs'. Any or all of these might legitimately be incorporated into many clinicians' concept of 'akathisia'. The descriptive detail the scale provides on these items would seem to be a bit like taking a microscope to describe the topography of an elephant!

Having struggled to record meticulously all disorder the scale affords one the opportunity to record, there remains the problem of analysis, to which we shall return. It may be, however, that the examiner's diligence in 'in-putting' may not be matched by a comparable ability to 'out-put', and much of the wisdom stored in complex multi-item scales of this sort may remain forever locked within, unamenable to ready analysis.

The Simpson or Rockland Scale has good statistical properties, nonetheless, and comes with full definitions of items and a description of recommended examination technique. It is valuable in establishing trends and typologies in very large at-risk populations – for those who have the stamina to undertake work of this sort! By contrast, it is also a useful tool for assessing change, for example in treatment trials with repeated measuring in small, manageable samples.

A smaller 'Abbreviated' version was developed concurrently by the same group 'for use in situations where such detail (as in the full scale) was not necessary'. This was felt to 'compliment' the full scale for use in screening for clinical trials. However, it is a somewhat uncomfortable mix of global and multi-item formats, the logic of which is unclear. The Abbreviated scale was used in several important, especially early, studies but did not find widespread favour, although this may, strangely, be changing somewhat.

Standardised rating scales for akathisia

The conceptual problems surrounding akathisia – in what way those with purely objective features are to be considered and where the disorder lies in relation to parkinsonism – have had a bearing on inhibiting development of recording scales, though probably a greater factor was the general neglect of the topic in research circles.

Several of the early combined scales included an akathisia item (e.g. van Putten in his 1974 scale) and we have already seen that the same is true of the TAKE, which conceptually views akathisia as part of the parkinson syndrome. As shall be seen, the modern combined scales also incorporate akathisia ratings.

The major development in recent years, however, has been the introduction of scales specifically dedicated to akathisia (Table 11.5). These are of two types. The first is the global approach enshrined in the Barnes Akathisia Scale (Barnes, 1989), which demands evaluation of the objective separate from the subjective component and includes a global impression rating for overall disorder. Definitions and instructions for examination are lucid and severity points well anchored and clinically relevant. The scale has established statistical properties. The advantages of this scale lie in its strong face validity and its practicality – one does not require to be a Philadelphia lawyer to use it with confidence.

The two other recent additions to the field do require somewhat greater expertise because both adopt a more molecular approach. The Hillside Rating Scale for Akathisia (HAS; Fleischhacker et al., 1989), comprises two subjective items – inner restlessness and urge to move – combined with a division of objective signs into three regional items – axial, upper limbs and lower limbs. Each of these five items is rated on a four-point continuum, with separate evaluations for the patient sitting, standing and lying. A final global evaluation for each item can also be recorded. The full scale allows the effect of activation procedures

Table 11.5. *Rating scales for akathisia*

Scale	Reference
Barnes Scale	Barnes (1989)
Hillside Akathisia Scale	Fleischhacker et al. (1989)
Prince Henry Hospital Akathisia Rating Scale	Sachdev (1994)

to be assessed, although this does not affect the basic scores, which are taken from the maximum disorder at any point in the examination. Global impression items for severity and improvement under treatment conditions are also provided.

The Prince Henry Hospital Akathisia (PHHA) Scale (Sachdev, 1994) was developed on the same premises as the Barnes Scale in that it utilised the same questionnaire items explored by Braude and colleagues (1983). However, Sachdev rejected the global approach of Barnes, which, he argued, 'disregards the richness of the clinical features'. The ten-item PHHA Scale comprises seven objectively evaluated items, four with the patient sitting and three with the patient standing, and three subjective items, all rated on a four-point scale. However, this continuum is somewhat different from that of most other scales in that point '1' is for mild but definite abnormality. The scale has good statistical properties and might be considered intermediate in complexity between the Barnes at one end and the Hillside at the other.

The comprehensiveness of these 'molecular' scales is of clear advantage in special projects, but also limits their use for routine purposes. It seems that the more global approach has, at the time of writing, gained the edge in terms of popularity.

Standardised rating scales for dystonia

The standardised recording of dystonia as a drug-related disorder, either acute or chronic, is a barren wilderness.

Acute dystonias do not lend themselves to this sort of formalised recording. The fact that their spectrum of symptomatology ranges from the purely subjective to the predominantly objective means that they cannot be appropriately accommodated in scales that are sign led. Furthermore, their pattern of sudden evolution and the considerable disability they engender act contrary to examination techniques that are cross-sectional or demand full patient participation.

Perhaps as a result – or perhaps as a consequence of the more general neglect of the topic as a legitimate field of research endeavour – no scales dedicated to the standardised rating of acute dystonias have been devised. The only systematic attempt to address this issue in recent years was incorporated in the Extrapyramidal Symptom Rating Scale (ESRS), though, as will be seen, this did not achieve an entirely happy outcome.

Several instruments dedicated to chronic dystonia have been devised. Fahn and Marsden published a series of scales for staging and recording the severity of, and functional disability associated with, 'torsion dystonia' (Marsden and Schachter, 1981), and a further effort was undertaken by Burke and colleagues (1985). Although not specifically developed for use in the setting of drug-related disorder, the former have been applied in this context (see van Harten et al., 1996). An alternative approach would be to rate patients on a sensitive multi-item scale for hyperkinetic disorders that incorporates dystonic items, such as the Rockland/Simpson Scale, and then extract post hoc movement with a dystonic typology. However, this is somewhat 'rough and ready'.

Combined rating scales

Nowadays, anything less than a comprehensive assessment of extrapyramidal status would be inadequate, even for routine clinical purposes. It might, therefore, be argued that the best method of recording is utilisation of a scale designed to embrace total symptomatology (Table 11.6). For those with expertise, this might be the case, but these scales are, in general, complex instruments that in routine situations may tax the skills – to say nothing of the patience – of the examiner. The roots of these scales are still firmly in the research sphere and hence in routine use they may not necessarily provide a mode of presenting data that has clinical meaning and allows of ready comparisons. Nonetheless, as they do pop up in the literature and may represent the shape of things to come, they demand an airing.

Whether the relationship between parkinsonism and tardive dyskinesia is one of association or reciprocity was hotly debated at one time, and Crane, in several variations of his tardive dyskinesia scale, reserved an item 'P' for parkinsonism. The first attempt at a comprehensive review of extrapyramidal symptomatology in antipsychotic-treated patients, however, was made by Kennedy, Hershon and McGuire (1971). These authors arbitrarily divided the body into 32 areas and examined these for the presence of any of five types of motor abnormality – tremor, rigidity, choreiform dyskinesia, restlessness and dystonia – each recorded on a five-point scale. In addition, these authors

Table 11.6. *Combined extrapyramidal disorder rating scales*

Scale	Reference
Scale with no name 1.	Kennedy et al. (1971)
Scale with no name 2.	Van Putten et al. (1974)
Smith Scale	Bell and Smith (1978)
Extrapyramidal Symptom Rating Scale (ESRS)	Chouinard et al. (1980)
St Hans Scale	Gerlach et al. (1993)

assessed functional impairment in relation to speech, dressing, gait, feeding and posture and included an objective motor test, namely, joining dots to form a square. This scale did have some idiosyncrasies, such as, for example, including both hypertonicity and bradykinesia in the definition of 'rigidity', and would have benefited from less regional and more symptom sensitivity. It was, nonetheless, ahead of its time and it is a source of regret that, as a comprehensive recording instrument, it was not developed further in its own right.

Van Putten (1974) also provided an early attempt at comprehensive recording, though as his focus was the 'acute' end of the EPS spectrum, this was relative. The scale is noteworthy for the particularly clear and clinically pertinent definitions of akathisia provided, though the author's concept of akinesia seems to incorporate rigidity as well as poverty of motor activity. Like the above example, this scale was never developed adequately.

The two major contenders in the combined category are the St Hans Scale and the ESRS. The former evolved through several incarnations from a number of methods of recording explored by Gerlach and colleagues in Denmark over some years and has now been streamlined from early versions that were impossibly complex. Items are rated on a seven-point scale. Dyskinetic disorder is rated for each of eight regional body divisions, which correspond to those of the AIMS except that 'head' and 'trunk' are considered separately. Two distinct ratings for passive and 'activated' movements are recommended, so either of these or a mean score can be derived. Eight parkinsonian features are also considered, though these represent a mix of 'core' features and manifestations of 'core' features. Thus, for example, 'facial expression', 'bradykinesia' and 'arm swing' are all rated separately. Both the subjective and objective features of akathisia can be accommodated, but dystonia is recorded only on a global impression basis.

This remains a complex instrument, but has two big advantages: its evolutionary development, which endows it with clinical wisdom, and statistical properties established with a diligence that others in the field must surely envy (Gerlach et al., 1993).

The ESRS is a unique instrument in including 12 questionnaire items to identify subjective symptomatology, a most important innovation in the field. Eight items are devoted to parkinsonian signs, under which is included akathisia (the subjective element is noted in the questionnaire), each rated on a seven-point continuum. This scale once again does not resolve the dilemma of whether it is 'core' symptomatology that should be the target of rating or regional manifestations of 'core' disorder. Thus, bradykinesia is rated conceptually, but so, too, are facial mask and arm swing on separate items.

An attempt to provide for specific ratings of both acute and chronic dystonia is laudable, but frankly does not work. The severity of acute dystonia appears to be judged on the basis purely of signs, which, as has been seen, is inadequate, and although in the original draft one could record dystonia (acute or chronic) of the lips, there was no provision for recording truncal disorder, though this has now been rectified. The major confusion, however, lies in the fact that a number of the descriptions of disorder to be rated under 'dyskinesias', which supposedly refers to non-dystonic hyperkinesias, are clearly dystonic.

The scale does bring a novel approach to the question of comparative judgement in rating hyperkinetic disorders. The question relates to the relative rating one gives mild but persistent disorder versus that for signs that are intermittent but moderate or marked in severity. The ESRS's solution is to recommend rating on the dual axes of frequency and amplitude. This has clear merit for tremor, but whether this extends to choreiform-type hyperkinesias is unclear. Furthermore, how disorder of internal musculature, such as of the larynx, can be graded by these principles is a mystery to the present author. The reasonable implication that this 'dual axis' method of rating will enhance reliability has not been established to date.

The ESRS is also a complex scale for regular use and not all its worthy efforts in the direction of innovation are satisfactory. Its statistical properties appear good but, somewhat surprisingly, these have not been established to quite the level one would expect of such a major instrument (Chouinard et al., 1980; 1984).

Learning disability

Several studies in the 1980s applied conventional scales to the evaluation of drug-related movement disorder in patients with learning disability. Throughout the 1980s, however, Sprague and colleagues, aware that many of the available scales lacked statistical credentials, developed a 34-item scale subsequently condensed to the 15-item Dyskinesia Identification System – Condensed User Scale, which abbreviates to the snappy acronym, DISCUS (Sprague and Kalachnik, 1991). This was specifically developed for use in those with developmentally based learning disabilities, and the opportunity is afforded to note 'other' types of disorder, including that which may 'assist in preventing mis-interpretation of movements'. Items are arranged under seven regional headings with a lingual bias, and rated on a five-point continuum with the provision on each item for noting where a defined movement could not be assessed. The subject's level of co-operation can also be recorded, and the scale comes with detailed definitions of terms and a clearly stated examination procedure.

The DISCUS emerged from a systematic piece of work that has resulted in a scale with established statistical properties and clinical relevance most evident in the population for whom it was primarily intended. However, it has been criticised on the basis that it still presents the same problems as conventional scales in rating those with profound learning disability. Its clinical as opposed to theoretical roots show in the syndromal overlap of its constituent items, and whether it is, indeed, better to avoid rating things that are difficult as opposed to insisting on a 'forced choice' in all cases is a matter of debate.

Some general issues

Statistical properties

The need to devise, and if necessary refine, rating scales on the basis of their statistical properties was not a consideration in many of the instruments currently available, though nowadays this would be required to be put at the forefront. Taking a commonly used scale and removing a couple of items, adding two or three more and altering the severity continuum on the basis of expediency is no longer acceptable. The aim of any rating scale is to provide data that are unbiased, reproducible and precise. To achieve this, any instrument must have established statistical properties. In choosing a scale, therefore, the clinician as well as the researcher should restrict their considerations to instruments with established statistical credentials.

Furthermore, it is necessary that those proposing to use recording schedules for routine as well as research purposes establish their own credentials by way of some, however rudimentary, reliability study.

Video recording

Rating scales possess in themselves no inherent validity nor have reliability that is referable to all circumstances. Drug-related movement disorders vary greatly between patients and within any patient over time, which can present major problems for routine clinical evaluation as well as for those wishing to establish the credentials for their recording schedule. Video recordings have been advocated as a suitable way of overcoming the influences of a number of modifying factors over which the examiner has little control.

There is no doubt that videos offer a number of advantages. They provide a permanent record in a cost-effective way and are especially suited to training and education. They also offer an invaluable method for establishing both test–retest and inter-rater reliability in relation to certain types of disorder. Furthermore, videos can be useful in conducting therapeutic trials for which random presentation of material can help maintain blindness.

They do have limitations too, however, such as the reduction in detail that results from the transposition of a three-dimensional situation into a two-dimensional image, a factor particularly at work in relation to hyperkinetic disorders of the tongue and some tremors. They are, furthermore, clearly of no use in evaluating disorder only detectable by contact, such as regional presentations of rigidity. It must also be remembered that, with extrapyramidal symptomatology, the very presence of a camera may impact on the patient sufficiently to alter the observable symptomatology.

The retention of videos for teaching and training purposes can be highly commended, but they must not in themselves be seen as a substitute for 'hands on' experience.

The role of context

In medicine, signs are the objective manifestations of disorder, but the clinical evaluation of these is never entirely objective. This is because clinical assessment occurs in a context. Simultaneous context refers to factors evident at the time of rating that are strictly irrelevant to the sign being rated, but may nonetheless bear down on the examiners perception of it. For example, the degree of distress that a patient with parkinsonism demonstrates in the execution of a particular task may influence the severity of disorder rated by the examiner; or ratings of dyskinesia in the hands may be influenced by involuntary activity in the feet.

Prior context refers to expectations of the patient's current status derived from past contact or, in a situation of rating groups of patients, a criterion bias operating as a 'hangover' from more severely or less severely affected subjects examined immediately before.

The intrusive influences of context are very difficult to overcome in practice and perhaps the best that can be expected is that awareness can be used to militate against them to some extent. The random scrambling of serial videos is an effective way of dealing with some of the influence of context in research studies.

Data analysis

In research environments, formal statistical analysis is a necessary consideration and, while for routine purposes this may be of lesser import, it is still important for the clinician to appreciate the issues in understanding the literature.

All standardised scales can harness considerable amounts of patient information, all of which has potential for the publication-hungry researcher. However, in the real world, acceptance that large amounts of such data will have to go is probably the key to a successful publication. The two major methods of analysis involve the use of total scores or those based on single symptom criteria.

Total scores (or means based on total scores) are now the most commonly utilised. This is certainly the easiest way to handle large amounts of data, especially from scales the majority of whose items will be rated zero. However, total scores are regionally insensitive and are prone to contamination. All scales (except the Prince Henry Hospital Akathisia Scale), in acknowledgement of the fact that cut-offs between normality and disorder are often not clear, include a '1' category for features that, although present, are by definition not considered pathological in either type or degree. These inevitably intrude into total scores, especially if the rater has used the category sloppily. Even the adoption of an arbitrary cut-off for normality still retains an inherent element of misclassification. A number of authors get round the problem by using only the global impression of total disorder for the purpose of analysis, but this is such an assault on sensitivity that it would seem to negate the very point of using a regionally ordered scale in the first place.

Single symptom criteria consider the sample in terms of the percentage rating at least one item at a predetermined level of severity – for example, the percentage scoring at least one item at '2' or at '3' etc. This eradicates contamination with non-pathological ratings but does risk underestimating total disorder. Thus, someone rating a '4' on one item only might, for the purposes of analysis, be considered the same as someone rating on several items at this level.

A sophisticated modification of a simple present/absent dichotomy has gained favour in recent years and this is defining 'caseness' in terms of operationally defined criteria, such as the Schooler and Kane criteria for tardive dyskinesia. This is mainly aimed at excluding doubtful cases at the mild end of the spectrum and represents a clean starting point for analysis. It is not useful for the exploration of issues surrounding severity.

The use of total scores is likely to continue to find favour, mainly because of the flexibility of the method and the amenability of data to a range of complex statistical manipulations, but an appreciation of its limitations is advised.

The choice of scale

This is to some extent the easiest issue for the author to address, for the answer comprises two simple parts: (1) it depends!, and (2) it's up to you!

Rating scales often seem to have been chosen on the basis of the most recent article that caught the doctor's attention, or some equally incidental reason. This is a mistake. For both routine and research purposes, the choice of recording instrument should depend on the purpose for which the information is sought. Indeed, in research investigations, the choice of scale *must* be a crucial and early part of the design phase. There is no point in undertaking a therapeutic trial using a scale of insufficient sensitivity to detect change, or in assessing side-effect liability of a new compound by rating only single aspects of the potential profile. Similarly, a highly sensitive multi-item scale may be inappropriately applied in a large epidemiological project, as too many data may be generated to handle conveniently. At the end of the day, sensitivity may have to be sacrificed in favour of practicality, with much wasted effort in the process. Also, of course, should formal analysis of data be required, it is worth remembering that large, complex scales in small, simple populations equals statistical disaster.

As has been emphasised, evaluation nowadays *must* be comprehensive, something that decisions about the choices for recording must take on board. Research studies should be influenced more directly by the specific issues above, and the greatest freedom of choice therefore lies with those wishing to use standardised methods for routine clinical situations. The combined scales offer comprehensiveness that is inbuilt, but carry with them the necessity for expertise, and hence are probably best reserved for their intended research clientele.

Accepting this, the jobbing clinician must select two or more instruments from the many available. While there is no hard and fast rule that can be offered in this regard, the author's fondness for the AIMS–TAKE package has already been noted. Whatever the choice, consideration needs to be given to the practicality of the instruments to routine situations, the adequacy of their statistical properties, and surety in their use by local training to establish reliabilities. The amount of effort implied in this is, in fact, slight and will soon be offset by savings in time that accrue from regular use. Also, think how smugly prepared one will be for whatever audit demands one's employers might make or whatever medicolegal attacks might be hurled against one!

12

Some medicolegal and quality-of-care issues

Introduction

There was a time, not so long ago, when reputations in medicine could be made on the basis of individualism. Indeed, for many of the 'great and good' of past generations, the key to professional standing lay less in adherence to a professional consensus or a nascent scientific literature than in idiosyncrasy of method and forcefulness of conviction. This was nowhere more evident than in psychiatry, which of course spawned one of the twentieth century's most pervasive philosophies on the back of just such principles.

The fact is, however, that the days of such 'individualism' are gone and all doctors, including psychiatrists, must operate within an escalating series of constraints. These emanate from many standpoints and include not just the obvious legal constraints of long standing, but also, increasingly, ethical considerations, professional practice guidelines, locally agreed contract standards and elements of 'user' satisfaction.

One area in which many of these constraints have the potential to coalesce is the one that has formed the particular focus of the present volume. To state it more specifically, the issue is the way in which the neurological adverse effect profiles of antipsychotic drugs should determine our perception of their place in the therapeutic armamentarium and the way in which they should be used. When one says 'our perception', one is not, of course, referring exclusively to the medical profession, for the wider society has the 'bottom line' role in sanctioning any interventions we may propose, which will in turn be influenced by the experiences of patients as well as doctors – and we have already seen the gulf that exists there!

The following is not intended as a comprehensive exposition – this would require a volume in itself – but is merely part of the overall aim of widening practitioners' perception. If, as is hoped, the 'carrot' for doctors acquiring knowledge and expertise is the stimulus of the clinical material, then what is to come might be viewed as the 'stick'.

'Informing' consent

The legal principle of 'consent' is fundamental to modern medical practice, certainly in developed countries, and there are very few circumstances in which it can be suspended. Such circumstances include medical emergency, patient waiver (if voluntarily and competently given), therapeutic privilege and patient incompetence.

Breeches of the requirements for consent clearly place doctors, including psychiatrists, beyond the law and at risk of prosecution, which in the UK may be under the common law of battery or, increasingly, may encompass questions of professional negligence. The arguments surrounding this are complex enough for psychiatry, and in Britain were aired in the debate on the potential impact of the Mental Health Act (1983) on research in the psychoses (Hirsch and Harris, 1988). The real dilemma arises from the requirement in recent years that consent should be informed.

The idea of 'informed consent' springs from the case of Salgo v. Leland Stanford University in 1957. It has been advocated for sound reasons that include the fact that it promotes patient autonomy, informs decision making by patients and, by empowering them, tends to some extent to equalise the doctor–patient relationship (Wettstein, 1988). The fact that it moves practice away from a specifically 'beneficence' model of care has been proposed as a further advantage.

Informed consent rests on three main planks (Meisel, Roth and Lidz, 1977):

> the information provided *to* the patient;
> voluntary decision making *by* the patient;
> competency *of* the patient.

It is ethically driven and, in fact, has no legal standing within any of the jurisdictions of the UK. Nonetheless, as far as professional guidelines – the standard by which doctors are now so frequently judged – are concerned, the legal and the ethical have unequivocally coalesced. In the language of the Mental Health Act (1983) Code of Practice, endorsed in the guidelines of the UK medical defence societies:

> 'Consent' is the voluntary and continuing permission of the patient to receive a particular treatment, based on an adequate knowledge of the purpose, nature, likely effects and risks of that treatment including the likelihood of its success and any alternatives to it.

The key word is clearly 'adequate', a principal component in 'informing' consent. 'Adequacy' covers specified areas, but they in their turn raise others. In providing information to patients' that is 'adequate' for the purpose of obtaining 'consent' that is 'informed', one might be obliged to cover a range of topics such as diagnosis, the nature and purpose of proposed interventions, their benefits, risks and likelihood of success, the availability of alternatives and the benefits, risks and likelihood of success of these, and the prognosis without intervention (Wettstein, 1988).

How does this principle translate into the practical use of antipsychotic drugs in their target populations? Of this list, it is perhaps only the question of alternatives to antipsychotics that can be dealt with fairly easily, for in schizophrenia, at least, there is good evidence that the alternatives, if considered, are very much of the second-best variety, not only in relation to short-term management but also in terms of long-term outcome. Indeed, it could be argued that very real ethical, and possibly legal, questions would arise if a diagnosis of schizophrenia were *not* now accompanied by a recommendation for the use of these drugs. Furthermore, an increasing body of research indicates strongly that the swifter a medication regime is implemented, the better for both symptomatic and long-term psychosocial/occupational outcomes. A policy of 'wait and see' is becoming more and more untenable.

As for the other questions, however, most are problematic. This is certainly the case with regard to the neurological risks of antipsychotic use.

As has been seen in the present volume, published figures of prevalence and incidence – the context in which risk can be quantified – vary widely for each of the main extrapyramidal syndromes. The physician aiming to 'inform' consent has to decide what is 'adequate' information from some pretty murky material. It is hardly conducive to a sound therapeutic relationship for the doctor to explain to his or her patient that on starting medication there is a 2.3–60 per cent risk of an acute dystonia, a 15–80+ per cent risk of parkinsonism, a 20–40 per cent risk of akathisia and, in the indeterminate future, a 20–60 per cent risk of tardive dyskinesia if treatment is maintained – and, in fact, the risk of developing a combination of any of these is unknown! Also, while the risk of some of these problems may be militated by additional medication, this is not itself without risks. One might then go on to explain what has been stated throughout the present text, namely, that such figures are so heavily dependent on a range of divergent variables that standing on their own they are in fact of dubious validity in the individual case.

They are, furthermore, far detached for the primary basis of most patients' concern: the impact of adverse experiences on functional capacity and quality of life. A doctor incorporating in his or her figures of risk a mild reduction in arm swing or slight labial pursing evident only on activation, is talking a different language from one whose concept is of embarrassing tremor or orofacial dyskinesia readily evident to the patient and the layman. And those whose practice is wedded to the use of high-potency compounds will have to recite a different litany from those of a more eclectic persuasion. In terms of quantifying functional impairment for the patient's information, one might as well recite 'The Owl and the Pussycat', as no sound data can be passed on from the professional literature. One might, of course, choose to enter into a discourse on the relative merits of the new versus the standard drugs, but the 'facts' one adopts are, at this stage, as likely to be impressions as immutable truths emanating from sound science.

All this will be unfolding in the context of illnesses whose symptomatology is likely to include an integral component of cognitive impairment afflicting concentration, attention and probably various aspects of memory as well. The somewhat surreal world into which this can lead the 'informer' is evident, and cognitive deficits in themselves have been highlighted as a major and poorly considered obstacle to the attainment of consent that is truly 'informed' in those acutely disturbed by virtue of psychotic illness (Jones, 1995).

Taken at its crudest level, the 'higher' ethical standard could be seen as being represented by the generation of information that is complex and multifaceted to aid decision making in an individual with an illness whose features include prominently perceptual 'overload', impaired decision-making processes and faulty mechanisms of storage and recall.

In fact, despite unqualified advocacy from many quarters that, as a matter of principle, patients ought to be provided with more information, this may not be entirely resonant with the wishes of patients themselves. A few years ago, the author conducted a survey of patients' attitudes to our service, one aspect of which concerned this issue. As Figure 12.1 illustrates, half the sample felt they had been given adequate information about their condition and its management, and only 10 per cent felt quite inadequately served in this regard. When those who stated that they would like to know more were further asked to specify, side-effects were certainly an issue (Fig. 12.2). However, the greatest percentage of patients who wished to know more wanted information on perhaps the one area for which psychiatrists have least valid information to provide – prognosis. Interestingly, only 13.5 per cent of the total sample of 333 admitted to having experienced difficulty in understanding what the doctors said to them, and in a third of instances this was simply because of 'information overload'. For these patients, the issue was not too little, but too much.

It must be seriously doubted whether the unadorned presentation of ultimately rather meaningless figures on neurological risk can be of value in informing patients' decision making with regard to treatment

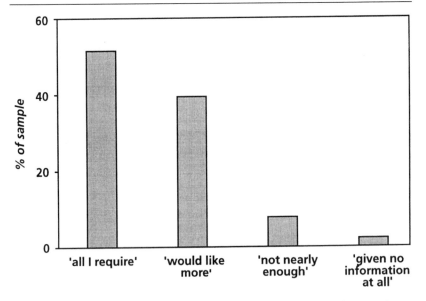

Fig. 12.1. Northwick Park Hospital outpatient survey: response to the question 'Do you feel you have been given enough information about your condition?'. (Response 300/333.)

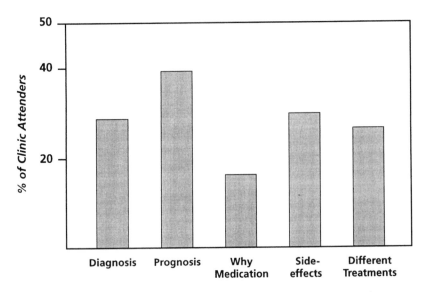

Fig. 12.2. Northwick Park Hospital outpatient survey: percentage attenders (n=333) who wished for more information in specific areas.

recommendations involving antipsychotic drugs. In order to 'adorn' them, one could perhaps go through the present volume together but even this is only likely to emphasise the limited predictions it is possible to put before the individual patient.

The fact is that extrapyramidal adverse effects are sometimes an unavoidable aspect of the necessary treatment for what are major medical disorders. That the problems of those afflicted by psychotic states are of an illness nature, in the treatment of which antipsychotic drugs play a crucial role, are facts that can now be disputed only by those whose perception is driven by petrified ideology and the luxury of never having had to witness the ravages of the untreated states. 'Informing' consent to the use of these treatments might therefore best start with advocacy of their benefits.

The medicolegal dimension

None of the above is, of course, a carte blanche for doctors to use these drugs without thought or care – quite the opposite. The fact of the drugs being necessary but yet possessed of sufficient neurological adverse effects to fill the present work is evidence enough for a greater recognition of the skill required in their use than perhaps even the profession has in the past been willing to acknowledge. The findings of Weiden et al. (1987) and Hoge et al. (1990) that we mentioned at the start of these pages are a sad indictment of psychiatry and a potent pointer to areas in which change *must* be forthcoming. Without that change from within, we shall find it forced upon us from without via any of the areas of constraint mentioned above.

If the reader has journeyed this far through the author's efforts, then the first and senior of the two mechanisms for bringing about change will have been oiled – awareness. Many of the problems that doctors encounter with patients who encounter EPS emanate from the simple fact that nobody has recognised what is going on. Awareness of the potential for neurological disturbance must be a number one priority for all those who prescribe and monitor the use of antipsychotics – and, of course, other relevant medications. This is encompassing an increasingly broad church, but is a particular requirement for psychiatrists, neurologists, geriatricians, primary care physicians and, ever more so, cardiologists. It should also nowadays be extended to involve nurses and other non-medical professionals who are adopting more of a front-line role in long-term supervision of patients of all types, though especially psychiatric.

This ought to be primarily a quality-of-care issue, but is regretfully becoming increasingly a legal one too. As yet, there is no case law established in the area of extrapyramidal adverse effects within the jurisdictions of the UK. In those cases in the USA highlighted in the medical literature in which liability has been found against physicians, a strong unifying theme has been failure of recognition (Tancredi, 1988). These cases have concerned tardive dyskinesia, no doubt reflecting a legal interest fuelled by the widely publicised prognostications of the medical profession, and while it is true that the avalanche of litigation on this topic predicted a decade ago may not have materialised, it would be a mistake to assume that there are not hordes of lawyers up the gullies shouting, stamping and yodelling for all their worth to make it happen.

In the author's personal experience of providing expert opinion, patients, their advocates and their legal advisors are all aware that the spectrum of potential concern is now considerably wider than just these late manifestations of disorder. An equal measure of awareness can be commended to doctors too.

The second mechanism to bring about the change that it is hoped will follow from awareness is acknowledgement of the impact of these adverse effects on the patients themselves, for it is only with such an acknowledgement that the impetus will come to explore the wider boundaries of the neurological symptomatology, the expertise to delineate this from other sources of similar disability, and the motivation to implement comprehensive management. Patients can forgive much of doctors and their recommendations provided they are persuaded that the problems these may foster are being taken seriously.

This is a further theme that emerges from cases brought before the American courts thus far: a perception that the matter, even if recognised, has not, in effect, been taken seriously enough (Tancredi, 1988). It is not considered a satisfactory standard to remain aware of such adverse effects but yet be seen to have attempted nothing to tackle them. It does not seem that the courts (at least in the USA) demand a perfect therapeutic outcome from such attempts – or necessarily *any* positive outcome – but the expectation remains of an attempt. Although tardive dyskinesia has again been the focus here, the author's recent experience of providing expert opinion in the UK would indicate that this legal expectation is extending to the range of EPS, as well it might with the greater availability of effective interventions for acute/intermediate disorders.

New drugs for old?

The argument may be put – and is likely to be increasingly put – that while the subject matter of the present volume is all very well, the thrust of it relates to yesterday's problems. There is now, after all, a new generation of antipsychotic compounds that render the present effort in effect a work of history. The future lies with these new drugs, which will free patients from the risks of such neurological nasties and doctors from the responsibility of acquiring skills in recognition and assessment (which most have never had but in rudimentary degree anyway). Psychiatrists, in particular, can return to the cosy world of unverifiable speculation.

It hardly need be stated that while the author would dearly love to share the optimism some commentators have expressed about this brave new psychopharmacological world, his perception of the situation is more phlegmatic. The new drugs, thanks largely to clozapine, have certainly stimulated a long overdue debate on the mechanisms of antipsychotic action that takes us beyond the strictures of the classical dopamine hypothesis and into diverse and – yes – exciting territory. The first realisations of this to translate into commercial products – the so-called SDAs – seem to be resulting in drugs that are indeed better tolerated neurologically and probably as a result more 'user friendly'. But to assume that the modest advantages thus far demonstrated, welcome as they are, represent a basis for liberating patients from risk or for absolving clinicians of their responsibilities for *comprehensive* patient care, is to fly in the face of good practice principles and over the rainbow to fantasy.

We are now likely to be seeing the first blasts of the trumpet on the ethical side of new drug use – with protagonists already arguing (to this mind, unconvincingly) that a first-line place for the new antipsychotics in the treatment of schizophrenia is an ethical imperative (Jones and Holliday, 1996). This case has been argued by experts from North America, which may be no coincidence because practitioners in that neck of the woods have conducted an intense, if not entirely monogamous, relationship with high-potency compounds for many years. Their affections have been particularly true to haloperidol, although had they heeded their peers, the profession may have been more circumspect. A powerful account of the stupefying effects of haloperidol in normal subjects who had volunteered to take it was influential in deterring normal volunteer studies with antipsychotics in general for the best part of a decade (Anderson, Reker and Cooper, 1981; King et al., 1995). It has always seemed to the author that a stout blow to the back of the head with a blunt object would flatten most people less than haloperidol. So, to those whose experience has for long been dominated by this compound and its ilk, *anything* must seem better!

However, to show that new compound 'X' is less extrapyramidally assaultive than, for example, haloperidol is merely to demonstrate how assaultive to extrapyramidal function haloperidol can be. Also, while demonstrating that compound 'X' produces no greater disturbance than placebo in patients long exposed to standard drugs may point to a lower likelihood of symptom induction, it cannot be interpreted as 'no liability'. Generalisations beyond this are speculative and must await appropriate comparisons.

A further plank to the 'ethical' argument is cost. It would, of course, be perverse to frame this in terms of absolute costs because the new-generation compounds are more expensive by several degrees of magnitude than standard drugs. What is suggested, however, is that *overall* health care costs can be reduced by, for example, shortening periods of inpatient care – a very attractive proposition in these times of squeezed health budgets worldwide. Indeed, some tentative evidence in this direction has been presented, though studies undertaken in the author's locality have not been confirmatory.

A great problem with work in this field relates to the infrequently explored effect of an optimistically received new treatment on the caregivers themselves and the way this alters practice. There are, for example, striking accounts in the literature of the beneficial effects of clozapine on long-term outcome as assessed on the Quality of Life Questionnaire (Meltzer et al., 1990; Meltzer, 1992). These accounts cannot fail to impress, but it must be appreciated that they emanate from open studies of a drug whose mode of administration is totally different from anything that has come before it. The mandatory monitoring procedures ensure a regular medical contact – however brief – that for many patients introduces a new dynamic into their long-term management. There is a further, albeit anecdotal, extension to this. The author has frequently observed the way in which clozapine's benefits can overflow into improved quality-of-life issues for *carers*. This in its turn may reflect in parameters of 'expressed emotion', thereby impacting on relapse and contributing to improvements in long-term outcome.

The point to be impressed is that, although at present the new antipsychotic agents look promising with regard to extrapyramidal tolerability, the evidence on which to gauge their relative place in management remains partial and it will be some years yet before many of the current speculations can be confirmed, modified – or rejected. In the interim, a very real concern is that an already underskilled profession may be seduced into a state of neurological 'apraxia' – knowing what they would like to do but simply unable to execute it – while the lawyers sharpen their knives!

There are, in addition, two 'markets' in which new-generation compounds are unlikely to impact for some time to come – if at all. The first is in depot formulations. American colleagues are frequently surprised to realise the extent to which this mode of administration has permeated practice in Britain, where over 50 per cent of patients with established recurrent schizophrenic disorder are managed this way – and even this figure is modest by some comparisons (see van Harten et al., 1996). In view of its favourable impact on compliance, this depot 'market' is unlikely to disappear overnight. Long-term safety issues will require thorough addressing before depot formulations of new drugs can be widely recommended if – and this is a formidable 'if' – their pharmacology permits.

The second 'market' is in developing nations. It is important for those whose working environments are the relatively well-heeled academic departments of affluent nations to bear in mind that 'ethical' and other arguments in favour of expensive new antipsychotic agents are, for most of the world (and hence most patients), ones that must await a future economic miracle – or radical pharmaceutical repricing! A similar argument might be extended to more affluent nations, where state or private purchasing authorities may place a ceiling on antipsychotic drug costs.

What if the new drugs turn out to be the answer to all, or most, of our tolerability prayers – are we then off the hook? I doubt it. In recent years, major changes have occurred in the organisation of health care delivery worldwide. These are exemplified by the introduction in the UK of an administrative split between those who provide services from those who purchase them. Deliverers of care, such as doctors, are now liable to maintain contract standards agreed (usually on their behalf) with purchasers. One thing purchasers are increasingly preoccupied with is outcome parameters, and in the author's experience they are particularly wedded to methods that provide these in numerical form – perhaps a warm reminder of the balance sheets to which they are so devoted! The pattern of adverse effects – actual or possible – and their impact on disability in local populations of the long-term psychiatrically ill would seem to this practitioner to be right up their street. Thus, regardless of the clinical impact of new-generation drugs, those who pay our salaries are quite likely to demand skills in EPS recognition and evaluation for some time to come.

Some practical suggestions

How, then, can the clinician satisfy these diverse constraints? This would, in fact, demand the squaring of a very obdurate circle. However, there is one crucial principle to hammer home, especially to junior doctors, and that is the central importance of the written record. Nowadays, it seems the concepts of 'case *notes* ' and 'case *records* ' are no longer synonymous, with the latter superseding the former. The written record must be a comprehensive account not only of decisions made and implemented, but also of decisions considered but not implemented – and why. Certainly, in legal contexts, notwithstanding statements and affidavits, the author has had it from senior counsel that matters of medical litigation are invariably swayed on the basis of the written record. Hence, the first step is the adequate recording of each set of considerations – the pros *and* the cons – out of which each management decision emerged.

The issue of consent would seem straightforward enough and, specifically with regard to our present discussion, that means consent to use antipsychotic drugs. This is required and, except in the circumstances mentioned above, should be sought (Brabbins, Butler and Bentall, 1996). The metamorphosis of consent to that which is 'informed' raises particular problems for psychiatry that have yet to be resolved. Adopting the literal approach outlined above is clearly a nonsense, but so too is avoiding necessary and effective treatment out of timidity or uncertainty. Seeking consent that is 'informed' from those with major psychiatric disorders need not be viewed as a 'stat' effort to be undertaken once only at the point of maximal mental state disturbance, and hence greatest difficulty in attaining, and abandoned thereafter. The on-going nature of the exercise, with the provision of information commensurate with the patient's ability to assimilate it, should be part of the doctor's continuing educational role and a crucial element in fostering a consensual approach to management. In this context, the author can strongly recommend the word 'recommend', which, with its authoritative but nonetheless advisory connotations and inherent element of choice, is one of the most useful words in the medical lexicon.

One point of specific relevance to the UK, may be worthy of general note. Psychiatric trainees in the UK often seem to labour under the misapprehension that detention under the assessment/short-term sections of the Mental Health Acts (MHAs) imparts an automatic authority to treat with drugs. This is incorrect. Such patients still have the right to refuse medical recommendations and have that decision respected, *provided* that the decision is competently arrived at. In the majority of cases in which compulsory powers have been implemented, there is likely to be sound reason to consider the patient incompetent in this regard. However, the author can but strongly advise that, for legal reasons, this should be stated in the record. Thus, if a patient detained under Sections 2 (MHA, 1983) or 26 (MH(Scotland)A, 1984) refuses a recommendation for drug treatment which is believed to be necessary, that refusal should be noted, along with the clinician's conclusion that, owing to the mental disorder from which the patient suffers, this decision is, in the clinician's opinion, incompetently derived and that in this situation the decision to administer necessary drug treatment will be implemented. The question of competency remains an essentially individual clinical decision, but in cases of doubt, a second opinion should be sought from a senior colleague.

The reason for emphasising this gets back to the point that any subsequent dispute is likely to be determined on the basis of the written record. The author has been advised by both legal counsel and eminent forensic psychiatric opinion that in such a scenario a court could well decide at a later date that, as the issue of competency was not recorded, the issue of consent was not properly considered as the law requires, and hence might conclude that any subsequent treatment was administered unlawfully. Although this point has a specific focus, it would seem to incorporate a general principle of merit for those operating in other jurisdictions.

The formats proposed for 'disclosures' on risk in relation to antipsychotics vary, and have included individual or small-group educational sessions. They may be solely verbal or combine verbal with written information. Some form of written information is frequently advocated, but the impact of mental state disturbance on comprehension during especially acute phases of illness would suggest that these may not withstand subsequent scrutiny, and hence run the risk of providing a false sense of comfort in a job well done.

In the USA several questionnaire formats have been proposed for obtaining informed consent, which would certainly have the advantage of introducing an element of standardisation into an otherwise fraught field. It does seem that while these may improve recall of consent procedures, current instruments have been criticised on the basis that they, in effect, tap into aspects of memory rather than understanding per se and hence may again be of limited value in the face of subsequent challenge. In general, it would seem at this stage preferable merely to record one's efforts individually for each individual case. The limited value in legal and other terms of any signed consent in the psychiatrically unwell must be emphasised, even if the practitioner feels that the question of competency has been covered.

In terms of conducting one's clinical practice, the soundest approach to patient care that can be recommended in order to accommodate all the various constraints to which psychiatrists (and others) are now subject is adoption of the legal principle of 'avoidance of avoidable cause'. To reiterate some points made previously in the present volume, the indications for use of antipsychotics should be strictly adhered to along the lines proposed above, as should recommended dose regimes. In addition, it would seem prudent to be circumspect in the use of high-potency standard compounds, particularly in high doses in the young or drug naive and the elderly, and in anyone for prolonged periods. Similarly, one might speculate (and speculate is the word) on the advisability of certain combinations, such as anti-psychotics and SSRIs, especially in vulnerable groups such as the elderly, until a clearer long-term picture emerges. It would further be helpful to maintain a structure to one's management plans such as was discussed earlier, which, by delineating the different phases of treat-ment, will help focus the aims of the plan in one's mind, and thereby help keep doses at their minimum, especially in long-term main-tenance.

It is, furthermore, important to be flexible in one's perception of the pharmacological tools available and to consider alternatives from different groups of antipsychotic, which on present evidence should, in the author's opinion, comprise a mix of standard and new-generation drugs – for the foreseeable future at least.

Most important of all, however, is the need for *regular* monitoring and a readiness to intervene when the clinical situation indicates. As has been stated, most of the standardised recording instruments in the field of drug-related movement disorders have traditionally had a strong research bias, both in their development and usage. Despite this, familiarity with a simple and comprehensive 'package' and its regular utilisation can be strongly commended to the clinician in routine prac-tice also, the reasons for which have already been set out. In the present context, it is also likely to satisfy the future requirements of not only health care purchasers but any who at some point may wish to scrutin-ise one's therapeutic endeavours.

The reader was forewarned that the issues raised in the present chapter were to some extent the 'stick' and, like all forms of flagellation, a degree of pain is inevitable. It may, indeed, be painful for the medical profession to address such questions, especially those of an ethical nature for which most of us are frankly ill-equipped. As one medical ethicist put it in response to a somewhat frustrated outburst from the author, 'We are here to raise the problems, not provide you with answers'.

It is easy when viewing psychiatry, and indeed medical practice in general, 'from the trenches' to see all of this as an infinite series of spuri-ous diversions that are downright unhelpful. But it would be a mistake to adopt such a battlefield mentality and detach ourselves from the debate – for a debate there is and will be, whether the profession wishes it or not.

The fact is our perception of the therapeutic modalities we recom-mend is inevitably one sided and, like that of all 'experts', distorted by familiarity, and it is necessary for the mirror to be held before us that we might see the blemishes. One of medicine's major tasks is to engage patients in our treatment recommendations and, whereas in former times, when society was less informed and more hierarchical, authoritarian individualism may have been an effective therapeutic method, nowadays a more consensual approach is expected.

At the end of the day, it is also more fun. If one's professional life feeds on knowledge, which that of doctors ought to, we cannot forget that ultimately it is the patients who tell us all we know.

References

Abse, W. (1966). *Hysteria and Related Mental disorders*. Bristol: John Wright.

Addonizio, G. & Alexopoulos, G.S. (1988). Drug-induced dystonia in young and elderly patients. *American Journal of Psychiatry*, **145**, 869–71.

Adler, L.A., Angrist, B., Weinreb, H. & Rotrosen, J. (1991). Studies on the time course and efficacy of beta-blockers in neuroleptic-induced akathisia and the akathisia of idiopathic Parkinson's disease. *Psychopharmacology Bulletin*, **27**, 107–11.

Adler, L.A., Peselow, E., Rosenthal, M. & Angrist, B. (1993d). A controlled comparison of the effects of propranolol, benztropine and placebo on akathisia – an interim analysis. *Psychopharmacology Bulletin*, **29**, 283–6.

Adler, L.A., Peselow, E., Rotrosen, J. et al. (1993b). Vitamin E treatment of tardive dyskinesia. *American Journal of Psychiatry*, **150**, 1405–07.

Aguilar, E.J., Keshavan, M.S., Martinez-Quiles, M.D., Hernandez, J., Gomez Beneyto, M. & Schooler, N. (1994). Predictors of acute dystonia in first-episode psychotic patients. *American Journal of Psychiatry*, **151**, 1819–21.

Alba, A., Trainor, F.S., Ritter, W. & Dasco, M.M. (1968). A clinical disability rating for parkinsonian patients. *Journal of Chronic Diseases*, **21**, 507–22.

Alexopoulos, G.S. (1979). Lack of complaints in schizophrenics with tardive dyskinesia. *Journal of Nervous and Mental Diseases*, **167**, 125–7.

Anden, N.E., Carlsson, A., Kerstell, J. et al. (1970). Oral L-dopa treatment in parkinsonism. *Acta Medica Scandinavica*, **187**, 247–55.

Anderson, B.G., Reker, D. & Cooper, T.B. (1981). Prolonged adverse effects of haloperidol in normal subjects. *New England Journal of Medicine*, **305**, 643–4.

Arana, G.W., Goff, D.C., Baldessarini, R.J. & Keepers, G.A. (1988). Efficacy of anticholinergic prophylaxis for neuroleptic-induced acute dystonia. *American Journal of Psychiatry*, **145**, 993–6.

Arblaster, L.A., Lakie, M., Mutch, W.J. & Semple, M. (1993). A study of the early signs of drug-induced parkinsonism. *Journal of Neurology, Neurosurgery and Psychiatry*, **56**, 301–03.

Aronson, T.A. (1985). Persistent drug-induced parkinsonism. *Bioligical Psychiatry*, **20**, 795–8.

Arthur, H., Dahl, M.L., Siwers, B. & Sjoqvist, F. (1995). Polymorphic drug metabolism in schizophrenic patients with tardive dyskinesia. *Journal of Clinical Psychopharmacology*, **15**, 211–16.

Arya, D.K. (1994). Extrapyramidal symptoms with selective serotonin reuptake inhibitors. *British Journal of Psychiatry*, **165**, 728–33.

Avissar, S. & Schreiber, G. (1989). Muscarinic receptor subclassification and G-proteins: significance for lithium action in affective disorders and for the treatment of the extrapyramidal side effects of neuroleptics. *Biological Psychiatry*, **26**, 113–30.

Avorn, J., Bohn, R.L., Mogun, H., et al. (1995). Neuroleptic drug exposure and treatment of parkinsonism in the elderly: a case control study. *American Journal of Medicine*, **99**, 48–54.

Ayd, F.J. (1961). A survey of drug-induced extrapyramidal reactions. *Journal of the American Medical Association*, **175**, 1054–60.

Ayd, F.J. (1967). Persistent dyskinesia: a neurologic complication of major tranquillisers. *Medical Science*, **18**, 32–40.

Ayd, F.J. (1974). Side-effects of depot fluphenazines. *Comprehensive Psychiatry*, **15**, 277–84.

Baldessarini, R.J., Katz, B. & Cotton, P. (1984). Dissimilar dosing with high-potency and low-potency neuroleptics. *American Journal of Psychiatry*, **141**, 748–52.

Barnes, T.R.E. (1989). A rating scale for drug-induced akathisia. *British Journal of Psychiatry*, **154**, 672–6.

Barnes, T.R.E. & Braude, W.M. (1985). Akathisia variants and tardive dyskinesia. *Archives of General Psychiatry*, **42**, 874–8.

Barnes, T.R.E. & Kidger, T. (1979). Tardive dyskinesia and problems of assessment. In *Current Themes in Psychiatry*, Vol. 2, ed. R. Gaind & B.L. Hudson, pp. 145–62. London: Macmillan.

Barnes, T.R.E. & Wiles, D.H. (1983). Variations in orofacial tardive dyskinesia during depot antipsychotic drug treatment. *Psychopharmacology*, **81**, 359–62.

Bates, L.D., Lampert, I., Prendergast, M. & Van Woerkom, A.E. (1996). Klazomania – the screaming tic. *Neurocase*, **2**, 31–3.

Bell, R.C.H. & Smith, R.C. (1978). Tardive dyskinesia: characterisation and prevalence in a statewide system. *Journal of Clinical Psychiatry*, **39**, 39–47.

Bennet, J.P., Landow, E.R., Dietrich, S. & Schuh, L.A. (1994). Suppression of dyskinesias in advanced Parkinson's disease: moderate daily clozapine doses provide long-term dyskinesia reduction. *Movement Disorders*, **9**, 409–14.

Bergen, J., Kitchin, R. & Berry, G. (1992). Predictors of the course of tardive dyskinesia in patients receiving neuroleptics. *Biological Psychiatry*, **32**, 580–94.

Bermanzohn, P.C. & Siris, S.G. (1992). Akinesia: a syndrome common to parkinsonism, retarded depression and negative symptoms of schizophrenia. *Comprehensive Psychiatry*, **33**, 221–32.

Bersani, G., Grispini, A., Marini, S., Pasini, A., Valducci, M. & Ciani, N. (1990).
5-HT2 antagonist ritanserin in neuroleptic-induced parkinsonism: a
double-blind comparison with orphenadrine and placebo. *Clinical
Neuropharmacology*, **13**, 500–06.

Bhugra, D. & Baker, S. (1990). State-dependent tardive dyskinesia. *Journal of
Nervous and Mental Diseases*, **178**, 720.

Bleuler, E. (1911). *Dementia Praecox or the Group of Schizophrenias*. Translated by
J. Zinkin. New York: International Universities Press, 1950.

Bocola, V., Fabbrini, G., Sollecito, A., Paladini, C. & Martucci, N. (1996).
Neuroleptic-induced parkinsonism: MRI findings in relation to clinical
course after withdrawal of neuroleptic drugs. *Journal of Neurology,
Neurosurgery and Psychiatry*, **60**, 213–16.

Bodfish, J.W., Newell, K.M., Sprague, R.L., Harper, V.N. & Lewis, M.H. (1996).
Dyskinetic movement disorder among adults with mental retardation:
phenomenology and co-occurrence with stereotypy. *American Journal of
Mental Retardation*, **101**, 118–29.

Brabbins, C., Butler, J. & Bentall, R. (1996). Consent to neuroleptic medication
for schizophrenia: clinical, ethical and legal issues. *British Journal of
Psychiatry*, **168**, 540–4.

Branchey, M. & Branchey, L. (1984). Patterns of psychotropic drug use and
tardive dyskinesia. *Journal of Clinical Psychopharmacology*, **4**, 41–5.

Brandon, S., McClelland, H.A. & Protheroe, C. (1971). A study of facial
dyskinesia in a mental hospital population. *British Journal of Psychiatry*,
118, 171–84.

Braude, W.M., Barnes, T.R.E. & Gore, S.M. (1983). Clinical characteristics of
akathisia: a systematic investigation of acute psychiatric inpatient
admissions. *British Journal of Psychiatry*, **143**, 139–50.

Breitbart, W., Marcotta, R.F. & Call, P. (1988). AIDS and neuroleptic malignant
syndrome. *Lancet*, ii, 1488–9.

Breitbart, W., Macotta, R., Platt, M.M. et al. (1996). A double-blind trial of
haloperidol, chlorpromazine and lorazepam in the treatment of delirium
in hospitalised AIDS patients. *American Journal of Psychiatry*, **153**, 231–7.

Brown, K.W. & White, T. (1991). Pseudoakathisia and schizophrenic negative
symptoms. *Acta Psychiatrica Scandinavica*, **84**, 107–09.

Brown, K.W. & White, T. (1992). Subsystems of tardive dyskinesia and some
clinical correlates. *Psychological Medicine*, **22**, 923–7.

Bruno, A. & Bruno, C. (1966). Effects of L-dopa on pharmacological
parkinsonism. *Acta Psychiatrica Scandinavica*, **42**, 264–71.

Burke, R.E., Fahn, S., Jankovic, J. et al. (1982). Tardive dystonia: late onset and
persistent dystonia caused by antipsychotic drugs. *Neurology*, **32**, 1335–46.

Burke, R.E., Fahn, S. & Marsden, C.D. (1986). Torsion dystonia: a double-blind
prospective trial of high dose trihexyphenidyl. *Neurology*, **36**, 160–4.

Burke, R.E., Fahn, S., Marsden, C.D., Bressman, S.B., Moskowitz, C. &
Friedman, J. (1985). Validity and reliability of a rating scale for the
primary torsion dystonias. *Neurology*, **35**, 73–7.

Burke, R.E. & Kang, U.J. (1988). Tardive dystonia: clinical aspects and
treatment. In *Advances in Neurology*, Vol 49: *Facial Dyskinesias*, ed. J.
Jankovic & E. Tolosa, pp. 199–210. New York: Raven Press.

Burke, R.E., Kang, U.J., Jankovic, J., Miller, L.G. & Fahn, S. (1989). Tardive akathisia: an analysis of clinical features and response to open therapeutic trials. *Movement Disorders*, **4**, 157–75.

Burn, D.J. & Brooks, D.J. (1993). Nigral dysfunction in drug-induced parkinsonism: an 18F-dopa study. *Neurology*, **43**, 552–6.

Caldwell, A.E. (1978). History of psychopharmacology. In *Principles of Psychopharmacology*, ed. W.G. Clark & J. del Giudice, pp. 9–40. New York, San Francisco, London: Academic Press.

Caligiuri, M.P., Barcha, H.S. & Lohr, J.B. (1989). Asymmetry of neuroleptic induced rigidity: development of quantitative methods and clinical correlates. *Psychiatry Research*, **30**, 275–84.

Caligiuri, M.P., Lohr, J.B. & Jeste, D.V. (1993). Parkinsonism in neuroleptic-naive schizophrenic patients. *American Journal of Psychiatry*, **150**, 1343–8.

Calne, D.B., Stern, G.M., Laurence, D.R., Sharkey, J. & Armitage, P. (1969). L-Dopa in post-encephalitic parkinsonism. *Lancet*, **1**, 744–6.

Campbell, M., Adams, P., Perry, R., Spencer, E.K. & Overall, J.E. (1988). Tardive and withdrawal dyskinesia in autistic children: a prospective study. *Psychopharmacology Bulletin*, **24**, 251–5.

Campbell, M., Anderson, L.T., Cohen, I.R. et al. (1982). Haloperidol in autistic children: effects on learning behavior and abnormal involuntary movements. *Psychopharmacology Bulletin*, **18**, 110–12.

Campbell, M., Perry, R., Bennett, W.G. et al. (1983). Long-term therapeutic efficacy and drug-related abnormal movements: a prospective study of haloperidol in autistic children. *Psychopharmacology Bulletin*, **19**, 80–3.

Campbell, M., Small, A.M., Green, W.H. et al. (1984). Behavioral efficacy of haloperidol and lithium carbonate: a comparison in hospitalised aggressive children with conduct disorders. *Archives of General Psychiatry*, **41**, 650–6.

Canter, C.J., De La Torre, R. & Mier, N. (1961). A method of evaluating disability in patients with Parkinson's disease. *Journal of Nervous and Mental Diseases*, **133**, 143–7.

Caradoc-Davies, G., Menkes, D.B., Clarkson, H.O. & Mullen, P. (1986). A study of need for anticholinergic medication in patients treated with long-term antipsychotics. *Australian and New Zealand Journal of Psychiatry*, **20**, 225–30.

Carpenter, W.T., Heinrichs, D.W. & Alphs, L.D. (1985). Treatment of negative symptoms. *Schizophrenia Bulletin*, **11**, 440–52.

Casey, D.E. (1989). Clozapine: neuroleptic-induced EPS and tardive dyskinesia. *Psychopharmacology*, **99**, S47–S53.

Casey, D.E. (1992). The rabbit syndrome. In *Movement Disorders in Neurology and Neuropsychiatry*, ed. A. Joseph & R. Young, pp. 139–42. Boston: Blackwell Scientific Publications.

Casey, D.E., Gerlach, J. & Bjorndal, N. (1982). Levodopa and receptor sensitivity modification in tardive dyskinesia. *Psychopharmacology*, **78**, 89–92.

Casey, D.E. & Rabins, P. (1978). Tardive dyskinesia as a life threatening illness. *American Journal of Psychiatry*, **135**, 486–8.

Cavanaugh, J.J. & Finlayson, A. (1984). Rhabdomyolysis due to acute dystonic reaction to antipsychotic drugs. *Journal of Clinical Psychiatry*, **45**, 356–7.

Chacko, R.C., Hurley, R.A. & Jankovic, J. (1993). Clozapine use in diffuse Lewy body disease. *Journal of Neuropsychiatry and Clinical Neuroscience*, **5**, 206–8.

Chadwick, D., Reynolds, E.H. & Marsden, C.D. (1976). Anticonvulsant-induced dyskinesias: a comparison with dyskinesias induced by neuroleptics. *Journal of Neurology, Neurosurgery and Psychiatry*, **39**, 1210–18.

Chakos, M.H., Alvir, J.M.J. Woerner, M.G. et al. (1996). Incidence and correlates of tardive dyskinesia in first episode of schizophrenia. *Archives of General Psychiatry*, **53**, 313–19.

Chakos, M.H., Mayerhoff, D.I., Loebel, A.D., Alvir, J. & Lieberman, J.A. (1992). Incidence and correlates of acute extrapyramidal symptoms in first episode of schizophrenia. *Psychopharmacology Bulletin*, **28**, 81–6.

Chatterjee, A., Chakos, M., Koreen, A. et al. (1995). The prevalence and clinical correlates of extrapyramidal signs and spontaneous dyskinesia in never-medicated schizophrenic patients. *American Journal of Psychiatry*, **152**, 1724–9.

Chiarello, R.J. & Cole, J.O. (1987). The use of psychostimulants in general psychiatry. *Archives of General Psychiatry*, **44**, 286–95.

Chiles, J.A. (1978). Extrapyramidal reactions in adolescents treated with high-potency antipsychotics. *American Journal of Psychiatry*, **135**, 239–40.

Chiorfi, M. & Moussaoui, D. (1985). Les schizophrenes jamais traites n'ont pas de movements abnormaux type dyskinesie tardive. *L'Encephale*, **11**, 263–5.

Chiu, H.F.K., Wing, Y.K., Kwong, P.K., Leung, C.M. & Lam, L.C.W. (1993). Prevalence of tardive dyskinesia in samples of elderly people in Hong Kong. *Acta Psychiatrica Scandinavica*, **87**, 266–8.

Chiu, L.P.W. (1989). Transient recurrence of auditory hallucinations during acute dystonia. *British Journal of Psychiatry*, **155**, 110–13.

Chouinard, G. (1995). The effects of risperidone in tardive dyskinesia: an analysis of the Canadian Multicenter Risperidone Study. *Journal of Clinical Psychopharmacology*, **15**, Suppl. 1, 36S–44S.

Chouinard, G., Annable, L., Mercier, P. & Ross-Chouinard, A. (1986). A five year follow-up study of tardive dyskinesia. *Psychopharmacology Bulletin*, **22**, 259–63.

Chouinard, G. & Jones, B.D. (1979). Early onset of tardive dyskinesia: case report. *American Journal of Psychiatry*, **136**, 1323–4.

Chouinard, G., Ross-Chouinard, A., Annable, L. & Jones, B.D. (1980). Extrapyramidal rating scale. *Canadian Journal of Neurological Science*, **7**, 233.

Chouinard, G. Ross-Chouinard, A., Gauthier, S., Annable, L. & Mercier, P. (1984). An extrapyramidal rating scale for idiopathic and neuroleptic-induced parkinsonism and dyskinesia. *Proceedings 14th CINP Congress, Florence, Italy, 19th–23rd June*, 16.

Christensen, A.V., Fjalland, B. & Nielson, I.M. (1976). On supersensitivity of dopamine receptors induced by neuroleptics. *Psychopharmacology*, **48**, 1–6.

Cole, J.D. & Davis, J.M. (1969). Antipsychotic drugs. In *The Schizophrenic Syndrome*, ed. L. Bellak & L. Loeb, pp. 478–568. New York: Grune and Stratton.

Comella, C.L. & Goetz, C.G. (1994). Akathisia in Parkinson's disease. *Movement Disorders*, **9**, 545–9.

Comella, C.L. & Tanner, C.M. (1992). The side effects of chronic treatment in Parkinson's disease. In *Movement Disorders in Neurology and Neuropsychiatry*, ed. A.B. Joseph & R.R. Young, pp. 236–46. Boston: Blackwell Scientific Publications.

Cook, P.E., Dermer, S.W. & McGurk, T. (1986). Fatal overdose with amantadine. *Canadian Journal of Psychiatry*, **31**, 757–8.

Cotzias, G.C., Papavasiliou, P.S., Fehling, C., Kaufman, B. & Mena, I. (1970). Similarities between neurological effects of L-dopa and apomorphine. *New England Journal of Medicine*, **282**, 31–3.

Crane, G.E. & Paulson, G. (1967). Involuntary movements in a sample chronic mental patients and their relation to treatment with neuroleptics. *International Journal of Neuropsychiatry*, **3**, 286–91.

Crane, G.E. & Naranjo, E.R. (1971). Motor disorders induced by neuroleptics. *Archives of General Psychiatry*, **24**, 179–84.

Crow, T.J. (1980). Molecular pathology of schizophrenia: more than one disease process? *British Medical Journal*, **280**, 66–8.

Crow, T.J., Johnstone, E.C. & McClelland, H.A. (1976). The co-incidence of parkinsonism and schizophrenia: some neurochemical implications. *Psychological Medicine*, **6**, 227–33.

Crow, T.J., Owens, D.G.C., Johnstone, E.C., Cross, A.J. & Owen, F. (1983). Does tardive dyskinesia exist? *Modern Problems of Pharmacopsychiatry*, **21**, 206–19.

Curson, D.A., Barnes, T.R.E., Bamber, R.W., Platt, S.D., Hirsch, S.R. & Duffy, J.C. (1985). Long-term depot maintenance of chronic schizophrenic out-patients: the seven year follow-up of the Medical Research Council Fluphenazine/placebo trial. II. The incidence of compliance problems, side-effects, neurotic symptoms and depression. *British Journal of Psychiatry*, **146**, 469–74.

Cutler, N.R., Post, R.M., Rey, A.C. & Bunney, W.E. (1981). Depression-dependent dyskinesias in two cases of manic–depressive illness. *New England Journal of Medicine*, **304**, 1088–9.

Daniel, J.R. & Mauro, V.F. (1995). Extrapyramidal symptoms associated with calcium channel blockers. *Annals of Pharmacotherapy*, **29**, 73–5.

Daras, M., Koppel, B.S. & Atos Radzion, E. (1994). Cocaine induced choreoathetoid movements ('crack dancing'). *Neurology*, **44**, 751–2.

Dave, M. (1994). Clozapine-related tardive dyskinesia. *Biological Psychiatry*, **35**, 886–7.

de Potter, R.W., Linkowski, P. & Mendlewicz, J. (1983). State-dependent tardive dyskinesia in manic–depressive illness. *Journal of Neurology, Neurosurgery and Psychiatry*, **46**, 666–8.

Dekret, J.J., Maany, I., Ramsey, R.A. & Mendels, J. (1977). A case of oral dyskinesia associated with imipramine treatment. *American Journal of Psychiatry*, **134**, 1297–8.

Delwaide, P.J. & Hurlet, A. (1980). Bromocriptine and buccolinguofacial dyskinesias in patients with senile dementia: a quantitative study. *Archives of Neurology*, **37**, 441–3.

DeVeaugh-Geiss, J. (1982). Prediction and prevention of tardive dyskinesia. In *Tardive Dyskinesia and Related Involuntary Movement Disorders*, ed. J. De Veaugh-Geiss, pp. 161–6. Boston, Bristol, London: John Wright.

Diamond, S.G. & Markham, C.H. (1983). Evaluating the evaluations: or how to weigh the scales of parkinsonian disability. *Neurology*, **33**, 1098–9.

DiMascio, A., Bernardo, D.L., Greenblatt, D.J. & Marder, J.E. (1976). A controlled trial of amantadine in drug-induced extrapyramidal disorders. *Archives of General Psychiatry*, **33**, 599–602.

Dinan, T.G. & Golden, T. (1990). Orofacial dyskinesia in Down's syndrome. *British Journal of Psychiatry*, **157**, 131–2.

Dixon, L., Weiden, P., Haag, G., Sweeney, J. & Frances, A.J. (1992). Increased tardive dyskinesia in alcohol abusing schizophrenics. *Comprehensive Psychiatry*, **33**, 121–2.

Donlon, P.T., Hopkin, J.T., Tupin, J.P., Wicks, J.J. & Wahba, M. (1980). Haloperidol for acute schizophrenic patients: an evaluation of three oral regimes. *Archives of General Psychiatry*, **37**, 691–5.

Dooneief, G., Mirabello, E., Bell, K., Marder, K., Stern, Y. & Mayeux, R. (1992). An estimate of the incidence of depression in idiopathic Parkinson's disease. *Archives of Neurology*, **49**, 305–7.

Double, D.B., Warren, G.C., Evans, M. & Rowlands, R.P. (1993). Efficacy of maintenance use of anticholinergic agents. *Acta Psychiatrica Scandinavica*, **88**, 381–4.

Drake, R.E. & Erlich, J. (1985). Suicide attempts associated with akathisia. *American Journal of Psychiatry*, **142**, 499–501.

Duane, D. (1988). Spasmodic torticollis. In *Advances in Neurology*, Vol. 49: *Facial Dyskinesias*, ed. J. Jankovic & E. Tolsa, pp. 135–50. New York: Raven Press.

Duvoisin, R.C. (1970). The evaluation of extrapyramidal disease. In *Monoamines, Noyaux Gris Centraux et Syndrome de Parkinson*, ed. J. Ajuriaguerra, pp. 313–25. Paris: Masson.

Egan, M.E., Hyde, T.M., Albers, G.W. et al. (1992). Treatment of tardive dyskinesia with vitamin E. *American Journal of Psychiatry*, **149**, 773–7.

Egan, M.F., Hyde, T.M., Tirschwell, D.L., Kleinman, J.E. & Weinberger, D.R. (1992b). Laterality of appendicular tardive dyskinesia in chronic schizophrenia. *Biological Psychiatry*, **31**, 1098–9.

Eldridge, M. (1970). The torson dystonias: literature review and genetic and clinical studies. *Neurology*, **20**, 1–78.

Elkashef, A., Ruskin, P.E., Bacher, N. & Barrett, D. (1990). Vitamin E in the treatment of tardive dyskinesia. *American Journal of Psychiatry*, **147**, 505–6.

Ellis, R.J., Caligiuri, M., Galasko, D. & Thal, L.J. (1996). Extrapyramidal motor signs in clinically diagnosed Alzheimer disease. *Alzheimer Disease and Associated Disorders*, **10**, 103–14.

Engelhardt, D.M. & Polizos, P. (1978). Adverse effects of pharmacotherapy in childhood psychosis. In *Psychopharmacology: A Generation of Progress*, ed. M.A. Lipton, A. Dimascio & K.F. Killam, pp. 1463–9. New York: Raven Press.

Erenberg, G., Cruse, R.P. & Rothner, A.D. (1985). Gilles de la Tourette syndrome: effect of stimulant drugs. *Neurology*, **35**, 1346–8.

Etzel, J.V. (1994). Diphenhydramine-induced acute dystonia. *Pharmacotherapy*, **14**, 492–6.

Factor, S.A., Podskalny, G.D. & Barron, K.D. (1994). Persistent neuroleptic induced rigidity and dystonia in AIDS dementia complex: a clinico-pathological case report. *Journal of Neurological Sciences*, **127**, 114–20.

Factor, S.A., Podskalny, G.D. & Molho, E.S. (1995). Psychogenic movement disorders: frequency, clinical profile and characteristics. *Journal of Neurology, Neurosurgery and Psychiatry*, **59**, 406–12.

Factor, S.A., Sanchez-Ramos, J.R. & Weiner, W.J. (1988). Cocaine and Tourette's syndrome. *Annals of Neurology*, **23**, 402–3.

Fahn, S. (1984). The varied clinical expressions of dystonia. *Neurologic Clinics*, **2**, 541–54.

Fahn, S., Elton, R.L. & Members of the UPDRS Development Committee (1987a). Unified Parkinson's Disease Rating Scale. In *Recent Developments in Parkinson's Disease*, ed. S. Fahn, C.D. Marsden, M. Goldstein & D.B. Calne, pp. 153–63. Florham Park, New Jersey: MacMillan.

Fahn, S., Marsden, C.D. & Calne, D.B. (1987b). Classification and investigation of dystonia. In *Movement Disorders II*, ed. C.D. Marsden & S. Fahn, pp. 332–58. London: Butterworths.

Fann, W.E., Sullivan, J.L. & Richman, B.W. (1976). Dyskinesia associated with tricyclic antidepressants. *British Journal of Psychiatry*, **128**, 490–3.

Farde, L., Norstrom, A.L., Wiesel, F.A., Pauli, S., Halldin, C. & Sedvall, G. (1992). Positron emission tomographic analysis of central D1 and D2 dopamine receptor occupancy in patients treated with classical neuroleptics and clozapine-relation to extrapyramidal side-effects. *Archives of General Psychiatry*, **49**, 538–44.

Farde, L., Nyberg, S., Oxenstierna, G., Nakashima, Y., Halldin, C. & Ericsson, B. (1995). Positron emission tomography studies on D2 and 5HT2 receptor binding in risperidone-treated schizophrenic patients. *Journal of Clinical Psychopharmacology*, **15** (Suppl. 1), 19S–23S.

Farren, C.K. & Dinan, T.G. (1994). Dyskinesia in mentally handicapped women: relationship to level of handicap, age, and neuroleptic exposure. *Acta Psychiatrica Scandinavica*, **90**, 210–13.

Faurbye, A., Rasch, P.J., Peterson, P.B., Brandborg, G. & Pakkenberg, G. (1964). Neurological symptoms in pharmacotherapy of psychoses. *Acta Psychiatrica Scandinavica*, **40**, 10–27.

Fayen, M., Goldman, M.B., Moulthrop, M.A. & Luchins, D.J. (1988). Differential memory function with dopaminergic versus anticholinergic treatment of drug-induced extrapyramidal symptoms. *American Journal of Psychiatry*, **145**, 483–6.

Fenton, W.S., Wyatt, R.J. & McGlashan, T.H. (1994). Risk factors for spontaneous dyskinesia in schizophrenia. *Archives of General Psychiatry*, **51**, 643–50.

Fernando, S.J.M. & Chir, B. (1966). Attack of chorea complicating oral contraceptive therapy. *Practitioner*, **197**, 210–11.

Feve, A., Angelcard, B., Fenelon, M., Logak, A., Guillard, A. & Saint-Guily, L. (1993). Post neuroleptic laryngeal dyskinesias: a cause of upper airway obstruction syndrome improved by local injections of botulinum toxin. *Movement Disorders*, **8**, 217–19.

Fitzgerald, P.M. & Jankovic, J. (1989). Tardive oculogyric crises. *Neurology*, **39**, 1434–7.

Flaherty, J.A. & Lahmeyer, H.W. (1978). Laryngeal–pharyngeal dystonia as a possible cause of asphyxia with haloperidol treatment. *American Journal of Psychiatry*, **135**, 1414–15.

Fleischhacker, W.W., Bergmann, K.J., Perovich, R. et al. (1989). The Hillside Akathisia Scale: a new rating instrument for neuroleptic-induced akathisia. *Psychopharmacology Bulletin*, **25**, 222–6.

Fleischhacker, W.W., Miller, C.H., Barnas, C. et al. (1993). The effect of activation procedures on neuroleptic-induced akathisia. *British Journal of Psychiatry*, **163**, 781–4.

Fleischhacker, W.W., Roth, S.D. & Kane, J.M. (1990). The pharmacologic treatment of neuroleptic-induced akathisia. *Journal of Clinical Psychopharmacology*, **10**, 12–21.

Fleming, P., Makar, H. & Hunter, K.R. (1970). Levodopa in drug-induced extrapyramidal disorders. *Lancet*, **ii**, 1186.

Freyhan, F.A. (1959). Therapeutic implications of differential effects of new phenothiazine compounds. *American Journal of Psychiatry*, **115**, 577–85.

Friedhoff, A.J. (1977). Receptor sensitivity modification (RSM); a new pradigm for the potential treatment of some hormonal and transmitter disturbances. *Comprehensive Psychiatry*, **18**, 309–17.

Friedman, J.H., Kucharski, L.T. & Wagner, R.L. (1987). Tardive dystonia in a psychiatric hospital. *Journal of Neurology, Neurosurgery and Psychiatry*, **50**, 801–3.

Friis, T., Christensen, T.R. & Gerlach, J. (1983). Sodium valproate and biperiden in neuroleptic induced akathisia, parkinsonism and hyperkinesia: a double-blind cross-over study with placebo. *Acta Psychiatrical Scandinavica*, **67**, 178–87.

Ganzini, L., Casey, D.E., Hoffman, W.F. & McCall, A.L. (1993). Prevalence of metoclopramide-induced tardive dyskinesia and acute extrapyramidal movement disorders. *Archives of Internal Medicine*, **153**, 1469–75.

Ganzini, L., Heintz, R.T., Hoffman, W.F. & Casey, D.E. (1991). The prevalence of tardive dyskinesia in neuroleptic-treated diabetics – a controlled study. *Archives of General Psychiatry*, **48**, 259–63.

Gardos, G. & Casey, D. (1984). *Tardive Dyskinesia and Affective Disorders*. Washington, DC: American Psychiatry Press.

Gardos, G., Casey, D.E., Cole, J.O. et al. (1994). Ten year outcome of tardive dyskinesia. *American Journal of Psychiatry*, **151**, 836–41.

Gardos, G. & Cole, J.O. (1980). Overview: public health issues in tardive dyskinesia. *American Journal of Psychiatry*, **137**, 776–81.

Gardos, G., Cole, J.O., Haskell, D., Marby, D., Paine, S.S. & Moore, P. (1988a). The natural history of tardive dyskinesia. *Journal of Clinical Psychopharmacology*, **8**, 31S–37S.

Gardos, G., Perenyi, A., Cole, J.O., Samu, I., Kocsis, E. & Casey, D.E. (1988b). Seven-year follow-up of tardive dyskinesia in Hungarian outpatients. *Neuropsychopharmacology*, **1**, 169–72.

Gardos, G., Teicher, M.H., Lipinski, J.F. Jr et al. (1992). Quantitative assessment of psychomotor activity in patients with neuroleptic-induced akathisia. *Progress in Neuropsychopharmacology and Biological Psychiatry*, **16**, 27–37.

Gattaz, W.F., Emrich, A. & Behrens, S. (1993). Vitamin E attenuates the development of haloperidol-induced dopaminergic hypersensitivity in rats: possible implications for tardive dyskinesia. *Journal of Neural Transmission (Genetics Section)*, **92**, 197–201.

Gerlach, J. (1977). Relationship between tardive dyskinesia, L-dopa-induced hyperkinesia and parkinsonism. *Psychopharmacology*, **51**, 259–63.

Gerlach, J. (1979). Tardive dyskinesia. *Danish Medical Bulletin*, **26**, 209–45.

Gerlach, J., Korsgaard, S., Clemmensen, P. et al. (1993). The St Hans Rating Scale for Extrapyramidal Syndromes: reliability and validity. *Acta Psychiatrica Scandinavica*, **87**, 244–52.

Gerlach, J. & Peacock, L. (1994). Motor and mental side-effects of clozapine. *Journal of Clinical Psychiatry*, **55**, 9 Suppl. B, 107–09.

Gerratt, B.R., Goetz, C.G. & Fisher, H.B. (1984). Speech abnormalities in tardive dyskinesia. *Archives of Neurology*, **41**, 273–6.

Gershanik, D.S. (1994). Drug-induced parkinsonism in the aged: recognition and prevention. *Drugs and Aging*, **5**, 127–32.

Gewirtz, G.R., Sharif, Z., Cadet, J.L., Sarti, P. & Gorman, J.M. (1993). Selegiline for neuroleptic-induced parkinsonism. *Pharmacopsychiatry*, **26**, 128–9.

Gibb, W.R. & Lees, A.J. (1986). The clinical phenomenon of akathisia. *Journal of Neurology, Neurosurgery and Psychiatry*, **49**, 861–6.

Gibb, W.R.G. & Lees, A.J. (1988). The relevance of the Lewy body to the pathogenesis of idiopathic Parkinson's disease. *Journal of Neurology, Neurosurgery and Psychiatry*, **51**, 745–52.

Gibson, A.C. (1981). Incidence of tardive dyskinesia in patients receiving depot neuroleptic injection. *Acta Psychiatrica Scandinavica*, **63**, 111–16.

Gilmour, C. & Bradford, J. (1987). The effect of medication on handwriting. *Journal of Canadian Society of Forensic Science*, **20**, 119–38.

Gimenez-Roldan, S., Mateo, D. & Bartolome, P. (1985). Tardive dyskinesia and severe tardive dystonia. *Acta Psychiatrica Scandinavica*, **71**, 488–94.

Glazer, W.M. & Morgenstern, H. (1988). Predictors of occurrence, severity and course of tardive dyskinesia in an outpatient population. *Journal of Clinical Psychopharmacology*, **8**, 10S–16S.

Glazer, W.M., Morgenstern, H. & Doucette, J.T. (1993). Predicting the long-term risk of tardive dyskinesia in outpatients maintained on neuroleptic medications. *Journal of Clinical Psychiatry*, **54**, 133–9.

Glazer, W.M., Morgenstern, H. & Doucette, J. (1994). Race and tardive dyskinesia among outpatients at a CMHC. *Hospital and Community Psychiatry*, **45**, 38–42.

Glazer, W., Morgenstern, H., Niedzwiecki, D. & Hughes, J. (1988). Heterogeneity of tardive dyskinesia: a multivariate analysis. *British Journal of Psychiatry*, **152**, 253–9.

Glenthoj, B., Hemmingsen, R., Allerup, P. & Bolwig, T.G. (1990). Intermittent versus continuous neuroleptic treatment in a rat model. *European Journal of Pharmacology*, **190**, 275–86.

Goldstein, J.M. (1995). Preclinical tests that predict clozapine-like atypical antipsychotic actions. In *Critical Issues in the Treatment of Schizophrenia*, 95th edn, ed. N. Brunello, G. Racagni, S.Z. Langer & J. Mendlewicz, pp. 95–101. Basel: Karger.

Greenberg, D.B. & Murray, G.B. (1981). Hyperventilation as a variant of tardive dyskinesia. *Journal of Clinical Psychiatry*, **42**, 401–03.

Gregory, R.P., Smith, P.T. & Rudge, P. (1992). Tardive dyskinesia presenting as severe dysphagia. *Journal of Neurology, Neurosurgery and Psychiatry*, **55**, 1203–04.

Gureje, O. (1989). The significance of sub-typing tardive dyskinesia: a study of prevalence and associated factors. *Psychological Medicine*, **19**, 121–8.

Guy, W. (1976), *ECDEU Assessment Manual for Psychopharmacology*. Washington, DC: Department of Health, Education and Welfare.

Halstead, S.M., Barnes, T.R.E. & Speller, J.C. (1994). Akathisia: prevalence and associated dysphoria in an inpatient population with chronic schizophrenia. *British Journal of Psychiatry*, **164**, 177–83.

Hammerstad, J.P., Elliott, K., Mak, E., Schulzer, M., Calne, S. & Calne, D.B. (1994). Tendon jerks in Parkinson's disease. *Journal of Neural Transmission (Parkinson's Disease Section)*, **8**, 123–30.

Hardie, R.J. & Lees, A.J. (1988). Neuroleptic-induced Parkinson's syndrome: clinical features and results of treatment with levodopa. *Journal of Neurology, Neurosurgery and Psychiatry*, **51**, 850–4.

Harrington, R.A., Hamilton, C.W., Brogden, R.H., Linkewich, J.A., Romankiewicz, J.A. & Heel, R.C. (1983). Metoclopramide: an updated review of its pharmacologie properties and clinical use. *Drugs*, **25**, 451–94.

Hausner, R.S. (1983). Neuroleptic induced parkinsonism and Parkinson's disease: differential diagnosis and treatment. *Journal of Clinical Psychiatry*, **44**, 13–16.

Hawkings, D.R. (1989). Successful prevention of tardive dyskinesia. *Journal of Orthomolecular Medicine*, **41**, 35–6.

Healy, D. (1996). *The Psychopharmacologists*. London: Chapman & Hall.

Hinkin, C.H., Van Gorp, W.G., Mandelkern, M.A. et al. (1995). Cerebral metabolic change in patients with AIDS: report of a 6 month follow-up using positron emission tomography. *Journal of Neuropsychiatry and Clinical Neurosciences*, **7**, 180–7.

Hirsch, S.R. & Harris, J. (1988). *Consent and the Incompetent Patient: Ethics, Law and Medicine*. London: Gaskell/Royal College of Psychiatrists.

Hoffman, W.F., Labs, S.M. & Casey, D.E. (1987). Neuroleptic-induced parkinsonism in older schizophrenics. *Biological Psychiatry*, **22**, 427–39.

Hoge, S.K., Appelbaum, P.S., Lawlor, T. et al. (1990). A prospective multicentre study of patients' refusal of antipsychotic medication. *Archives of General Psychiatry*, **47**, 949–56.

Hollister, L.E. (1957). Unexpected asphyxial death and tranquiliser drugs. *American Journal of Psychiatry*, **114**, 366–7.

Hriso, E., Kuhn, T., Masdeu, J.C. & Grundman, M. (1991). Extrapyramidal symptoms due to dopamine-blocking agents in patients with AIDS encephalopathy. *American Journal of Psychiatry*, **148**, 1558–61.

Hughes, A.J., Daniel, S.E., Kilford, L. & Lees, A.J. (1992). Accuracy of clinical diagnosis of idiopathic Parkinson's disease: a clinical pathological study of 100 cases. *Journal of Neurology, Neurosurgery and Psychiatry*, **55**, 181–4.

Huttunen, M. (1995). The evolution of the serotonin–dopamine antagonist concept. *Journal of Clinical Psychopharmacology*, **15** Suppl. 1, 4S–10S.

Hyde, T.M., Egan, M.F., Brown, R.J., Weinberger, D.R. & Kleinman, J.E. (1995). Diurnal variation in tardive dyskinesia. *Psychiatry Research*, **56**, 53–7.

Iager, A-C., Kirch, D.G., Jeste, D.V. & Wyatt, R.J. (1986). Defect symptoms and abnormal involuntary movement in schizophrenia. *Biological Psychiatry*, **21**, 751–5.

Inada, T., Yagi, G., Kamijima, K. et al. (1990). A statistical trial of subclassifications for tardive dyskinesia. *Acta Psychiatrica Scandinavica*, **82**, 404–07.

Jelliffe, S.E. (1929). Psychologic components in postencephalitic oculogyric crisis. *Archives of Neurology and Psychiatry*, **21**, 491–532.

Jellinek, T. (1977). Mood elevating effect of trihexyphenidyl and biperiden in individuals taking antipsychotic medication. *Diseases of the Nervous System*, **38**, 353–5.

Jeste, D.V., Caligiuri, M.P., Paulson, J.S. et al. (1995). Risk of tardive dyskinesia in older patients: a prospective longitudinal study of 266 outpatients. *Archives of General Psychiatry*, **52**, 756–65.

Jeste, D.V., Lohr, J.B., Clark, K. & Wyatt, R.J. (1988). Pharmacological treatments of tardive dyskinesia in the 1980s. *Journal of Clinical Psychopharmacology*, **8** Suppl. 4, 38S–48S.

Jeste, D.V., Potkin, S.G., Sinha, S., Feder, S. & Wyatt, R.J. (1979). Tardive dyskinesia: reversible and persistent. *Archives of General Psychiatry*, **36**, 585–90.

Jeste, D.V. & Wyatt, R.J. (1979). In search of treatment for tardive dyskinesia: review of the literature. *Schizophrenia Bulletin*, **5**, 251–93.

Jeste, D.V. & Wyatt, R.J. (1981a). Dogma disputed: is tardive dyskinesia due to postsynaptic dopamine receptor supersensitivity? *Journal of Clinical Psychiatry*, **42**, 455–7.

Jeste, D.V. & Wyatt, R.J. (1981b). The changing epidemiology of tardive dyskinesia: an overview. *American Journal of Psychiatry*, **138**, 297–309.

Johnstone, E.C., Crow, T.J., Ferrier, I.N. et al. (1983). Adverse effects of anticholinergic medication on positive schizophrenic symptoms. *Psychological Medicine*, **13**, 513–27.

Johnstone, E.C., MacMillan, J.F., Frith, C.D., Benn, D.K. & Crow, T.J. (1990). Further investigation of the predictors of outcome following first schizophrenic episodes. *British Journal of Psychiatry*, **157**, 182–9.

Johnstone, E.C, Owens, D.G.C., Bydder, G.M., Coulter, N., Crow, T.J. & Frith, C.D. (1989). The spectrum of structural brain change in schizophrenia. *Psychological Medicine*, **19**, 91–103.

Jones, B.D. & Holliday, S.G. (1996). The use of antipsychotic medication: some ethical considerations. In *Schizophrenia: Breaking Down the Barriers*, ed. S.G. Holliday, R.J. Ancill & A. MacEwan, pp. 111–35. Chichester: Wiley.

Jones, G.H. (1995). Informed consent in chronic schizophrenia? *British Journal of Psychiatry*, **167**, 565–8.

Joyce, R. & Gunderson, C. (1980). Carbamazepine-induced orofacial dyskinesia. *Neurology*, **30**, 133–4.

Jungmann, E. & Schoffling, K. (1982). Akathisia and metoclopramide. *Lancet*, **2**, 221.

Jus, K., Jus, A. & Villeneuve, A. (1973). Polygraphic profile of oral tardive dyskinesia and of rabbit syndrome: for quantitative and qualitative evaluation. *Diseases of the Nervous System*, **34**, 27–32.

Kalachnik, J.E. (1984). Tardive dyskinesia and the mentally retarded: a review. In *Advances in Mental Retardation and Developmental Disabilities*, ed. S. Bruening, J. Atson & R. Barrett, pp. 329–56. Greenwich, Connecticut: JAI Press Inc.

Kalra, S., Bergeron, C. & Lang, A.E. (1966). Lewy body disease and dementia. *Archives of Internal Medicine*, **156**, 487–93.

Kaminer, Y., Munitz, H. & Wijsenbeek, H. (1982). Trihexyphenidyl (Artane) abuse: euphoriant and anxiolytic. *British Journal of Psychiatry*, **140**, 473–4.

Kane, J.M., Honigfeld, G., Singer, J. & Meltzer, H.Y. (1988). Clozapine and the treatment-resistant schizophrenic: a double-blind comparison with chlorpromazine. *Archives of General Psychiatry*, **45**, 789–96.

Kane, J.M. & Smith, J.M. (1982). Tardive dyskinesia: prevalence and risk factors, 1959–1979. *Archives of General Psychiatry*, **39**, 473–81.

Kane, J.M., Wegner, J., Stenzler, S. & Ramsey, P. (1980). The prevalence of presumed tardive dyskinesia in psychiatric in-patients and out-patients. *Psychopharmacology*, **69**, 247–51.

Kane, J.M., Woerner, M.G., Pollack, S., Zafferman, A.Z. & Lieberman, J.A. (1993). Does clozapine cause tardive dyskinesia? *Journal of Clinical Psychiatry*, **54**, 327–30.

Kane, J.M., Woerner, M., Weinhold, P., Wegner, J. & Kinon, B. (1982). A prospective study of tardive dyskinesia development: preliminary results. *Journal of Clinical Psychopharmacology*, **2**, 345–9.

Kang, U.J., Burke, R.E. & Fahn, S. (1986). Natural history and treatment of tardive dystonia. *Movement Disorders*, **1**, 193–208.

Kaplan, S.R. & Murkovsky, C. (1978). Oral–buccal dyskinesia symptoms associated with low-dose benzodiazepine treatment. *American Journal of Psychiatry*, **135**, 1558–9.

Karson, K.N., Jeste, D.V., LeWitt, P.A. & Wyatt, R.J. (1984). A comparison of two iatrogenic dyskinesias. *American Journal of Psychiatry*, **140**, 1504–06.

Kastrup, O., Gastpar, M. & Schwartz, M. (1994). Acute dystonia due to clozapine. *Journal of Neurology, Neurosurgery and Psychiatry*, **57**, 119.

Keegan, D.L. & Rajput, A.H. (1973). Drug-induced dystonia tarda – treatment with L-dopa. *Diseases of the Nervous System*, **38**, 167–9.

Keepers, G.A. & Casey, D.E. (1986). Prediction of neuroleptic-induced dystonia. *Journal of Clinical Psychopharmacology*, **7**, 342–4.

Keepers, G.A., Clappison, V.J. & Casey, D.E. (1983). Initial anticholinergic prophylaxis for neuroleptic-induced extrapyramidal syndromes. *Archives of General Psychiatry*, **40**, 1113–17.

Kendler, K.S. (1976). A medical student's experience with akathisia. *American Journal of Psychiatry*, **133**, 454.

Kennedy, P.F., Hershon, H.I. & McGuire, R.J. (1971). Extrapyramidal disorders after prolonged phenothiazine therapy, including a factor analytic study of clinical features. *British Journal of Psychiatry*, **118**, 509–18.

Khanna, R., Das, A. & Damodaran, S.S. (1992). Prospective study of neuroleptic-induced dystonia in mania and schizophrenia. *American Journal of Psychiatry*, **149**, 511–13.

Kidger, T., Barnes, T.R.E., Trauer, T. & Taylor, P.J. (1980). Subsyndromes of tardive dyskinesia. *Psychological Medicine*, **10**, 513–20.

King, D.J., Burke, M. & Lucas, R.A. (1995). Antipsychotic drug-induced dysphoria. *British Journal of Psychiatry*, **167**, 480–2.

Ko, G.N., Zhang, L.D., Yan, W.W. et al. (1989). The Shanghai 800: prevalence of tardive dyskinesia in a Chinese psychiatric hospital. *American Journal of Psychiatry*, **146**, 387–9.

Kolbe, H., Clow, A., Jenner, P. & Marsden, C.D. (1981). Neuroleptic-induced acute dystonic reactions may be due to enhanced dopamine release on to supersensitive postsynaptic receptors. *Neurology (NY)*, **31**, 434–9.

Korczyn, A.D. & Goldberg, G.J. (1972). Intravenous diazepam in drug-related dystonic reactions. *British Journal of Psychiatry*, **121**, 75–7.

Kraepelin, E. (1919). *Dementia Praecox and Paraphrenia*. Translated by R.M. Barclay. New York: R.E. Krieger.

Kucharski, L.T., Smith, J.M. & Dunn, D.D. (1980). Tardive dyskinesia and hospital discharge. *Journal of Nervous and Mental Diseases*, **168**, 215–18.

Kurz, M., Hummer, M., Oberbauer, H. & Fleischhacker, W.W. (1995). Extrapyramidal side-effects of clozapine and haloperidol. *Psychopharmacology*, **118**, 52–6.

La Hoste, G.J., O'Dell, S.J., Widmark, C.B., Shapiro, R.M., Potkin, S.G. & Marshall, J.F. (1991). Differential changes in dopamine and serotonin receptors induced by clozapine and haloperidol. In *Advance in Neuropsychiatry and Psychopharmacology*, Vol. 1: *Schizophrenia Research*, ed. C.A. Tamminga & S.C. Schultz, pp. 351–62. New York: Raven Press.

Lang, A.E. & Johnson, K. (1987). Akathisia in idiopathic Parkinson's disease. *Neurology*, **37**, 477–81.

Langston, J.W., Ballard, P., Tetrud, J.W. & Irwin, I. (1983). Chronic parkinsonism in humans due to a product of meperidine-analog synthesis. *Science*, **219**, 979–80.

Lapierre, Y.D. & Anderson, K. (1983). Dyskinesia associated with amoxapine antidepressant therapy: a case report. *American Journal of Psychiatry*, **140**, 493–4.

Larsen, T.A., Calne, S. & Calne, D.B. (1984). Assessment of Parkinson's disease. *Clinical Neuropharmacology*, **7**, 165–9.

Laska, E., Varga, E., Wanderling, J., Simpson, G.M., Logemann, G.W. & Shah, B.K. (1973). Patterns of psychotropic drug use for schizophrenia. *Diseases of the Nervous System*, **34**, 294–305.

Lazarus, A.L. & Toglia, J.U. (1985). Fatal myoglobinuric renal failure in a patient with tardive dyskinesia. *Neurology*, **35**, 1055–7.

Lees, A.J. & Smith, E. (1983). Cognitive deficits in the early stages of Parkinson's disease. *Brain*, **106**, 257–70.

Lehmann, H.E., Ban, T.A. & Saxena, B.M. (1970). A survey of extrapyramidal manifestations in the inpatient population of a psychiatric hospital. *Laval Medical*, **41**, 909–16.

Leigh, R.J., Foley, J.M., Remler, B.F. & Civil, R.H. (1987). Oculogyric crisis: a syndrome of thought disorder and ocular deviation. *Annals of Neurology*, **22**, 13–17.

Lidsky, T.I. (1995). Re-evaluation of the mesolimbic hypothesis of antipsychotic drug action. *Schizophrenia Bulletin*, **21**, 67–74.

Lieberman, A. (1974). Parkinson's disease: a critical review. *American Journal of Medical Science*, **267**, 66–80.

Lieberman, A., Dziatolowki, M., Gopinathan, G., Kopersmith, M., Neophytides, A. & Korein, J. (1980). Evaluation of Parkinson's disease. In *Ergot Compounds and Brain Function: Neuroendocrine and Neuropsychiatric Aspects*, M. Goldstein, pp. 277–86. New York: Raven Press.

Lieberman, J.A., Kane, J.M. & Alvir, J. (1987). Provocative tests with psychostimulant drugs in schizophrenia. *Psychopharmacology*, **91**, 415–33.

Lieberman, J.A. & Saltz, B.L. (1992). Tardive Tourette's: tardive dyskinesia form fruste or a distinct clinical syndrome? In *Movement Disorders in Neurology and Neuropsychiatry*, ed. A.B. Joseph & R.R. Young, pp. 134–8. Boston: Blackwell Scientific Publications.

Lieberman, J.A., Saltz, B.L., Johns, C.A., Pollack, S., Borenstein, M. & Kane, J.M. (1991). The effects of clozapine on tardive dyskinesia. *British Journal of Psychiatry*, **158**, 503–10.

Lipinski, J.F., Zubenko, G.S., Barreira, P. & Cohen, B.M. (1983). Propranolol in the treatment of neuroleptic-induced akathisia. *Lancet*, **2**, 685–6.

Locascio, J.J., Malone, R.P., Small, A.M. et al. (1991). Factors related to haloperidol response and dyskinesias in autistic children. *Psychopharmacology Bulletin*, **27**, 119–25.

Lohr, J.B. (1991). Oxygen radicals and neuropsychiatric illness. *Archives of General Psychiatry*, **48**, 1097–106.

Lohr, J.B. & Caligiuri, M.P. (1996). A double-blind placebo-controlled study of vitamin E treatment of tardive dyskinesia. *Journal of Clinical Psychiatry*, **57**, 167–73.

Lowe, T.L., Cohen, D.J., Detlor, J., Kremenitzer, M.W. & Shaywitz, B.A. (1982). Stimulant medications precipitate Tourette's syndrome. *Journal of the American Medical Association*, **247**, 1729–31.

Luchins, D.J., Freed, W.J. & Wyatt, R.J. (1980). The role of cholinergic supersensitivity in the medical symptoms associated with withdrawal of antipsychotic drugs. *American Journal of Psychiatry*, **137**, 1395–8.

Luijckx, G., Nieuwhof, C., Troost, J. & Weber, W.E.J. (1995). Parkinsonism in alcohol withdrawal. *Clinical Neurology and Neurosurgery*, **97**, 336–9.

Lyskowski, J., Nasrallah, H.A., Dunner, F.J. & Bucher, K. (1982). A longitudinal survey of side-effects in a lithium clinic. *Journal of Clinical Psychiatry*, **43**, 284–6.

Magliozzi, J.R., Gillespie, H., Lombrozo, L. & Hollister, L.E. (1985). Mood alteration following oral and intravenous haloperidol and relationship to drug concentration in normal subjects. *Journal of Clinical Pharmacology*, **25**, 285–90.

Malone, R.P., Ernst, M., Godfrey, K.A., Locascio, J.J. & Campbell, M. (1991). Repeated episodes of neuroleptic-related dyskinesias in autistic children. *Psychopharmacology Bulletin*, **27**, 113–17.

Manos, N., Gkiouzepas, J. & Logothetis, J. (1981). The need for continuous use of antiparkinsonian medication with chronic schizophrenic patients receiving long-term neuroleptic therapy. *American Journal of Psychiatry*, **138**, 184–8.

Marder, S.R., Hubbard, J.W., Van Putten, T. & Midha, K.K. (1989). Pharmacokinetics of long-acting injectable neuroleptic drugs: clinical implications. *Psychopharmacology*, **98**, 433–9.

Marjama, J., Troster, A.I. & Koller, W.C. (1995). Psychogenic movement disorders. *Neurologic Clinics*, **13**, 283–97.

Marsden, C.D. (1976). Dystonia: the spectrum of the disease. In *The Basal Ganglia*, ed. M.D. Yahr, pp. 351–67. New York: Raven Press.

Marsden, C.D. & Jenner, P. (1980). The pathophysiology of extrapyramidal side-effects of neuroleptic drugs. *Psychological Medicine*, **10**, 55–72.

Marsden, C.D., Marion, M.H. & Quinn, N. (1984). The treatment of severe dystonia in children and adults. *Journal of Neurology, Neurosurgery and Psychiatry*, **47**, 1166–73.

Marsden, C.D., Mindham, R.H.S. & Mackay, A.V.P. (1986). Extrapyramidal movement disorders produced by antipsychotic drugs. In *The Psychopharmacology and Drug Treatment of Schizophrenia*, ed. P.B. Bradley & S.R. Hirsch, pp. 340–402. Oxford: Oxford University Press.

Marsden, C.D. & Schachter, M. (1981). Assessment of extrapyramidal disorders. In *Methods in Clinical Pharmacology – Central Nervous System*, ed. M.H. Lader & A. Richens, pp. 89–111. London: MacMillan.

Marsden, C.D., Tarsy, D. & Baldessarini, R.J. (1975). Spontaneous and drug-induced movement disorders in psychotic patients. In *Psychiatric Aspects of Neurological Disease*, ed. D.F. Benson & D. Blumer, pp. 219–66. New York, San Francisco, London: Grune and Stratton.

Mattson, R.H. & Calverley, J.R. (1968). Dextroamphetamine sulphate-induced dyskinesias. *Journal of the American Medical Association*, **204**, 400–02.

Mazurek, M.F. & Rosebush, P.I. (1996). Circadian pattern of acute neuroleptic-induced dystonic reactions. *American Journal of Psychiatry*, **153**, 708–10.

McClelland, H.A., Dutta, D., Metcalf, A. & Kerr, T.A. (1986). Mortality and facial dyskinesia. *British Journal of Psychiatry*, **148**, 310–16.

McCowan, P.K. & Cook, L.C. (1928). Oculogyric crises in chronic epidemic encephalitis. *Brain*, **51**, 285–309.

McCreadie, R.G., Hall, D.J., Berry I.J., Robertson, L.J., Ewing, J.I. & Geals, M.F. (1992a). The Nithsdale Schizophrenia Surveys X: obstetric complications, family history and abnormal movements. *British Journal of Psychiatry*, **161**, 799–805.

McCreadie, R.G., MacDonald, E., Wiles, D., Campbell, G. & Paterson, J.R. (1995). The Nithsdale Schizophrenia Surveys XIV: plasma lipid peroxide and serum vitamin E levels in patients with and without tardive dyskinesia, and in normal subjects. *British Journal of Psychiatry*, **167**, 610–17.

McCreadie, R.G. & Ohaeri, J.U. (1994). Movement disorder in never and minimally treated Nigerian schizophrenic patients. *British Journal of Psychiatry*, **164**, 184–9.

McCreadie, R.G., Robertson, L.J. & Wiles, D.H. (1992b). The Nithsdale Schizophrenia Surveys. IX. Akathisia, parkinsonism, tardive dyskinesia and plasma neuroleptic levels. *British Journal of Psychiatry*, **161**, 793–9.

McCreadie, R.G., Thara, R. Kamath, S. et al. (1996). Abnormal movements in never medicated Indian patients with schizophrenia. *British Journal of Psychiatry*, **168**, 221–6.

McDowall, F., Lee, J.E., Swift, T., Sweet, R.D., Ogsbury, J.S. & Tessler, J.T. (1970). Treatment of Parkinson's disease with dihydroxyphenylalanine (Levodopa). *Annals of Internal Medicine*, **72**, 29–35.

McEvoy, J.F. (1987). A double-blind comparison of antiparkinson drug therapy: amantadine versus anticholinergics in 90 normal volunteers, with an emphasis on differential effects on memory function. *Journal of Clinical Psychiatry*, **48** Suppl. 9, 20–3.

McKeith, I., Fairbairn, A.F., Bothwell, R.A. et al. (1994). An evaluation of the predictive validity and inter-rater reliability of clinical diagnostic criteria for senile dementia of Lewy body type. *Neurology*, **44**, 872–7.

McKeith, I., Fairbairn, A.F., Perry, R., Thompson, P. & Perry, E. (1992). Neuroleptic sensitivity in patients with senile dementia of Lewy body type. *British Medical Journal*, **305**, 673–8.

McKeith, I., Galasko, D., Wilcock, G.K. & Byrne, E.J. (1995). Lewy body dementia – diagnosis and treatment. *British Journal of Psychiatry*, **167**, 709–17.

McKenna, P.J., Lund, C.E., Mortimer, A.M. & Biggins, C.A. (1991). Motor, volitional and behavioral disorders in schizophrenia: the 'conflict of paradigms' hypothesis. *British Journal of Psychiatry*, **158**, 328–36.

McPherson, R. & Collis, R. (1992). Tardive dyskinesia: patient's lack of awareness of movement disorder. *British Journal of Psychiatry*, **160**, 110–12.

Mehta, D., Mallya, A. & Volavka, J. (1978). Mortality of patients with tardive dyskinesia. *American Journal of Psychiatry*, **136**, 371–2.

Meisel, A., Roth, L.H. & Lidz, C.W. (1977). Toward a model of the legal doctrine of informed consent. *American Journal of Psychiatry*, **134**, 285–9.

Meiselas, K.D., Spencer, E.K., Oberfield, R., Peselow, E.D., Angrist, B. & Campbell, M. (1989). Differentiation of stereotypes from neuroleptic-related dyskinesias in autistic children. *Journal of Clinical Psychopharmacology*, **9**, 207–9.

Meltzer, H.Y. (1992). Dimensions of outcome with clozapine. *British Journal of Psychiatry*, **160** Suppl. 17, 46–53.

Meltzer, H.Y., Burnett, S., Bastani, B. & Ramirez, L.F. (1990). Effects of 6 months clozapine treatment on the quality of life of chronic schizophrenic patients. *Hospital and Community Psychiatry*, **41**, 892–7.

Meltzer, H.Y., Matsubara, S. & Lee, J.C. (1989). Classification of typical and atypical antipsychotic drugs on the basis of dopamine D1, D2 and serotonin 2 pKi values. *Journal of Pharmacology and Experimental Therapeutics*, **251**, 238–46.

Meltzer, H.Y., Young, M., Metz, J., Fang, V.S., Schyve, P.M. & Arora, R.C. (1979). Extrapyramidal side effects and increased serum prolactin following fluoxetine, a new antidepressant. *Journal of Neural Transmission,* **45,** 165–75.

Messiha, F.S. (1993). Fluoxetine: adverse effects and drug–drug interactions. *Journal of Toxicology – Clinical Toxicology,* **31,** 603–30.

Metzer, W.S., Newton, J.E.O., Steele, R.W. et al. (1989). HLA antigens in drug-induced parkinsonism. *Movement Disorders,* **4,** 121–8.

Micheli, F., Paradaz, M.F., Gatto, M. et al. (1987). Flunarizine and cinnarizine-induced extrapyramidal reactions. *Neurology,* **37,** 881–4.

Miller, C.H., Fleischhacker, W.W., Ehrmann, H. & Kane, J.M. (1990). Treatment of neuroleptic-induced akathisia with the 5-HT2 antagonist ritanserin. *Psychopharmacology Bulletin,* **26,** 373–6.

Mindham, R.H.S. (1976). Assessment of drug-induced extrapyramidal reactions and of drugs given for their control. *British Journal of Clinical Pharmacology,* **3,** 395–400.

Mindham, R.H.S., Gaind, R., Anstee, B.H. & Rimmer, L. (1972). Comparison of amantadine, orphenadrine and placebo in the control of phenothiazine induced parkinsonism. *Psychological Medicine,* **2,** 406–13.

Modell, J.G., Tandon, R. & Beresford, T.D. (1989). Dopaminergic activity of the antimuscarinic antiparkinsonian agents. *Journal of Clinical Psychopharmacology,* **9,** 347–51.

Moleman, P., Janzen, G., Von Bargen, B., Kappers, E.J., Pepplinkhuizen, L. & Schmitz, P.I.M. (1986). Relationship between age and parkinsonism in psychiatric patients treated with haloperidol. *American Journal of Psychiatry,* **143,** 232–4.

Moller, H.J. (1993). Neuroleptic treatment of negative symptoms in schizophrenic patients: efficacy, problems and methodological difficulties. *European Neuropsychopharmacology,* **3,** 1–11.

Montastruc, J.L., Llau, M.E., Rascol, O. & Senard, J.M. (1994). Drug-induced parkinsonism – a review. *Fundamental and Clinical Pharmacology,* **8,** 293–306.

Morgenstern, H. & Glazer, W.M. (1993). Identifying risk factors for tardive dyskinesia among long-term outpatients maintained with neuroleptic medications. *Archives of General Psychiatry,* **50,** 723–33.

Mullin, P.J., Kershaw, P.W. & Bolt, J.W.M. (1970). Choreoathetotic movement disorder in alcoholism. *British Medical Journal,* **4,** 278–81.

Muscettola, G., Pampallona, S., Barbato, G., Casiello, M. & Bollini, P. (1993). Persistent tardive dyskinesia: demographic and pharmacological risk factors. *Acta Psychiatrica Scandinavica,* **87,** 29–36.

Narabayashi, H. (1995). The neural mechanisms and progressive nature of symptoms of Parkinson's disease – based on clinical, neurophysiological and morphological studies. *Journal of Neural Transmission (Parkinson's Disease Section),* **10,** 63–75.

Nath, A., Jankovic, J. & Pettigrew, L.C. (1987). Movement disorders and AIDS. *Neurology,* **37,** 37–41.

National Institute of Mental Health Psychopharmacology and Service Center Collaborative Study Group (1964). Phenothiazine treatment in acute schizophrenia. *Archives of General Psychiatry,* **10,** 246–61.

Nausieda, P.A., Koller, W.C., Weiner, W.J. & Klawans, H.L. (1979). Clinical and experimental studies of phenytoin-induced hyperkinesias. *Journal of Neural Transmission*, **45**, 291–305.

Neale, R., Gerhardt, S. & Liebman, J.M. (1984). Effects of dopamine agonists, catecholamine depletors, and cholinergic and gaba-ergic drugs on acute dyskinesias in squirrel monkeys. *Psychopharmacology*, **82**, 20–6.

Newton-John, H. (1988). Acute upper airway obstruction due to supraglottic dystonia induced by a neuroleptic. *British Medical Journal*, **297**, 964–5.

Nordic Dyskinesia Study Group (1986). Effect of different neuroleptics in tardive dyskinesia and parkinsonism. A video-controlled multicentre study with chlorprothixene, perphenazine, haloperidol and haloperidol + biperiden. *Psychopharmacology*, **90**, 423–9.

Obeso, J.A., Rothwell, J.C., Lang, A.E. & Marsden, C.D. (1983). Myoclonic dystonia. *Neurology (Cleveland)*, **33**, 825–30.

O'Callaghan, E.O., Larkin, C., Kinsella, A. & Waddington, J.L. (1990). Obstetric complications, the putative familial-sporadic distinction and tardive dyskinesia in schizophrenia. *British Journal of Psychiatry*, **157**, 578–84.

Ogren, S.O., Florvall, L., Hall, H., Magnusson, O. & Angeby-Moller, K. (1990). Neuropharmacological and behavioral properties of remoxipride in the rat. *Acta Psychiatrica Scandinavica*, **82** Suppl. 358, 21–6.

Owens, D.G.C. (1990). Dystonia: a potential psychiatric pitfall. *British Journal of Psychiatry*, **156**, 620–34.

Owens, D.G.C. (1994). Extrapyramidal side-effects and tolerability of risperidone: a review. *Journal of Clinical Psychiatry*, **55** Suppl. 5, 29–35.

Owens, D.G.C. (1995). Drug-related movement disorders. In *Movement and Allied Disorders in Childhood*, ed. M.M. Robertson & V. Eapen, pp. 199–236. Chichester: John Wiley & Son.

Owens, D.G.C. (1996). Adverse effects of antipsychotic agents – do newer agents offer advantages? *Drugs*, **51**, 895–930.

Owens, D.G.C. & Johnstone, E.C. (1980). The disabilities of chronic schizophrenia: their nature and factors contributing to their development. *British Journal of Psychiatry*, **136**, 384–95.

Owens, D.G.C., Johnstone, E.C. & Frith, C.D. (1982). Spontaneous involuntary disorders of movement: their prevalence, severity and distribution in chronic schizophrenics with and without treatment with neuroleptics. *Archives of General Psychiatry*, **39**, 452–61.

Padrell, M.D., Navarro, M., Faura, C.C. & Horga, J.F. (1995). Verapamil-induced parkinsonism. *American Journal of Medicine*, **99**, 436.

Parkes, J.D., Zilkaj, K.J., Calver, D.M. & Knill-Jones, R.P. (1970). Controlled trial of amantadine hydrochloride in Parkinson's disease. *Lancet*, **1**, 259–62.

Perenyi, A., Bagdy, G., Arato, M. & Frecska, E. (1984). Biochemical markers in the study of clinical effects and extrapyramidal side effects of neuroleptics. *Psychiatry Research*, **13**, 119–27.

Perry, R., Campbell, M., Green, W.H. et al. (1985). Neuroleptic-related dyskinesias in autistic children: a prospective study. *Psychopharmacology Bulletin*, **21**, 140–3.

Peuskins, J. & Risperidone Study Group (1995). Risperidone in the treatment of patients with chronic schizophrenia: a multinational, multicentre, double-blind, parallel group study versus haloperidol. *British Journal of Psychiatry*, **166**, 712–26.

Poewe, W.H., Lees, A.J. & Stern, G.M. (1988). Dystonia in Parkinson's disease: clinical and pharmacological features. *Annals of Neurology*, **23**, 73–8.

Pohl, R., Yeragani, V.K. & Ortiz, A. (1986). Response of tricyclic-induced jitteriness to a phenothiazine in two patients. *Journal of Clinical Psychiatry*, **47**, 427.

Polizos, P. & Engelhardt, D.M. (1978). Dyskinetic phenomena in children treated with psychotropic medications. *Psychopharmacology Bulletin*, **14**, 65–8.

Prien, R.F., Haber, P.A. & Caffey, E.M. (1975). The use of psychoactive drugs in elderly patients with psychiatric disorders: survey conducted in 12 Veterans Administration hospitals. *Journal of the American Geriatric Society*, **23**, 104–12.

Quinn, N. (1995). Parkinsonism – recognition and differential diagnosis. *British Medical Journal*, **310**, 447–52.

Quitkin, F., Rifkin, A. & Klein, D.F. (1976). Neurological soft signs in schizophrenia and character disorders. *Archives of General Psychiatry*, **33**, 845–53.

Radford, J.M., Brown, T.M. & Borison, R.L. (1995). Unexpected dystonia while changing from clozapine to risperidone. *Journal of Clinical Psychopharmacology*, **15**, 225–6.

Rainier-Pope, C.R. (1979). Treatment with diazepam of children with drug-induced extrapyramidal symptoms. *South African Medical Journal*, **55**, 328–30.

Rajput, A.H., Offord, K.P. & Beard, C.M. (1987). A case-controlled study of smoking habits, dementia and other illness in idiopathic Parkinson's disease. *Neurology*, **37**, 226–32.

Rich, M.W. & Radwany, S.M. (1994). Respiratory dyskinesia: an under-recognised phenomenon. *Chest*, **105**, 1826–32.

Richardson, M.A., Haugland, G. & Craig, T.J. (1991). Neuroleptic use, parkinsonian symptoms, tardive dyskinesia and associated factors in child and adolescent psychiatric patients. *American Journal of Psychiatry*, **148**, 1322–8.

Richardson, M.A., Haugland, M.A., Pass, R. & Craig, T.J. (1986). The prevalence of tardive dyskinesia in a mentally retarded population. *Psychopharmacology Bulletin*, **22**, 243–9.

Rifkin, A., Quitkin, F., Kane, J.M., Struve, F. & Klein, D.F. (1978). Are prophylactic antiparkinson drugs necessary? A controlled study of procyclidine withdrawal. *Archives of General Psychiatry*, **35**, 483–9.

Rifkin, A., Quitkin, F. & Klein, D.F. (1975). Akinesia: a poorly recognised drug-induced extrapyramidal behavioral disorder. *Archives of General Psychiatry*, **32**, 672–4.

Rogers, D. (1985). The motor disorders of severe psychiatric illness: a conflict of paradigms. *British Journal of Psychiatry*, **47**, 221–32.

Rogers, D., Karki, C., Bartlett, C. & Pocock, P. (1991). The motor disorders of mental handicap: an overlap with the motor disorders of severe psychiatric illness. *British Journal of Psychiatry*, **158**, 97–102.

Rogers, D., Lees, A.J., Smith, E., Trimble, M. & Stern, G.M. (1987). Bradyphrenia in Parkinson's disease and psychomotor retardation in depressive illness. *Brain*, **110**, 761–76.

Rosen, A.M., Mukherjee, S., Olarte, S., Varia, V. & Cardenas, C. (1982). Perception of tardive dyskinesia in out-patients receiving maintenance neuroleptics. *American Journal of Psychiatry*, **139**, 372–3.

Rupniak, N.M.J., Jenner, P. & Marsden, C.D. (1986). Acute dystonia induced by neuroleptic drugs. *Psychopharmacology*, **88**, 403–19.

Sachdev, P. (1993a). Clinical characteristics of 15 patients with tardive dystonia. *American Journal of Psychiatry*, **150**, 498–500.

Sachdev, P. (1993b). Risk factors for tardive dystonia: a case-control comparison with tardive dyskinesia. *Acta Psychiatrica Scandinavica*, **88**, 98–103.

Sachdev, P. (1994). A rating scale for drug-induced akathisia: development, reliability and validity. *Biological Psychiatry*, **35**, 263–71.

Sachdev, P. (1995a). *Akathisia and Restless Legs*. Cambridge, New York, Melbourne: Cambridge University Press.

Sachdev, P. (1995b). The epidemiology of drug-induced akathisia. Part I: Acute akathisia. *Schizophrenia Bulletin*, **21**, 431–49.

Sachdev, P. (1995c). The development of the concept of akathisia: a historical overview. *Schizophrenia Research*, **16**, 33–45.

Sachdev, P. (1995d). The epidemiology of drug-induced akathisia: Part II: Chronic, tardive and withdrawal akathisias. *Schizophrenia Bulletin*, **21**, 451–61.

Sachdev, P. & Kruk, J. (1994). Clinical characteristics and predisposing factors in acute drug-induced akathisia. *Archives of General Psychiatry*, **51**, 963–74.

Sachdev, P. & Loneragan, C. (1993). Intravenous challenges of benztropine and propranolol in acute neuroleptic-induced akathisia. *Clinical Neuropharmacology*, **16**, 324–31.

Sachdev, P. & Tang, W.M. (1992). Psychotic symptoms preceding ocular deviation in a patient with tardive oculogyric crises. *Australian and New Zealand Journal of Psychiatry*, **26**, 666–70.

Sarwer-Foner, G.J. (1960). Recognition and management of drug-induced extrapyramidal reactions and 'paradoxical' behavioural reactions in psychiatry. *Canadian Medical Association Journal*, **83**, 312–18.

Sasso, E., Delsoldato, S., Negrotti, A. & Mancia, D. (1994). Reversible valproate-induced extrapyramidal disorders. *Epilepsia*, **35**, 391–3.

Scherer, J., Tatsch, K., Schwarz, J., Oertel, W.H., Konjarczyk, M. & Albus, M. (1994). D2-dopamine receptor occupancy differs between patients with and without extrapyramidal side-effects. *Acta Psychiatrica Scandinavica*, **90**, 266–8.

Schonecker, M. (1957). Ein eigentumliches syndrom im oralen bereich bei megaphenapplikation. *Nervenartz*, **28**, 35.

Schooler, N.R. & Kane, J.M. (1982). Research diagnoses for tardive dyskinesia. *Archives of General Psychiatry*, **39**, 486–7.

Schulte, J.R. (1985). Homicide and suicide associated with akathisia and haloperidol. *American Journal of Forensic Psychiatry*, **6**, 3–7.

Schwab, R.S. & England, A.C. (1969). Projection technique for evaluating surgery in Parkinson's disease. In *Third Symposium on Parkinson's Disease*, ed. F.J. Gillingham & I.M.L. Donaldson, pp. 152–7. Edinburgh: E. & S. Livingstone.

Schwartz, G. Gosenfeld, L., Gilderman, A., Jiwesh, J. & Ripple, R.E. (1986). Akathisia associated with carbamazepine therapy. *American Journal of Psychiatry*, **143**, 1190–1.

Sethi, K.D. & Zamrini, E.Y. (1990). Asymmetry in clinical features of drug-induced parkinsonism. *Journal of Neuropsychiatry*, **2**, 64–6.

Shackman, D.R., Van Putten, T. & May, P.R.A. (1979). Micrographia and akinesia. *American Journal of Psychiatry*, **136**, 839–40.

Shader, R.I. & Greenblatt, D.J. (1971). Uses and toxicity of belladonna alkaloids and synthetic anticholinergics. *Seminars in Psychiatry*, **3**, 449–76.

Shear, M.K., Frances, A. & Weiden, P. (1983). Suicide associated with akathisia and depot fluphenazine treatment. *Journal of Clinical Psychopharmacology*, **3**, 235–6.

Shedlack, K.J., Soldato-Couture, C. & Swanson, C.L. (1994). Rapidly progressive tardive dyskinesia in AIDS. *Biological Psychiatry*, **35**, 147–8.

Shriqui, C., Bradwejn, J., Annable, L. & Jones, B. (1992). Vitamin E in the treatment of tardive dyskinesia: a double-blind placebo controlled study. *American Journal of Psychiatry*, **149**, 391–3.

Sigwald, J., Bouttier, D., Raymond, C. & Piot, C. (1959). Quatre cas de dyskinesie facio-bucco-linguo-masticatice a evolution prolongee secondaire a un traitement par les neuroleptiques. *Revue Neurologique (Paris)*, **100**, 751–5.

Silver, H. & Geraisy, N. (1995). Effects of biperiden and amantadine on memory in medicated schizophrenic patients, a double-blind cross-over study. *British Journal of Psychiatry*, **166**, 241–3.

Silver, H., Geraisy, N. & Schwartz, M. (1995). No difference in the effect of biperiden and amantadine on parkinsonism- and tardive dyskinesia-type involuntary movements. *Journal of Clinical Psychiatry*, **56**, 167–70.

Simpson, D.M.I., Ramos, F. & Ramirez, L.F. (1988). Death in a psychiatric patient from amantadine poisoning. *American Journal of Psychiatry*, **145**, 267–8.

Simpson, G.M., Amuso, D., Blair, J.H. & Farkas, T. (1964). Phenothiazine-produced extrapyramidal system disturbance. *Archives of General Psychiatry*, **10**, 127–36.

Simpson, G.M. & Angus, J.W.S. (1970). A rating scale for extrapyramidal side effects. *Acta Psychiatrica Scandinavica*, Suppl. 212, 11–19.

Simpson, G.M., Lee, L.H., Zoubok, B. & Gardos, G. (1979). A rating scale for tardive dyskinesia. *Psychopharmacology*, **64**, 171–9.

Simpson, G.M. & Meyer, J.M. (1996). Dystonia while changing from clozapine to risperidone. *Journal of Clinical Psychopharmacology*, **16**, 260–1.

Simpson, G.M., Varga, E., Lee, J.H. & Zoubok, B. (1978). Tardive dyskinesia and psychotropic drug history. *Psychopharmacology*, **58**, 117–24.

Singh, H., Levinson, D.F., Simpson, G.M., Lo E.E.S. & Friedman, E. (1990). Acute dystonia during fixed-dose neuroleptic treatment. *Journal of Clinical Psychopharmacology*, **10**, 389–96.

Smith, J.M. (1980). Abuse of the antiparkinson drugs: a review of the literature. *Journal of Clinical Psychiatry*, **41**, 351–4.

Smith, J.M., Kucharski, L.T., Eblen, C., Knutsen, E. & Linn, C. (1979a). An assessment of tardive dyskinesia in schizophrenic outpatients. *Psychopharmacology*, **64**, 99–104.

Smith, J.M., Kucharski, L.T., Oswald, W.T. & Waterman, L.J. (1979b). A systematic investigation of tardive dyskinesia in inpatients. *American Journal of Psychiatry*, **136**, 918–22.

Solomon, K. (1977). Phenothiazine-induced bulbar palsy-like syndrome and sudden death. *American Journal of Psychiatry*, **134**, 308–11.

Spencer, E.K., Kafantaris, V., Padron-Gayol, M.V., Rosenberg, C.R. & Campbell, M. (1992). Haloperidol and schizophrenic children: early findings from a study in progress. *Psychopharmacology Bulletin*, **28**, 183–6.

Sprague, R.L. & Kalachnik, J.E. (1991). Reliability, validity and a total score cutoff for the Dyskinesia Identification System: Condensed User Scale (DISCUS). *Psychopharmacology Bulletin*, **27**, 51–8.

Sramek, J.J., Simpson, G.M., Morrison, R.L. & Heiser, J.F. (1986). Anticholinergic agents for prophylaxis of neuroleptic-induced dystonic reactions: a prospective study. *Journal of Clinical Psychiatry*, **47**, 305–09.

Stacy, M., Cardoso, F. & Jankovic, J. (1993). Tardive stereotypy and other movement disorders in tardive dyskinesias. *Neurology*, **43**, 937–41.

Stacy, M. & Jankovic, J. (1992). Differential diagnosis of Parkinson's disease and the parkinsonism plus syndromes. *Neurologic Clinics*, **10**, 341–5.

Steck, H. (1954). Le syndrome extrapyramidal et diencephalique au cours des traitements au Largatil et au Serpasil. *Annales Medico-Psychologiques*, **112**, 737–44.

Stephen, P.J. & Willamson, J. (1984). Drug-induced parkinsonism in the Elderly. *Lancet*, **ii**, 1082–3.

Stone, R.K., Alvarez, W.F. & May, J.E. (1988). Dyskinesia, antipsychotic drug exposure and risk factors in a developmentally disabled population. *Pharmacology Biochemistry and Behavior*, **29**, 45–51.

Stones, M., Kennedy, D.C. & Fulton, J.D. (1990). Dystonic dysphagia associated with fluspirilene. *British Medical Journal*, **301**, 668–9.

Sutcher, H.D., Underwood, R.B., Beatty, R.A. & Sugar, O. (1971). Orofacial dyskinesia: a dental dimension. *Journal of the American Medical Association*, **216**, 1459–63.

Swazey, J.P. (1974). *Chlorpromazine in Psychiatry – A Study of Therapeutic Innovation*. Boston, MA: MIT Press.

Swett, C. (1975). Drug-induced dystonia. *American Journal of Psychiatry*, **132**, 532–4.

Szymanski, S., Lieberman, J.A., Safferman, A. & Galkowski, B. (1993). Rib fractures as an unusual complication of severe tardive dyskinesia. *Journal of Clinical Psychiatry*, **54**, 160.

Tamminga, C.A., Thaker, G.K., Moran, M., Kakigi, T. & Gao, X.M. (1994). Clozapine in tardive dyskinesia – observations from human and animal model studies. *Journal of Clinical Psychiatry*, **55** Suppl. 9B, 102–06.

Tamminga, C.A., Thaker, G.K. & Nguyen, J.A. (1989). Gaba-mimetic treatments for tardive dyskinesia: efficacy and mechanism. *Psychopharmacology Bulletin*, **25**, 43–6.

Tan, C.H., Chiang, P.C., Ng, L.L. & Chee, K.T. (1994). Oculogyric spasm in Asian psychiatric in-patients on maintenance medication. *British Journal of Psychiatry*, **165**, 381–3.

Tan, C.H. & Tay, L.K. (1991). Tardive dyskinesia in elderly psychiatric patients in Singapore. *Australian and New Zealand Journal of Psychiatry*, **25**, 119–22.

Tancredi, L.R. (1988). Malpractice and tardive dyskinesia: a conceptual dilemma. *Journal of Clinical Psychopharmacology*, **8**, 71S–76S.

Thach, B.T., Chase, T.N. & Bosma, J.F. (1975). Oral facial dyskinesia associated with prolonged use of antihistaminic decongestants. *New England Journal of Medicine*, **293**, 486–7.

Thornton, A. & McKenna, P.J. (1994). Acute dystonic reactions complicated by psychotic phenomena. *British Journal of Psychiatry*, **164**, 115–18.

Tominaga, H., Fukuzako, H., Izumi, K. et al. (1987). Tardive myoclonus. *Lancet*, **1**, 322.

Treciokas, L.J., Ansel, R.D. & Markham, C.H. (1971). One–two years treatment of Parkinson's disease with levodopa. *California Medicine*, **114**, 7–16.

Tune, L. & Coyle, J.T. (1981). Acute extrapyramidal side-effects: serum levels of neuroleptics and anticholinergics. *Psychopharmacology*, **75**, 9–15.

Turner, T.H. (1989). Schizophrenia and mental handicap: a historical review with implications for further research. *Psychological Medicine*, **19**, 301–14.

Uhrbrand, L. & Faurbye, A. (1960). Reversible and irreversible dyskinesia after treatment with perphenazine, chlorpromazine, reserpine and ECT. *Psychopharmacologia*, **1**, 408–18.

Uitti, R.J., Snow, B.J., Shinotoh, H. et al. (1994). Parkinsonism induced by solvent abuse. *Annals of Neurology*, **35**, 616–19.

UK Bromocriptine Research Group (1989). The Self-Care Scale. Bromocriptine in Parkinson's disease: a double blind study comparing 'low–slow' and 'high–fast' introductory dosage regimes in de novo patients. *Journal of Neurology, Neurosurgery and Psychiatry*, **52**, 77–82.

Van Bogaert, L. (1934). Ocular paroxysms and palilalia. *Journal of Nervous and Mental Diseases*, **80**, 48–61.

Van Gorp, W.G., Mandelkern, M.A., Gee, M. et al. (1992). Cerebral metabolic dysfunction in AIDS: findings in a sample with and without dementia. *Journal of Neuropsychiatry and Clinical Neurosciences*, **4**, 280–7.

Van Harten, P.N. (1992). Pisa syndrome – a confusing term. *British Journal of Psychiatry*, **160**, 424–5.

Van Harten, P.N., Matroos, G.E., Hoek, H.W. & Kahn, R.S. (1996). The prevalence of tardive dystonia, tardive dyskinesia, parkinsonism and akathisia: the Curacao Extrapyramidal Syndromes Study I. *Schizophrenia Research*, **19**, 195–203.

Van Putten, T. (1974). Why do schizophrenic patients refuse to take their drugs? *Archives of General Psychiatry*, **31**, 67–72.

Van Putten, T. (1975). The many faces of akathisia. *Comprehensive Psychiatry*, **16**, 43–7.

Van Putten, T. & Marder, S.R. (1987). Behavioural toxicity of antipsychotic drugs. *Journal of Clinical Psychiatry*, **48** Suppl., 13–19.

Van Putten, T. & May, P.R.A. (1978). 'Akinetic depression' in schizophrenia. *Archives of General Psychiatry*, **35**, 1101–07.

Van Putten, T., May, P.R. & Marder, S.R. (1984). Akathisia with haloperidol and thiothixene. *Psychopharmacology Bulletin*, **20**, 114–17.

Van Putten, T., Mutalipassi, L.R. & Malkin, M.D. (1974). Phenothiazine-induced decompensation. *Archives of General Psychiatry*, **30**, 13–19.

Villeneuve, A. (1972). The rabbit syndrome – a peculiar extrapyramidal reaction. *Canadian Psychiatric Association Journal*, **17**, 69–72.

Vreeling, F.W., Verhey, F.R.J., Houx, P.J. & Jolles, J. (1993). Primitive reflexes in Parkinson's disease. *Journal of Neurology, Neurosurgery and Psychiatry*, **56**, 1323–6.

Waddington, J.L., O'Callaghan, E.O., Buckley, P. et al. (1995). Tardive dyskinesia in schizophrenia: relationship to minor physical anomalies, frontal lobe dysfunction and cerebral structure on magnetic resonance imaging. *British Journal of Psychiatry*, **167**, 41–4.

Waddington, J.L. & Youssef, H.A. (1986). Late onset involuntary movements in chronic schizophrenia: relationship of 'tardive' dyskinesia to intellectual impairment and negative symptoms. *British Journal of Psychiatry*, **149**, 616–20.

Waddington, J.L., Youssef, H.A. & Kinsella, A. (1990). Cognitive dysfunction in schizophrenia followed up over 5 years and its longitudinal relationship to the emergence of tardive dyskinesia. *Psychological Medicine*, **20**, 835–42.

Wasserman, S. & Yahr, M.D. (1980). Choreic movements induced by the use of methadone. *Archives of Neurology*, **37**, 727–8.

Waziri, R. (1980). Lateralisation of neuroleptic-induced dyskinesia indicates pharmacologic asymmetry in the brain. *Psychopharmacology*, **68**, 51–3.

Webster, D.D. (1968). Critical analysis of the disability in Parkinson's disease. *Modern Treatment*, **5**, 257–82.

Wechsler, I.S. & Brock, S. (1922). Dystonia musculorum deformans with special reference to a myostatic form and the occurrence of decerebrate rigidity phenomena: a study of six cases. *Archives of Neurology and Psychiatry*, **8**, 538–52.

Wegner, J.C., Catalano, F., Gibralter, J. & Kane, J.M. (1985). Schizophrenics with tardive dyskinesia – neuropsychological deficit and family psychopathology. *Archves of General Psychiatry*, **42**, 860–5.

Weiden, P.J., Mann, J.J., Hass, G., Mattson, M. & Frances, A. (1987). Clinical nonrecognition of neuroleptic-induced movement disorders: a cautionary study. *American Journal of Psychiatry*, **144**, 1148–53.

Weiner, W.J., Goetz, C.G., Nauseida, P.A. & Klawans, H.L. (1978). Respiratory dyskinesia: extrapyramidal dysfunction and dyspnoea. *Annals of Internal Medicine*, **88**, 327–31.

Weiss, D., Aizenberg, D., Hermesh, H. et al. (1995). Cyproheptadine treatment in neuroleptic-induced akathisia. *British Journal of Psychiatry*, **167**, 483–6.

Wettstein, R.M. (1988). Informed consent and tardive dyskinesia. *Journal of Clinical Psychopharmacology*, **8**, 65S–69S.

Wilbur, R. & Kulik, A.V. (1983). Propranolol for akathisia. *Lancet*, **2**, 917.

Wilson, J.A., Primrose, W.R. & Smith, R.G. (1987). Prognosis of drug-induced Parkinson's disease. *Lancet*, **i**, 443–4.

Wilson, R.L., Waziri, R., Nasrallah, H.A. & McCalley-Whitters, M. (1984). The lateralisation of tardive dyskinesia. *Biological Psychiatry*, **19**, 629–35.

Wilson, S.A.K. (1940). Epidemic encephalitis. In *Neurology*, ed. A. Ninian Bruce, pp. 99–144. London: Edward Arnold.

Woerner, M.G., Kane, J.M., Lierberman, J.A. et al. (1991). The prevalence of tardive dyskinesia. *Journal of Clinical Psychopharmacology*, **11**, 34–42.

Wohlfart, G., Ingvar, D.H. & Hellberg, A-M. (1961). Compulsory shouting (Benedek's 'klazomania') associated with oculogyric spasms in chronic epidemic encephalitis. *Acta Psychiatrica Scandinavica*, **36**, 369–77.

Wojcik, J.D., Gelenberg, A.J., LaBrie, R.A. & Mieske, M. (1980). Prevalence of tardive dyskinesia in an outpatient population. *Comprehensive Psychiatry*, **21**, 370–9.

World Health Organisation (1990). Heads of Centres Collaborating in WHO Co-Ordinated Studies on Biological Aspects of Mental Illness. Prophylactic use of anticholinergics in patients on long-term neuroleptic treatment: a consensus statement. *British Journal of Psychiatry*, **156**, 412.

Yaryura-Tobias, J.A., Wolpert, A., Dana, L. & Malis, S. (1973). Action of L-dopa on drug-induced extrapyramidal syndromes. *Diseases of the Nervous System*, **31**, 60–3.

Yassa, R. & Ananth, J. (1981). Familial tardive dyskinesia. *American Journal of Psychiatry*, **138**, 1618–19.

Yassa, R., Camille, Y. & Belzile, L. (1987). Tardive dyskinesia in the course of antidepressant therapy: a prevalence study and review of the literature. *Journal of Clinical Psychopharmacology*, **7**, 243–6.

Yassa, R. & Jeste, D.V. (1992). Gender differences in tardive dyskinesia – a critical review of the literature. *Schizophrenia Bulletin*, **18**, 701–15.

Yassa, R. & Nair, N.P.V. (1984). Incidence of tardive dyskinesia in an outpatient population. *Psychosomatics*, **25**, 479–81.

Yassa, R. & Nair, N.P.V. (1987). The effect of tardive dyskinesia on body weight. *Acta Psychiatrica Scandinavica*, **75**, 209–11.

Yassa, R., Nair, V. & Dimitry, R. (1986a). Prevalence of tardive dystonia. *Acta Psychiatrica Scandinavica*, **73**, 629–33.

Yassa, R., Nair, V. & Schwartz, G. (1986b). Early versus late onset of psychosis and tardive dyskinesia. *Biological Psychiatry*, **21**, 1291–7.

Yassa, R. & Samarthji, L. (1986). Prevalence of the rabbit syndrome. *American Journal of Psychiatry*, **143**, 656–7.

Youssef, H.A. & Waddington, J.L. (1987). Morbidity and mortality in tardive dyskinesia: associations in chronic schizophrenia. *Acta Psychiatrica Scandinavica*, **75**, 74–7.

Index